Clinical Manual for Management of PTSD

Clinical Manual for Management of PTSD

Edited by

David M. Benedek, M.D., D.F.A.P.A.

Gary H. Wynn, M.D.

Senior Advisory Board

Richard A. Bryant, Ph.D.

Arieh Y. Shalev, M.D.

Robert J. Ursano, M.D., D.F.A.P.A.

Simon A. Wessely, M.D., F.R.C.P., F.R.C.Psych.

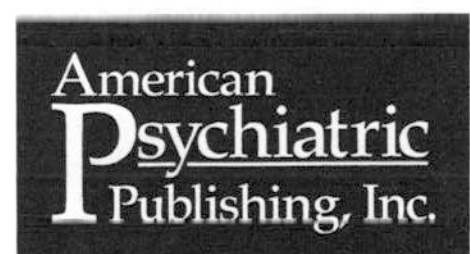

Washington, DC
London, England

Note: The authors have worked to ensure that all information in this book is accurate at the time of publication and consistent with general psychiatric and medical standards, and that information concerning drug dosages, schedules, and routes of administration is accurate at the time of publication and consistent with standards set by the U.S. Food and Drug Administration and the general medical community. As medical research and practice continue to advance, however, therapeutic standards may change. Moreover, specific situations may require a specific therapeutic response not included in this book. For these reasons and because human and mechanical errors sometimes occur, we recommend that readers follow the advice of physicians directly involved in their care or the care of a member of their family.

Books published by American Psychiatric Publishing, Inc., represent the views and opinions of the individual authors and do not necessarily represent the policies and opinions of APPI or the American Psychiatric Association.

The views and assertions contained herein are the private views of the authors and are not to be construed as official, or reflecting policies or positions of the Deployment Health Clinical Center, Defense and Veterans Brain Injury Center, Walter Reed Army Medical Center, Walter Reed Army Institute of Research, Uniformed Services University of the Health Sciences, Department of Defense, Department of Veterans Affairs, or the United States Government.

Manufactured in Canada on acid-free paper
13 13 12 11 10 5 4 3 2 1
First Edition
Typeset in Adobe AGaramond and Formata.

American Psychiatric Publishing, Inc.
1000 Wilson Boulevard
Arlington, VA 22209-3901
www.appi.org

Library of Congress Cataloging-in-Publication Data
Clinical manual for management of PTSD / edited by David M. Benedek, Gary H. Wynn. -- 1st ed.
p. ; cm.
Includes bibliographical references and index.
ISBN 978-1-58562-359-4 (alk. paper)
1. Post-traumatic stress disorder. 2. Post-traumatic stress disorder--Treatment. I. Benedek, David M. II. Wynn, Gary H., 1958-
[DNLM: 1. Stress Disorders, Post-Traumatic. WM 172 C64182 2011]
RC552.P67C56 2011
616.85'21--dc22

2010012310

British Library Cataloguing in Publication Data
A CIP record is available from the British Library.

If you would like to buy between 25 and 99 copies of this or any other APPI title, you are eligible for a 20% discount; please contact APPI Customer Service at appi@psych.org or 800-368-5777. If you wish to buy 100 or more copies of the same title, please e-mail us at bulksales@psych.org for a price quote.

Thanks to mom and dad for role modeling the art of balancing professional obligations and scholarship with the responsibilities and joys of parenthood; to my boss for continuing to provide me with opportunities to explore my interests and expand my knowledge; and to my wonderful wife and children for the love, support, and patience that provide me with daily reminders that I am truly a fortunate guy. —D.M.B.

For my mom and dad, who have always been my biggest fans.
—G.H.W.

Contents

PART II

Therapeutics and Management

PART III

Special Topics

Contributors

Sunday Adewuyi, M.B.B.S.
Assistant Instructor, Department of Psychiatry, University of Texas Southwestern Medical Center, Dallas, Texas

Margret E. Bell, Ph.D.
Staff Psychologist, Women's Health Sciences Division, National Center for PTSD, VA Boston Healthcare System, Boston, Massachusetts

David M. Benedek, M.D., D.F.A.P.A.
Professor, Deputy Chair, and Associate Director and Senior Scientist, Center for the Study of Traumatic Stress, Department of Psychiatry, Uniformed Services University of the Health Sciences, Bethesda, Maryland

Richard A. Bryant, Ph.D.
Scientia Professor and ARC Laureate Fellow, School of Psychology, University of New South Wales, Sydney, New South Wales, Australia

Kathleen F. Carlson, Ph.D.
Core Investigator, Center for Chronic Disease Outcomes Research, Minneapolis VA Medical Center; Assistant Professor, Department of Medicine, University of Minnesota, Minneapolis, Minnesota

Stephen J. Cozza, M.D.
Professor of Psychiatry, Associate Director, Center for the Study of Traumatic Stress, Uniformed Services University of the Health Sciences, Bethesda, Maryland

Jo Ann Difede, Ph.D.
Associate Professor, Department of Psychiatry, Weill Cornell Medical College, New York, New York

Charles C. Engel, M.D., M.P.H.
Director, Deployment Health Clinical Center, Walter Reed Army Medical Center, Washington, D.C.; Associate Professor and Associate Chair (Research), Department of Psychiatry, Uniformed Services University of the Health Sciences, Bethesda, Maryland

Michael C. Freed, Ph.D., E.M.T.-B.
Clinical Research Psychologist, Deployment Health Clinical Center, Walter Reed Army Medical Center, Washington, D.C.; Research Assistant Professor, Uniformed Services University of the Health Sciences, Bethesda, Maryland

Louis M. French, Psy.D.
Chief, TBI Service, Department of Orthopedics and Rehabilitation and Defense and Veterans Brain Injury Center, Walter Reed Army Medical Center, Washington, D.C.; Department of Neurology, Uniformed Services University of the Health Sciences, Bethesda, Maryland

Matthew J. Friedman, M.D., Ph.D.
Executive Director, National Center for PTSD, U.S. Department of Veterans Affairs, VA Medical Center, White River Junction, VT; Professor of Psychiatry and Pharmacology and Toxicology, Dartmouth Medical School, Hanover, New Hampshire

Kristie L. Gore, Ph.D.
Associate Director of Research, Deployment Health Clinical Center, Walter Reed Army Medical Center, Washington, D.C.; Research Assistant Professor of Research, Department of Psychiatry, Uniformed Services University of the Health Sciences, Bethesda, Maryland

Geoffrey G. Grammer, M.D.
Chief, Inpatient Psychiatry Service, Department of Psychiatry, Walter Reed Army Medical Center, Washington, D.C.

Thomas A. Grieger, M.D., D.F.A.P.A.
Professor, Department of Psychiatry, Uniformed Services University of the Health Sciences, Bethesda, Maryland

Jennifer M. Guimond, Ph.D.
Research Assistant Professor, Center for the Study of Traumatic Stress, Department of Psychiatry, Uniformed Services University of the Health Sciences, Bethesda, Maryland

Charles W. Hoge, M.D.
Director, Division of Psychiatry and Neuroscience, Walter Reed Army Institute of Research, Silver Spring, Maryland

Grant L. Iverson, Ph.D.
Professor, Department of Psychiatry, University of British Columbia; Director, Neuropsychology Outcome Assessment Laboratory, British Columbia Mental Health and Addictions Services, Vancouver, British Columbia, Canada

Katherine M. Iverson, Ph.D.
Postdoctoral Fellow, Women's Health Sciences Division, National Center for PTSD, VA Boston Healthcare System, Department of Psychiatry, Boston University, Boston, Massachusetts

Douglas C. Johnson, Ph.D.
Science Officer, Warfighter Performance, Naval Health Research Center, San Diego, California; Assistant Professor in Psychiatry, University of California–San Diego School of Medicine, La Jolla, California

Laurence J. Kirmayer, M.D., F.R.C.P.C.
James McGill Professor and Director, Division of Social and Transcultural Psychiatry, Department of Psychiatry, McGill University; Director, Culture and Mental Health Research Unit, Jewish General Hospital, Montreal, Quebec, Canada

John H. Krystal, M.D.
Robert L. McNeil, Jr. Professor of Translational Research, Chair, Department of Psychiatry, Yale University School of Medicine; Director, Clinical Neuroscience Division, VA National Center for PTSD, West Haven, Connecticut

Kristin M. Lester, Ph.D.
Clinical Psychologist, Women's Health Sciences Division, National Center for PTSD, VA Boston Healthcare System, Boston, Massachusetts

Toby Measham, M.D., M.Sc.
Lecturer and Assistant Professor, Division of Social and Transcultural Psychiatry, Department of Psychiatry, McGill University, Montreal, Quebec, Canada

Scott C. Moran, M.D.
Psychiatry Residency Training Director, National Capitol Consortium, Walter Reed Army Medical Center, Washington, D.C.

Alexander Neumeister, M.D.
Associate Professor of Psychiatry, Department of Psychiatry, Mount Sinai School of Medicine, New York, New York

Carol S. North, M.D., M.P.E.
The Nancy and Ray L. Hunt Chair in Crisis Psychiatry, Director, Program in Trauma and Disaster, Dallas VAMC; Professor, Departments of Psychiatry and Surgery, Division of Emergency Medicine, UT Southwestern Medical Center, Dallas, Texas

C. Beth Ready
Psychology Research Technician, Women's Health Sciences Division, National Center for PTSD, VA Boston Healthcare System, Boston, Massachusetts

Patricia A. Resick, Ph.D.
Director, Women's Health Sciences Division, National Center for PTSD, VA Boston Healthcare System, Professor of Psychiatry and Psychology, Boston University, Boston, Massachusetts

Albert Rizzo, Ph.D.
Associate Director, Institute for Creative Technologies; Research Professor, Department of Psychiatry and School of Gerontology, University of Southern California, Marina del Rey, California

Barbara O. Rothbaum, Ph.D., A.B.P.P.
Professor in Psychiatry, Director, Trauma and Anxiety Recovery Program, Emory University School of Medicine, Atlanta, Georgia

Cécile Rousseau, M.D., M.Sc.
Associate Professor, Division of Social and Transcultural Psychiatry, Department of Psychiatry, McGill University. Montreal, Quebec, Canada

Michael J. Roy, M.D., M.P.H.
Director, Division of Military Internal Medicine, Professor of Medicine, Uniformed Services University of the Health Sciences, Bethesda, Maryland

Nina A. Sayer, Ph.D.
Research Director, Polytrauma and Blast-Related Injuries QUERI, Investigator, Center for Chronic Disease Outcomes Research, Minneapolis VA Medical Center, Minneapolis, Minnesota

Paula P. Schnurr, Ph.D.
Deputy Executive Director, National Center for PTSD, White River Junction, Vermont; Research Professor of Psychiatry, Dartmouth Medical School, Hanover, New Hampshire

Arieh Y. Shalev, M.D.
Professor of Psychiatry, Hadassah and the Hebrew University School of Medicine; Head, Department of Psychiatry, Hadassah University Hospital, Jerusalem, Israel

Murray B. Stein, M.D., M.P.H.
Professor of Psychiatry and Family and Preventive Medicine, University of California–San Diego School of Medicine, La Jolla, California

Amy E. Street, Ph.D.
Staff Psychologist, Women's Health Sciences Division, National Center for PTSD, VA Boston Healthcare System; Assistant Professor, Department of Psychiatry, Boston University School of Medicine, Boston, Massachusetts

Alina M. Suris, Ph.D., A.B.P.P.
Clinical Director, Mental Health Trauma Services, Dallas VAMC, Associate Professor of Psychiatry, Department of Psychiatry, UT Southwestern Medical Center, Dallas, Texas

Robert J. Ursano, M.D., D.F.A.P.A.
Chairman, Department of Psychiatry, Uniformed Services University of the Health Sciences, Bethesda, Maryland

Espen Walderhaug, Ph.D.
Postdoctoral Fellow, Clinical Neuroscience Division, Department of Psychiatry, Yale University School of Medicine, West Haven, Connecticut

Simon A. Wessely, M.D., F.R.C.P., F.R.C.Psych.
Professor of Epidemiological and Liaison Psychiatry, King's College London, and Director, King's Centre for Military Health Research, Institute of Psychiatry, London, United Kingdom

Joshua E. Wilk, Ph.D.
Clinical Research Psychologist, Division of Psychiatry and Neuroscience, Walter Reed Army Institute of Research, Silver Spring, Maryland

Gary H. Wynn, M.D.
Assistant Chief, Inpatient Psychiatry Service, Walter Reed Army Medical Center, Washington, D.C.; Assistant Professor of Psychiatry, Uniformed Services University of the Health Sciences, Bethesda, Maryland

Disclosure of Interests

The contributors listed below have indicated a financial interest in or other affiliation with a commercial supporter, a manufacturer of a commercial product, a provider of a commercial service, a nongovernmental organization, and/or a government agency, as follows:

Charles C. Engel, M.D., M.PH.—*Research Support:* Department of Defense Congressionally Directed Medical Research Program, National Institute of Mental Health (NIMH).

Geoffrey G. Grammer, M.D.—*Consulting:* Eli Lilly and Company speakers' bureau.

Katherine M. Iverson, Ph.D.—*Grants/Research Support:* The author's contribution to Chapter 7 was supported by NIMH training grant T32 MH019836, awarded to Terence M. Keane.

John H. Krystal, M.D.—*Grants/Research Support:* Work on Chapter 3 was supported by a grant from the Department of Veterans Affairs (VA) to the VA National Center for PTSD and VA Alcohol Research Center, as well as by National Institute on Alcohol Abuse and Alcoholism (NIAAA) Grants 5 AA14906-04 and 2P50 AA012870-07 to Dr. Krystal. *Consulting:* Eli Lilly, scientific consultant on PTSD.

Alexander Neumeister, M.D.—*Grants/Research Support:* Department of Veterans Affairs, as described above for Dr. Krystal.

Carol S. North, M.D., M.P.E.—*Grants/Research Support:* Assisi Foundation of Memphis; National Center for PTSD (REDMH); NIAAA; and NIMH Grant MH068853.

Barbara O. Rothbaum, Ph.D.—*Consulting/Equity Ownership:* The author is a consultant to and owns equity in Virtually Better, Inc., which is developing products related to virtual reality research; however, Virtually Better did not create the Virtual Iraq environment described in this volume in Chapter 9. The terms of this arrangement have been reviewed and approved by Emory University in accordance with its conflict of interest policies.

Arieh Y. Shalev, M.D.—*Grants/Consulting (investigator-initiated):* Lundbeck Pharmaceuticals.

Espen Walderhaug, Ph.D.—*Grants/Research Support:* Department of Veterans Affairs, as described above for Dr. Krystal. *Fellowship:* Postdoctoral fellowship grant, Research Council of Norway, Division for Science.

The following contributors stated that they had no competing interests during the year preceding manuscript submission:

Sunday Adewuyi, M.B.B.S.
Margret E. Bell, Ph.D.
David M. Benedek, M.D.
Richard A. Bryant, Ph.D.
Kathleen F. Carlson, Ph.D.
Stephen J. Cozza, M.D.
Jo Ann Difede, Ph.D.
Michael C. Freed, Ph.D., E.M.T.-B.
Louis M. French, Psy.D.
Matthew J. Friedman, M.D., Ph.D.
Kristie L. Gore, Ph.D.
Thomas A. Grieger, M.D.
Jennifer M. Guimond, Ph.D.
Charles W. Hoge, M.D.
Grant L. Iverson, Ph.D.
Douglas C. Johnson, Ph.D.
Laurence J. Kirmayer, M.D.
Kristin M. Lester, Ph.D.
Toby Measham, M.D., M.Sc.
Scott C. Moran, M.D.
C. Beth Ready
Patricia A. Resick, Ph.D.
Albert Rizzo, Ph.D.
Cécile Rousseau, M.D., M.Sc.
Michael J. Roy, M.D., M.P.H.
Nina A. Sayer, Ph.D.
Paula P. Schnurr, Ph.D.
Murray B. Stein, M.D., M.P.H.
Amy E. Street, Ph.D.
Alina M. Suris, Ph.D.
Robert J. Ursano, M.D.
Simon A. Wessely, M.D.
Joshua E. Wilk, Ph.D.
Gary H. Wynn, M.D.

Preface

Traumatic events, disasters, and war are all too common in everyday life. Therefore, posttraumatic stress disorder must be anticipated as part of the life of many. Across modern history societies have also become more complex and interconnected. As a result, nations have become increasingly aware of—and involved in—the challenges and conflicts affecting other nations around the globe.

This century has brought tremendous international advances in technology, in medicine, and in our understanding of the pathophysiology and neurobiology of psychological and neuropsychiatric disorders. Despite this progress, we must confront the inescapable reality that our world is—and will continue to be—ravaged by traumatic events including violence, injury, war, disaster, death, and destruction. The psychological and behavioral consequences of traumatic events, disaster, and war have been observed and recorded for millennia.

Recent decades have seen an explosion of interest in understanding, mitigating, and preventing the consequences of exposure to the horrors of large and small disasters including physical or sexual assault, motor vehicle accident, industrial accident, military combat, terrorist attack, flood, hurricane, tsunami, and earthquake. Academic and professional circles have struggled with precise and accepted definitions of traumatic events for individuals and as part of disasters, war, and terrorism. The descriptions and definitions of the syndromes experienced by those who develop severe pathological reactions to exposure have evolved over centuries. They are now captured in the diagnostic criteria for posttraumatic stress disorder (PTSD) and several additional neuropsychiatric and behavioral disorders.

DSM-5 and ICD-11 will doubtless continue the process of diagnostic refinement and will continue to spark nosological debate. What cannot be debated is that while the majority of survivors will not develop severe psychological reactions, a proportion of those exposed to traumatic events will experience debilitating symptoms of intrusion, reexperiencing, hyperarousal, and avoidance. Although the subtleties of case definition may vary from year to year and society to society, clinicians cannot afford to wait for international consensus or the harmonization of terms. As we write this we are only just into 2010, and already global attention has focused on earthquakes in Haiti and Chile, on terrorist attacks in the Middle East and Europe and the United States, and on continuing military conflicts in Iraq, Afghanistan, other nations around the world. As in any year in modern history, there have been multiple plane and commuter train crashes and countless physical assaults, rapes, and community tragedies involving motor vehicle accidents. More than ever before, clinicians are now expected to join those who assess, manage, and treat the survivors and family members manifesting symptoms resulting from exposure to these most unfortunate realities of the human experience.

In this volume, world leaders in translational research surrounding epidemiology, neurobiology, psychotherapy, psychopharmacology, and other somatic therapies outline the most current evidence-based approaches to the assessment, diagnosis, treatment, and management of patients with PTSD. Our approach to the diagnosis, treatment, and rehabilitation of persons suffering from the consequences of traumatic experience will also evolve over time. However, societies and individuals will continue to experience social, interpersonal, behavioral, and psychological consequences in the aftermath of trauma, and clinicians will be called on to address these consequences.

For the moment, clinicians may take solace in the notion that the interventions outlined in this volume, although targeted at PTSD as currently defined, represent approaches at the forefront of our current understanding of the most severe medical consequences of exposure to traumatic events. They represent approaches likely to transcend many of the obstacles imposed by the ever-changing and complex interactions between trauma, the self, and society and by the artificial boundaries established by the changing nature of diagnostic criteria for posttraumatic stress disorder. The clinical approaches that we recommend are strongly dependent on survivors' natural supports, will not serve as a replacement for those, and should be applied with the highest sensitivity to how and what the survivor's physical, social, and psychological environment allows him or her to achieve. Building systems of care that incorporate these sensitivities and caring interventions is a challenge worthy of substantial effort.

Robert J. Ursano, M.D., D.F.A.P.A., *Chair*
Richard A. Bryant, Ph.D.
Arieh Y. Shalev, M.D.
Simon Wessely, M.D., F.R.C.P., F.R.C.Psych.

Senior International Editorial Advisory Board
Clinical Manual for Management of PTSD

PART I

Introduction and Overview

1

Introduction

David M. Benedek, M.D., D.F.A.P.A.
Gary H. Wynn, M.D.

Posttraumatic stress disorder (PTSD) has garnered considerable attention over the past decade from mental health professionals, the medical community at large, and other sources such as the media. Since the inclusion of PTSD three decades ago in the *Diagnostic and Statistical Manual of Mental Disorders* 3rd Edition (DSM-III; American Psychiatric Association 1980), controversy and debate have surrounded the diagnosis. Controversial aspects of the diagnosis have included the very existence of the disorder, the validity of each of the criteria, the biological and psychological bases for symptoms, and the efficacy of various treatment modalities. Despite these uncertainties, the diagnosis has received increasing public support and attention. This focus has come primarily from observations and reports regarding the psychological impact of several large-scale natural disasters (e.g., Hurricane Katrina in the southern United States, the tsunami in the Indonesian province of Aceh) and the armed conflicts in Iraq and Afghanistan. Although these large-scale trauma exposures may garner the greatest media attention, traumas resulting in high rates of PTSD also include individual exposures, such as sexual and physical assault (Kessler et al. 1995). As military conflicts, natural disasters, and various other traumas occur at the individual and population levels, this manual comes at a time of continued risk for PTSD as well as heightened opportunity for new insight into the clinical phenomenology, neurobiology, and treatment of PTSD.

A Brief History of PTSD

The history of humanity is rife with incidents of mass exposure to danger, chaos, violence, and social disruption. Descriptions of the psychopathological consequences of trauma appear in some of the earliest known literature (e.g., Homer's *Iliad*). Although the nature of the descriptions has changed throughout the millennia, the core concept of a trauma having negative psychological consequences has remained constant.

In the United States, the earliest conceptualization of the psychological impact of trauma was the condition termed *nostalgia*. Primarily referring to settlers on the western front and soldiers in the Civil War, *nostalgia* was adapted from the European concept of nostalgia as excessive homesickness. According to Calhoun (1864), the four primary causes of nostalgia were hasty enlistments, expectations of a short war, service far from home, and writing letters when far from home. To combat the impact of nostalgia on military effectiveness, Calhoun recommended regularly scheduled leave for soldiers rather than furloughs for emergencies or serious injury only. Shortly after the end of the American Civil War in 1865, the concept of nostalgia faded from medical literature.

In the same time frame, Da Costa (1871) described "irritable heart" as a syndrome of fatigue, palpitations, dizziness, left-sided chest pain, and dyspnea with minimal exertion in several hundred American Civil War soldiers. More commonly known as "soldier's heart," this syndrome was also termed *neurocirculatory asthenia* and *cardiovascular neurosis*. Although this syndrome considerably predates the formulation of the diagnosis of PTSD, it fits the model of increased somatic complaints and anxiety seen in those with the current-day diagnosis.

During World War I, trench warfare brought about another descriptive syndrome of the psychological impact of trauma. Shell shock or battle fatigue was a short-term response to the horrors of war, resulting in fatigue, delayed responsiveness, and a generalized disconnection from one's surroundings. This syndrome likely represents one of the earliest descriptions of acute stress disorder, given the focus on disconnection shortly after the traumatic exposure.

Although numerous other descriptions of the psychological impact of trauma have been published over the years, the current formulation was formally recognized as PTSD in DSM-III in 1980. The diagnostic criteria established in DSM-III represented an effort to reconcile aspects of the posttrauma syndromes described throughout history. PTSD was conceptualized as a disorder that might occur after a broad range of traumatic exposures (i.e., beyond combat), and a range of symptoms specifying criteria for the disorder was provided. In the three decades since the introduction of PTSD, the original construct has undergone changes. Most notably, the original requirement that the traumatic event be "outside the range of normal human experience" has been eliminated. This change further broadened the scope of potentially traumatic experiences that might precipitate the disorder. Currently, some researchers and clinicians call for the removal of the diagnostic requirement of a sense of "fear, hopelessness, or horror" in response to the trauma. Others suggest that PTSD be removed from the anxiety disorders section of the next DSM edition and be included instead in a new classification of event-related disorders. Although further changes in the conceptualization of PTSD are inevitable, we hope this manual will provide a solid foundation of current understanding of the nature of response to traumatic exposures that clinicians must address, as well as effective strategies for diagnostic assessment, management, and treatment.

The Purpose of This Manual

The origins of this manual are rooted in the recognition of a burgeoning population of individuals with PTSD and a perceived need for a text specifically geared toward clinicians. In the three decades since the introduction of PTSD in DSM-III, a significant amount of research has been published regarding the etiology, manifestations, and treatment of PTSD. With recent increased interest and support for research and validation of therapeutic intervention, the field has moved even faster in recent years. This clinical manual is an effort to bridge the gap between the research community and the clinician by providing an easy-to-use, up-to-date resource of clinically relevant information on PTSD. Clinicians are often overburdened with their patient panels and have limited time to pursue every area of any given topic of interest. We intend to provide clinicians with a consolidated and thoughtful reference useful to everyday practice. Finally, in recognition of the controversy regarding a number of aspects of PTSD, we attempt to present viewpoints summarizing and synthesizing the research to date. This manual is an attempt not to argue one point of view, but rather to summarize the current state of knowledge, point out gaps in understanding, and address clinically relevant issues.

How to Use This Manual

This clinical manual can be used in multiple ways. Clinicians may find it useful as a desktop reference and read only those parts pertinent to some aspect of daily practice. As a complete text, this manual can be an ideal starting point for clinicians moving into more work with patients who have PTSD. Alternatively, experienced clinicians with years of work with PTSD may find this volume helpful in updating their knowledge of more recent research and treatment modalities. For residents and students, this manual can provide a solid understanding of PTSD and the various manifestations and treatment modalities available in current practice.

This clinical manual is designed to be a practical guide—a reference used at the bedside, on rounds, in the classroom, or in the office. For simple use and ease of reference, this text is divided into several sections.

Part I, "Introduction and Overview," is a clinician-oriented review of the "basics" of PTSD. This section is intended to provide a framework for understanding the nature and clinical meaning of the diagnosis of PTSD.

Epidemiology is covered in Chapter 2, with a focus on clinical relevance and impact. Beyond simply a detailed review of the current epidemiological data, a thorough discussion of the relationship of epidemiology to clinical practice is provided. Additional information on the course and persistence of PTSD symptoms as well as the disease impact is reviewed.

The biological basis of PTSD is reviewed in detail in Chapter 3. This chapter covers a wide range of topics, which include heritability and environment, various neurobiological systems involved in PTSD, and neuroimaging.

In Chapter 4, diagnosis and initial assessment of PTSD are reviewed, with detailed explanations of various instruments and methods currently available. This chapter provides a solid grounding in the basic diagnostic assessment of PTSD and is a helpful learning tool for younger practitioners and a good review for seasoned clinicians.

This section concludes with a review of the comorbidities of PTSD. PTSD almost always has comorbidities, and it is often difficult to separate one disorder from another. Chapter 5 addresses PTSD both as a separate diagnosis from its comorbidities and as a manifestation in conjunction with other diagnoses.

Part II, "Therapeutics and Management," covers general concepts for the treatment of PTSD. This section (Chapters 6–10) provides large amounts of specific information on a wide array of treatments. In addition, this section covers clinically pertinent aspects of management, such as dealing with a violent patient, efficacy of various types of therapies, pharmacological management, and management of functional impairments.

In Part II, numerous tables are provided to help summarize the available data and allow the clinician to reference material in an easier fashion. This section will likely be consulted often by those providers who are familiar with PTSD and desire quick information on specifics of management. Each chapter in this section stands on its own regarding the understanding of specific issues that, in total, constitute the management of PTSD.

Part III, "Special Topics," covers topics that are specific to subpopulations of PTSD patients. Despite the nearly universal risk of exposure to traumatic events, various subgroups may demonstrate particular manifestations of PTSD and may bring different needs and issues to their clinician.

In Chapter 11, children and adolescents are covered in detail, with attention to their unique PTSD risks and experiences. In addition to providing a detailed review of childhood PTSD, the chapter authors evaluate alternate views of responses to trauma. The unique needs and challenges confronting providers treating younger PTSD patients are then covered. The psychotherapeutic modalities available in current practice are covered, followed by a discussion of psychopharmacology in children and adolescents.

Current estimates suggest that as many as 1 in 5 women and 1 in 12 men in the United States experience some form of sexual assault or coercion during their lifetime. Given that being the victim of sexual assault carries a significant risk of developing PTSD and that there are a number of unique factors to this population, a detailed review is provided in Chapter 12.

Human history has been rife with conflict, and the history of the psychological consequences of trauma has often focused on the experience of veterans of conflict. Because of the continued armed conflict around the world and the large numbers of veterans suffering from PTSD, military and veteran populations are covered in detail in Chapter 13.

With increasing life expectancy, the geriatric population of the world has grown significantly in the past few decades. Given the physiological alterations occurring with age, as well as the possibility of either being traumatized during later years or having lived with PTSD for many decades, geriatrics is covered as a separate topic in Chapter 14.

Head injury has received a great deal of media and scientific attention lately resulting from observations of head injuries incurred in the wars in Iraq and Afghanistan as well as in sports. Of particular interest is the issue of traumatic brain injury (TBI) and postconcussive syndrome. Given that trauma is the source of TBI, the question of causation or the synergistic impact with PTSD is an important area of research. Additionally, understanding these two disorders and their potential intertwining nature can be vital to effective management of TBI and PTSD. In light of this important topic, the authors of Chapter 15 address the issue of TBI as it relates to PTSD.

Large-scale tragedies and armed conflicts result in psychological impact on a cultural scale and often bring different cultures into contact with one another. In Chapter 16, the authors' review of cultural aspects of PTSD strives to make clinicians aware of some of the sociocultural issues that may be important when interacting with specific ethnicities or cultures (e.g., immigrants, refugees, asylum seekers).

Finally, we remind the reader that each individual with PTSD is just that—an individual. Although the majority of concepts and therapeutic modalities presented in this manual are supported by convincing research, a robust evidence basis for efficacy should not be a replacement for clinical experience, therapeutic alliance, and a thorough understanding of an individual patient's concerns and needs. Clinicians are encouraged to make use of their understanding of the individual patient, take into account the context of any treatment, and supplement with further individualized inquiry when considering any therapy discussed in this text.

References

American Psychiatric Association: Diagnostic and Statistical Manual of Mental Disorders, 3rd Edition. Washington, DC, American Psychiatric Association, 1980

Calhoun JT: Nostalgia as a disease of field service. The Medical and Surgical Reporter 11:130–132, 1864

Da Costa JM: On irritable heart: a clinical study of a form of functional cardiac disorder and its consequences. Am J Med Sci 61:18–52, 1871

Kessler RC, Sonnega A, Bromet E, et al: Posttraumatic stress disorder in the National Comorbidity Survey. Arch Gen Psychiatry 52:1048–1060, 1995

2

Epidemiology

Michael C. Freed, Ph.D., E.M.T.-B.
Kristie L. Gore, Ph.D.
Charles C. Engel, M.D., M.P.H.

Relationship of Epidemiology to Clinical Practice

Epidemiologists concern themselves with the health of populations, whereas clinicians mainly concern themselves with the health of individual patients. Generally speaking, epidemiology attempts to improve the public health through policies and public health surveillance and population health indicators. Epidemiologists help policy makers and health care planners establish population-based priorities within their unique beneficiary populations. They provide information about illness occurrence and related health outcomes to inform decisions about the type, amount, and distribution of necessary medical resources.

The authors would like to acknowledge the help of Phoebe Kuesters.

Epidemiologists use many tools, research designs, and quantitative parameters to assess illness dynamics in populations of interest, most importantly the general population. For example, epidemiologists may calculate the incidence, prevalence, relative risk, odds ratio, and mortality associated with a particular disease (see Table 2–1). They may also investigate the outcomes of illness in patients. The clinician, by comparison, attempts to improve individuals' health through direct patient care and patient-level health indicators (e.g., laboratory results or a mental status examination finding).

Clinical epidemiology has often been described as the basic science of clinical medicine, because it equips clinicians with tools for determining the utility of various treatments, diagnostic tests, and health risk factors (see Table 2–2) in a way that the biological and behavioral sciences alone typically cannot. Clinical epidemiology describes the distribution of diseases in efforts to identify their determinants (i.e., statistically associated factors that may be causes of the diseases), rates of incidence (i.e., new-onset cases in a given time frame), prevalence, and risk and protective factors (reported in Zatzick and Galea 2007). Clinical epidemiology still focuses on populations rather than individuals, but the emphasis is on populations and issues of greatest concern to the clinician. Clinical epidemiologists assess patient populations, such as those in primary care and various specialty settings (e.g., outpatient or inpatient mental health services).

One might ask why a chapter on the epidemiology of posttraumatic stress disorder (PTSD) is included in a book that is geared toward clinicians, or might wonder what population-level research can tell clinicians about their individual patients. The epidemiology of PTSD is relevant to the clinician in several ways. As discussed in the following subsections, it provides 1) evidence of disease base rates, risk factors, and correlates; 2) normative screening data; 3) real-world support for interventions to assist the health care practitioner; and 4) rates of detection and treatment and patterns of medical utilization in those with the disease. This evidence also informs health policy decisions for resource allocation.

Evidence of Disease Base Rates, Risk Factors, and Correlates

Epidemiology "has done much to clarify the legitimacy of PTSD" (McFarlane 2004, p. 874). Epidemiology of PTSD has provided evidence of the preva-

Table 2–1. Definitions of key epidemiological terms

Key term	Definition
Incidence	Number of new cases occurring in a population over a specified time period—that is, the cases per person per time. For example, an incidence of 100 per 100,000 people per year is the same as 1% per year. Incidence is a *rate*.
Prevalence	Proportion of people in a sample at a point in time who have the illness in question. Often referred to as the "point prevalence," prevalence is a *proportion*, not a rate. Prevalence = incidence × duration.
Relative risk	Ratio of two incidence rates, usually the incidence of the illness in exposed individuals divided by the incidence of the illness in nonexposed individuals. The relative risk can also be used to compare cohorts. For example, if the incidence of disease A is 5 cases per 100,000 in men but 10 cases per 100,000 in women, then the relative risk of the disease is 10÷5, or 2; the risk of developing disease A in women is twice that of men.
Odds ratio	An approximation of relative risk, using a statistical technique called logistic regression, but the interpretation is slightly different. For example, disease B kills 1 woman but leaves 2 alive (i.e., odds against dying are 0.5, or 1:2; relative risk of death is 33%). In contrast, disease B kills 5 men but leaves 1 alive (i.e., odds in favor of death are 5:1; relative risk of death is 80% in men). Thus, the odds of death are 10-fold greater for men than for women.
Mortality	Incidence of death.

Table 2–2. Clinical issues and questions addressed by epidemiologists

Clinical issue	Clinical question
Etiology	Can putative risk factor A cause condition B?
	My patient has major depression. What are the chances it is caused by his war experience?
Treatment	If I use new treatment B for condition X, how many patients will I treat before I get one more responder than I would have using the old treatment A?
	If I use trauma-focused cognitive-behavioral therapy for PTSD, how many patients will I treat before I get one more patient "better" than I would have using traditional psychodynamic approaches?
Diagnosis	What is the likelihood that my patient has condition A given test value B?
	What is the likelihood that my patient has PTSD given that he is jumpy, experiences nightmares about the trauma, and avoids talking about the event?
Prognosis	What is the chance that my patient with condition A will have outcome B over period C?
	Ms. Smith was in a horrible car accident 1 month ago and now meets criteria for PTSD. What are the chances that her symptoms will improve over the next year if she does not receive treatment?
Harm	What is the likelihood that treatment A will cause side effect B?
	My patient has no history of high blood pressure. If I give her prazosin to treat combat-related nightmares, what are the chances that she will fall from a rapid drop in blood pressure?

lence, longitudinal course, and risk and resilience factors associated with both trauma exposure and subsequent PTSD symptom onset. See Figure 2–1 for an epidemiological perspective on PTSD.

Clinician observation of the individual with PTSD is confounded with other issues epidemiology can help sort out (McFarlane 2004). For example, after World War I, "traumatic neurosis" in veterans was attributed to early developmental experiences, and not the impact of war. Another perspective held that a social system supportive of financial compensation for trauma-exposed individuals was the major contributor to subsequent disability. Current epidemiological findings (DeViva and Bloem 2003), however, suggest that the relationship between compensation seeking and symptom exaggeration is more complicated than was once thought. Thus, epidemiology provides empirically based knowledge about how clinicians can and should think about determinants of the disorder. This knowledge may conflict with unsupported clinician bias. Further support for the existence of PTSD as a diagnostic category comes from large population-based studies that administered mental health diagnostic interviews to a random sample of households in the United States (e.g., Kessler et al. 1995, 2005).

Normative Data on Screening Instruments to Help Providers Interpret Test Results

Brief PTSD screening measures exist that are usable in primary care (e.g., Gore et al. 2008; Prins et al. 2004) and other settings. PTSD screens can be flexibly used, depending on patient demographics, PTSD prevalence, and clinic needs, to maximally identify patients with PTSD and minimize errors (Yeager et al. 2007). Screening instruments can only be tailored by using population data. When a screen is administered to a specific patient, providers interpret the results in the context of the setting and the patient characteristics. However, the ideal cutoffs of these measures can differ greatly depending on the population. When a 4-item PTSD screen (Prins et al. 2004) is used, for example, a cutoff score of 2 appears to be optimally efficient for patients in military primary care clinics (Gore et al. 2008), whereas a cutoff of 3 is optimally efficient when that same 4-item PTSD screen is used in Veterans Affairs primary care clinics (Prins et al. 2004).

Information to Help With the Implementation of Research-Based Interventions in Real-World Settings

Epidemiology can be used to guide trauma-focused interventions in a manner complementary to how basic science research guides efficacy research, the so-called bench-to-bedside paradigm (Zatzick and Galea 2007). Basic science often serves as the precursor to efficacy trials, which are then either implemented or evaluated as part of an effectiveness trial. This paradigm is incomplete because it often fails to account for contextual variables, which were controlled for or excluded in highly internally valid efficacy trials.

For example, in a review of 34 studies, Spinazzola et al. (2005) reported that the predominant reason for participant exclusion was severe comorbid psychopathology, despite the fact that co-occurrence of another mental health condition is the norm rather than the exception (e.g., 87% of the veterans with PTSD in Magruder et al.'s [2005] study were also diagnosed with a co-occurring mood, substance use, or anxiety disorder). Also, as reported by Wang et al. (2005), only 7% of persons with PTSD seek treatment within the first year of symptom onset, with a 12-year (median) delay to seeking treatment. Spinazzola et al. (2005, p. 426) wrote, "There is perhaps no other Axis I disorder for which the issue of comorbidity is more relevant than PTSD." Thus, epidemiology provides information about the real-world correlates of PTSD (e.g., negative correlation with physical health associated with frequent use of primary care services; Deykin et al. 2001) and their potential impact on efficacy-based treatments. This knowledge serves to identify large gaps in current research such that early intervention strategies may consider targeting a broad array of symptoms rather than solely symptoms of PTSD.

Information to Assist in Provider Recognition and Use of Health Services

Epidemiologists have demonstrated that PTSD is underdiagnosed in medical settings. Magruder et al. (2005) reported that less than half of patients with a research diagnosis of PTSD had a diagnosis of PTSD in their medical record. This discrepancy is a problem because untreated PTSD is associated with impairments in multiple domains of life (Davidson et al. 2004), high rates of physical and medical comorbidity (Kessler et al. 1995, 2005; Magruder et al.

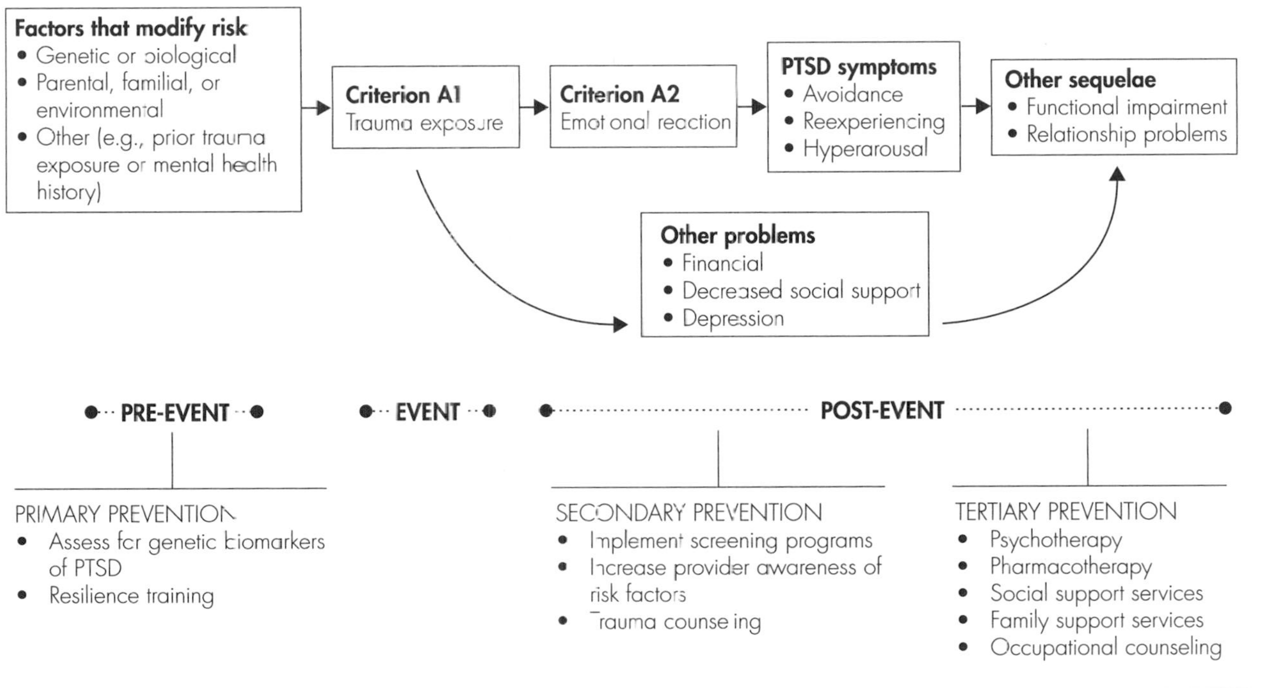

Figure 2–1. Longitudinal progression of PTSD and potential points of clinical intervention.

2005; Stein et al. 2000), and increased health service utilization (Schnurr et al. 2000; Stein et al. 2000). Recently traumatized individuals are more likely to present to primary care than to specialty mental health settings. For example, one study found that following a sexual assault, 72.6% of the victims sought medical treatment within a year, whereas only 19.1% sought mental health care (Kimerling and Calhoun 1994).

Information That Can Be Used for Advocacy of Better Resource Allocation

Epidemiology can be used to determine how PTSD affects health at the population level. Disease burden and population-level health metrics account for mortality, longitudinal course (i.e., persistence), severity (i.e., symptom severity or impact on quality of life), and pervasiveness (i.e., prevalence and incidence). These population-level health metrics for PTSD can then be compared with metrics for other diseases, with the goal of better prioritizing where to direct resources. Clinicians can also use these metrics to better advocate for the resources needed to treat their patients.

Summary of Relationship to Clinical Practice

We wrote this chapter keeping in mind the aforementioned purposes of epidemiology in PTSD. This chapter is not meant to be an exhaustive review of the literature. Rather, we reference hallmark and commonly cited articles, as well as those that are most current to date. The remainder of the chapter is divided into eight parts. We define PTSD diagnostic criteria, rates of trauma exposure, and rates of PTSD development following specific trauma exposures. We describe data on the course of illness in those with PTSD; risk factors, correlates, and consequences; and the impact on the health care system and on society. We then discuss the application of epidemiological findings to the clinical management of PTSD and provide concluding thoughts.

What Is PTSD?

According to the *Diagnostic and Statistical Manual of Mental Disorders*, 4th Edition, Text Revision (DSM-IV-TR; American Psychiatric Association 2000), PTSD is an anxiety disorder with symptoms divided into three categories: reexperiencing (Criterion B), avoidance (Criterion C), and hyperarousal (Criterion D). Symptoms occur following a traumatic event in which "an individual experienced, witnessed, or was confronted with an event or events that involved actual or threatened death or serious injury, or a threat to the physical integrity of self or others" (Criterion A1, p. 467). Also, the individual's emotional response to the traumatic event involved "intense fear, helplessness, or horror" (Criterion A2, p. 467). For a patient to be diagnosed with PTSD, his or her symptoms must be present for at least 1 month (Criterion E) and be clinically significant (Criterion F).

PTSD was forged, in part, out of political policy stemming from the unpopularity of the Vietnam War (Jones and Wessely 2007). Although a more thorough discussion of the diagnostic criteria is provided in Chapter 4, "Assessment and Diagnosis of PTSD," the definition of *trauma* has been refined from the first time PTSD appeared in DSM-III (American Psychiatric Association 1980) to the current definition in DSM-IV-TR (American Psychiatric Association 2000)

Defining Criterion A and developing a universal standard has been difficult (Davidson and Foa 1991). With each change in definition, comparability of rates of PTSD and other population characteristics (e.g., response to treatment or risk moderators) between DSM versions may be suspect. For example, a trauma that meets Criterion A1 in DSM-IV-TR may be too broad for "an event that is outside the range of usual human experience and that would be markedly distressing to almost anyone," as defined in DSM-III-R (American Psychiatric Association 1987).

Epidemiology of Criterion A

The majority of adults are exposed to some traumatic event(s) in their lifetime (see Table 2–3), with women generally reporting fewer exposures than men. In the U.S. general population, rates of exposure to one or more traumas have ranged from 39% (Breslau et al. 1991) to as high as 90% (Breslau et al. 1998). Ten percent of men and 6% of women reported being exposed to at least four events (Kessler et al. 1995). In Switzerland, exposure to potentially traumatic events was 28% (Hepp et al. 2006), and in Australia, rates of exposure were 49.5% for women and 64.6% for men (Creamer et al. 2001). Other subpopulations, such as combat troops, are at particularly high risk of exposure. For example, Hoge et al. (2004) reported that 95% of U.S. Army and Marine service members who served in the Iraq war and 84% of Army service members who served in Afghanistan were exposed to combat (i.e., life-threatening circumstances that would meet Criterion A1). Likewise, disaster workers or populations living in regions prone to natural disasters may be repeatedly exposed to traumatic events. Clinicians therefore need to be cautious about presuming a PTSD diagnosis based solely on trauma exposure.

Traumatic exposure and a reaction of intense fear, helplessness, or horror are necessary for Criterion A. The conditional probability (i.e., the chance) of experiencing Criterion A2 differs according to sex and trauma type (Breslau and Kessler 2001). For example, research demonstrated the conditional probability of endorsing A2 after experiencing military combat is 33.8%, which is relatively low compared with other A1 events. Rape (for women) and a potentially life-threatening car accident result in conditional probabilities of 93.3% and 73.2%, respectively. The sex difference was most pronounced for being shot or stabbed (92.3% females vs. 29.1% males). In general, the conditional probability of endorsing A2 was 85.7% for females versus 69.0% for males, a statistically significant difference. The researchers examined differences in conditional probabilities by race, education, and broad event type (e.g., assaultive violence, other injury/shock, sudden unexpected death of a loved one, or learning about trauma), and found significant differences in the likelihood of developing PTSD following specific traumatic events.

The inclusion of Criterion A2 marginally attenuates the prevalence of PTSD, in the absence of including A2 in the diagnosis (Weathers and Keane 2007). That is, A2 is a weak predictor of PTSD, but the absence of A2 is a strong indicator of no PTSD. The relationship among A1, A2, and subsequent PTSD may be further complicated by preparedness, particularly in emergency and military personnel (Adler et al. 2008). Adler et al. (2008) acknowledged the role of A2 but suggested that the fear, helplessness, or horror reaction may not reflect the reaction of persons in certain occupations. Interview data from 202 military service members returning from combat and meeting Criterion A1 revealed that 80% of the sample did not endorse A2 as written in DSM-IV-TR. Despite this difference, service members endorsing or not endorsing A2 reported similar rates of reexperiencing symptoms, hyperarousal symptoms, functional impairment, PTSD symptom criteria with referral for follow-up, and PTSD symptom criteria with functional impairment.

Table 2–3. Relation of traumatic event exposure to PTSD

	Rate			
	Men		Women	
Traumatic event type	Exposure	PTSD	Exposure	PTSD
Any trauma	61%	8%	51%	20%
Multiple traumas (>1)	35%	—	25%	—
Accidents	25%	6%	14%	9%
Threatened with weapon	19%	2%	7%	33%
Natural disaster with fire	19%	4%	15%	6%
Shock[a]	11%	4%	12%	10%
Physical attack	11%	2%	7%	21%
Combat	6%	39%	—	—
Physical abuse	3%	22%	5%	49%
Molestation	3%	12%	12%	27%
Neglect	2%	24%	3%	20%
Rape	1%	65%	9%	46%
Other	2%	13%	<1%	33%

[a]An endorsement of shock was coded when a respondent indicated an affirmative answer to the following question: "You suffered a great shock because one of the events on this list happened to someone close to you."

Source. Adapted from Kessler RC, Sonnega A, Bromet E, et al.: "Posttraumatic Stress Disorder in the National Comorbidity Survey." *Archives of General Psychiatry* 52:1048–1060, 1995, pp. 1052 and 1053.

Service members who endorsed A2, compared with those who did not, were more likely to meet the avoidance criteria (41% vs. 23%), meet criteria for PTSD based on the three symptom clusters (without endorsing functional impairment; 31% vs. 18%), and report higher levels of symptom distress (Adler et al. 2008). Of the sample of service members who met PTSD diagnostic criteria and received a referral for treatment, 16% did not report a qualifying A2 emotional response. Most participants (62%) reported that they responded to the A1 stressor with occupationally relevant reactions (e.g., like a soldier, based on training). The work of Adler et al. (2008) suggests that clinicians need to be mindful of their patients' training, because some occupational groups may be seeking help (and could arguably benefit from treatment) even though they report no Criterion A2 reactions.

Epidemiology of PTSD Following Traumatic Events

Despite these high rates of traumatic exposure, relatively few people develop PTSD (see Table 2–3). Using DSM-III-R criteria for PTSD, Breslau et al. (1991) reported a lifetime prevalence of 11% in women (31% of trauma-exposed women) and 6% in men (14% of trauma-exposed men). Kessler et al. (1995) reported a lifetime prevalence of 7.8%, with women more than twice as likely to meet criteria (10.4%) compared with men (5%), despite the increased exposure rate for men. Kessler et al. (1999) reported a 12-month prevalence of 3.9%, and more recently of 3.5% with approximately one-third of the cases being serious, moderate, and mild (severity determined by functional status and self-injury risk factors; Kessler et al. 2005). According to Hoge et al. (2004), rates of PTSD (determined by a self-report screening checklist) in combat-exposed troops ranged from 4% to 20%. No respondents in a Swiss cohort met the full DSM-IV-TR criteria (Hepp et al. 2006), and in an Australian group (Creamer et al. 2001), the 12-month prevalence was 1.2%.

Not surprisingly, a relationship exists among characteristics of the A1 event (e.g., type, severity, frequency) and the development of PTSD. Kessler et al. (1995) reported the conditional risk of PTSD by trauma type in a U.S. sample. In men, rape and combat exposure in a war were associated with the highest risk of developing PTSD (65% and 39%, respectively). Being threatened with a weapon or being physically attacked was associated with the lowest risk (1% and 2%, respectively). In women, rape (46%) and being threatened with a weapon (33%) were associated with the highest risk, whereas exposure to a natural disaster (5%) was the lowest. Kessler et al. argued that in general, interpersonal violence, more so than other traumas, is associated with the highest risk of PTSD development. In Tables 2–4, 2–5, and 2–6, we present the prevalence of PTSD in three special populations: children, disaster workers and survivors, and combat troops, respectively.

Kessler (2000) and McNally (2003) summarized findings from several other international studies (including refugees and children exposed to war trauma) and concluded that the conditional risk of PTSD is substantially higher among people exposed to horrific ongoing traumas in developing countries. Consistent with scope and intentionality of the trauma, rates of PTSD following natural disasters are lower than from technological (e.g., mining accident) or manmade disasters (e.g., religious uprising; Neria et al. 2008). There is a relationship between proximity to disaster site and rates of PTSD, such that victims of a natural disaster with direct exposure have the highest rates, followed by rescue workers, with the general population having the lowest rates. Similarly, factors such as degree of physical injury, risk to life, fatalities, and severity of property destruction are important to consider and are predictive of high rates of PTSD (Neria et al. 2008). However, at extreme ends of the dose-response curve, the relationship between exposure and symptoms becomes muddled. McNally (2003) suggested that once traumatic exposure reaches some maximum level, there is no more effect on PTSD symptom severity.

At the opposite end of the spectrum, Mol et al. (2005) and Bodkin et al. (2007) reported that symptoms of PTSD (Criteria B, C, and D) are often met without Criterion A1. Mol et al. (2005) distinguished stressful (e.g., divorce with no abuse) from traumatic events and found that self-reported PTSD symptoms were higher for stressful events. Bodkin et al. (2007) examined PTSD symptoms in patients seeking pharmacological treatment for major depression. Seventy-eight percent of participants who experienced a trauma met criteria for PTSD, and 78% of participants who did not experience a Criterion A1 event met the same PTSD symptom criteria. These findings are

Table 2–4. PTSD in children

Population/event	Exposure to trauma	Prevalence of PTSD	Risk moderators
Community sample ages 9, 11, and 13 followed until age 16	54%–68%	0.1%–0.4%	• Violent or sexual trauma • Exposure to two or more traumas • Age • Prior anxiety or depression • Environmental adversity • Parenting problems
Previously healthy children unexpectedly referred to a pediatric intensive care unit	All	14% (at 3 months postdischarge) 18% (at 9 months postdischarge)	• Maternal PTSD • New stressful events • Avoidance symptoms
Children who witnessed or survived a fire	All	19% (at 9 months postfire)	• Maternal PTSD • New stressful events • Avoidance symptoms

Source. Bronner et al. 2008; Copeland et al. 2007.

Table 2–5. PTSD or symptoms of PTSD in survivors and disaster workers after large-scale natural and manmade events

Type of event and cohort	Prevalence	Comments
Natural		
Buffalo Creek Dam collapse	44% and 28%	After event and 14 years postdisaster, respectively
Firefighter responders to Australian bushfires	32%, 27%, 30%	Consistent prevalence rates at 4, 11, and 29 months postdisaster, respectively
Police responders to Hurricane Katrina	19%	PTSD risk factors included recovering bodies, assault, injury to a family member, and crowd control
Manmade		
Refugees who resettled in Western countries	3%–50% or more	9% prevalence is associated with better-designed studies; variation is due to wide variation in reviewed studies
Terrorist attacks (review)	28%	Wide variation among samples
New York City residents after 9/11 attacks	8%–20%	Highest rates of PTSD based on proximity
9/11 disaster workers and volunteers in NYC[a]		Bimodal distribution of prevalence[a]
Studies finding highest prevalence	81%–100% (2 studies)	Authors included PTSD treatment studies, where prevalence estimates were not population based
All other reviewed studies	8%–22.5% (9 studies)	8% (transit workers) to 22.5% (disaster workers)

[a]Bills et al. (2008) did not comment specifically on this wide difference in prevalence. However, the researchers suggested that differences in prevalence could be due to rates of exposure, proximity to and duration of exposure to the disaster, and type of job associated with exposure (e.g., a transit worker with a more peripheral role in disaster response may have a lower risk of PTSD than a first responder). Also, the two studies with the highest prevalence were designed to assess either response to treatment or likelihood of seeking treatment. Thus the population from which these samples were drawn was likely not to be representative of a general exposed disaster worker population because the participants were more likely to be symptomatic upon entry into the studies.

Source. Bills et al. 2008; Keane et al. 2006; West et al. 2008.

Table 2–6. PTSD in combat-exposed military service members and veterans

War	Prevalence in deployers	Odds of PTSD if deployed vs. not deployed
Vietnam war	9%–19%	3
Gulf war	2%–24%	3
Iraq war	13%–18%	2–3
Afghanistan war	6%–12%	1

Source. Adapted from Magruder KM, Yeager DE: "The Prevalence of PTSD Across War Eras and the Effect of Deployment on PTSD: A Systematic Review and Meta-Analysis." *Psychiatric Annals* 39:778–788, 2009. Copyright © 2009 SLACK Inc. Used with permission.

incongruent with a dose-response model of PTSD and suggest that the symptoms are not "caused" by trauma. Thus, findings from epidemiological studies that rely on self-reported symptoms without an adequate evaluation of Criterion A might be misleading.

Course of Illness and Symptom Persistence

Delayed Onset

Of persons who develop PTSD, many experience delayed onset of symptoms (i.e., symptom onset occurs at least 6 months following exposure to the traumatic event; American Psychiatric Association 2000). In a sample of Vietnam veterans (Schnurr et al. 2003), symptom onset occurred an average of 1.34 years after entry into Vietnam; 40% of the sample reported that symptoms first occurred 2 or more years after entering Vietnam. McFarlane (2004) discussed delayed-onset PTSD and presented findings from several studies using civilian and veteran populations. Most striking is that some people experience latency periods of decades. Grieger et al. (2006) reported that the majority (78.8%) of injured soldiers who reported PTSD and depression symptoms at 7 months reported no symptoms at 1 month following hospitalization. Other researchers reported an increase in prevalence from 7.6% at 3 months to 10% at 12 months postinjury, with nearly half of all 12-month cases being delayed onset (Carty et al. 2006).

Persistence of Symptoms

PTSD is chronic for many patients, with symptoms lasting as long as 50 or more years in some cases (Magruder et al. 2005). In Vietnam veterans, average symptom duration was 18.5 years, with 92.5% of veterans experiencing symptoms for more than 5 years, and 40.2% of veterans reporting a duration of 20 or more years (Schnurr et al. 2003). Kessler et al. (1995) found that 60% of patients with PTSD reached spontaneous remission in 72 months, but type of trauma affected time to remission. Citing a personal communication with Kessler, McFarlane (2004) reported that time from combat to remission was 85 months (7 years). Even with treatment, approximately one-third of respondents in Kessler's 1995 study did not remit at 120 months, suggesting that these people with treatment-refractory PTSD will experience lifelong symptoms. In a U.S. burden of disease study (Michaud et al. 2006), researchers estimated PTSD to last 4 years for males and 5 years for females. Researchers have argued that the development and course of PTSD can be moderated by risk and resilience factors, such as intensity, frequency, and duration of trauma; social support; family history of mental illness; ethnicity; and sex (Friedman 2006; Hoge et al. 2004; Institute of Medicine 2006; Kessler 2000).

Factors That Modify Risk

Causation and the Language Used to Describe Risk Factors

Researchers have identified factors that may modify the risk of PTSD development, but the mechanisms are poorly understood. To date, most researchers have identified *correlates*, which are factors that consistently vary according to criteria of PTSD. For example, women are more likely to develop PTSD than men (Kessler et al. 1995). However, a correlate says nothing about causation or the directionality of the relationship. For that, we (the present authors) use the term *determinant* or *consequence*.

Correlates are easier to identify because researchers can use cross-sectional data collection designs without having to rely on retrospective memory. Only with longitudinal studies and/or randomization can researchers be more confident in assessing determinants or consequences of PTSD. We focus on the causal relationship between trauma exposure and subsequent symptom development (see Table 2–7). In theory, Criterion A is the *determinant* of PTSD symptoms, and the symptoms are a *consequence* of traumatic exposure. As seen in the table and discussed elsewhere in this chapter, however, the relationship is not straightforward, and other factors may moderate or mediate symptom distress after traumatic exposure (see Table 2–8). Awareness of these factors can help clinicians better identify who may need treatment, who may need more intensive treatment, and what areas treatment might target to improve functioning.

Factors modifying risk are often confusing and can be misleading if one does not look "beneath the variable" (Ursano et al. 2008) at the complex relationship among these variables to identify determinants and consequences of PTSD. Additionally, such information must be useful to the clinician. Clinicians assess and treat individuals, not populations. Population-level epidemiological data would need to meaningfully inform and change clinical practice to be useful to the clinician.

Specific Factors

In a thorough review, Keane et al. (2006) distinguished among three categories of PTSD correlates. First, individual-specific preexisting correlates include sex, age, race, mental health history, marital status, and prior traumas. Second, event-specific correlates include aspects such as trauma severity, frequency, duration, intentionality, perceived threat, and the individual's emotional response. Third, posttrauma factors consist of elements such as social support. Other posttrauma factors in the literature include financial difficulties, social stressors (Galea et al. 2008), negative appraisals of the trauma and actions of others, avoidance coping, and hypervigilant safety behaviors (Brewin 2008). All these correlates have demonstrated at least modest predictive value in the development and maintenance of PTSD (Keane et al. 2006). However, studies find different correlates and risk factors in different populations, and some disagreement exists about the relevance of these variables.

Researchers have long argued whether peritraumatic dissociation at the time of exposure is a risk factor for PTSD. Current findings to date (van der Velden and Wittmann 2008) suggest that no empirical consensus exists regarding peritraumatic dissociation as a predictor of symptom development. Other correlates following major physical trauma include chronic illness, blaming others, an unsettled compensation claim, unemployment, and use of a lawyer (Harris et al. 2008). In intensive care unit survivors (Davydow et al.

Table 2–7. Considerations in the assessment of causation

	Theoretical question	Examples
Strength of association	Do traumatic events lead to the development of PTSD more so than other problems (e.g., depression)?	Is the association strong for a given patient (e.g., sudden severe depression after a traumatic event in someone with no previous psychiatric history)?
Consistency of association	Is the association consistent across multiple studies using different designs and measures?	Is the association consistent for a given patient over time (e.g., exacerbations in PTSD usually precede depression and suicidality)?
Biological plausibility	Does the research finding make sense given current theory? Are changes evident in neurobiology, neurophysiology, or behavior?	Following exposure to a trauma, does the patient reexperience the event, avoid reminders, and demonstrate hypervigilant behaviors?
Dose-response relationship	Do studies find that increased dose of exposure and the likelihood of outcome follow a logical dose-response pattern? (Severity and duration of trauma increases likelihood of PTSD.)	Can a provider expect that a soldier who once heard a mortar attack one-quarter mile from his location will experience the same level of distress as a soldier who was involved in multiple firefights and hand-to-hand combat?
Temporal sequence	Which is the cart and which is the horse? Did exposure to trauma cause PTSD, and can PTSD from index trauma A increase the likelihood of PTSD from index trauma B?	Did a traumatic event precede the PTSD symptoms? Did the patient experience anxiety symptoms (e.g., panic disorder with agoraphobia, general anxiety disorder, and depression) without trauma exposure? Did the patient experience anxiety symptoms prior to trauma exposure?

Table 2–8. Factors that modify risk of PTSD and PTSD severity

Preexisting and individual-specific	Trauma or response to trauma	Posttrauma
Mental health history	Trauma type, severity, and proximity to event (more severe, manmade, and violent with the highest risk)	Perceived lack of social support
Sex (female)	Perceived life threat	Subsequent life stress
Personality (external locus of control)	Peritraumatic emotions or dissociation	Stigma
Lower socioeconomic status	Negative cognitions about self and world	Community-level supports
Lower education level	Traumatic brain or other physical injury	Parenting practices (in children and adolescents), such as being too controlling or too protective
Race (minority status)		
Previous traumatic exposure (cumulatively increases risk)		
Family psychiatric history (family environment more so than genetic factors)		
Age (very young and very old more at risk)		
Pretrauma catastrophic thinking		
Poor social support		
Epigenetic factors such as maternal or parental PTSD		

Source. Bisson et al. 2007; Bokszczanin 2008; Keane et al. 2006; King 2008; Yehuda et al. 2008.

2008), prior psychopathology, greater benzodiazepine administration, and distressing memories about the intensive care unit were associated with a postinjury PTSD diagnosis.

Existing research clearly shows that PTSD co-occurs frequently with other mental disorders (Kessler et al. 1995; Magruder et al. 2005); however, another mental disorder may be a determinant, consequence, or both. By way of retrospective reporting, researchers have demonstrated that preexisting mental health conditions, such as depression, anxiety disorders, substance use disorders, and conduct disorders (Breslau 2002), increase the likelihood of PTSD development. More recently, Koenen et al. (2008) reported in a longitudinal sample that 100% of those diagnosed with PTSD in the past year, and 94% of those with lifetime PTSD, met criteria for another mental disorder between ages 11 and 21 years. The authors reported the odds (adjusted odds ratio) of having had a mental disorder by age 15 were 5.5 times greater for participants who developed PTSD than for those who experienced a trauma but did not develop PTSD. These findings suggest that a prior mental health history is a likely determinant of PTSD.

Other findings suggest that a mental disorder may also be a consequence of traumatic exposure. Copeland et al. (2007) followed cohorts of children for 4–7 years to assess traumatic exposure and pretrauma and posttrauma mental health functioning. They found that children exposed to trauma had almost double the rates of mental health disorders compared with those not exposed. They also found that higher rates of posttraumatic stress symptoms (most of their sample did not meet full criteria for PTSD) were associated with higher rates of mental health diagnoses. These results were mediated by the number of trauma exposures, because number of exposures greater than one was associated with poorer functioning. The statistical models from Copeland et al. (2007) demonstrated that age, prior anxiety, and previous trauma exposure are important determinants of trauma response in the next year.

The effects of trauma exposure appear to be cumulative, especially in women, such that exposures sensitize individuals to the effects of subsequent traumas, even if those subsequent events are of lesser magnitude (Breslau and Anthony 2007). As briefly reviewed by Keane et al. (2006), one explanation of the sensitization hypothesis is based in biology; that is, if normal stress hormones are activated over long periods (like during repeated exposures), brain physiology may be altered.

It is important to recognize the complex relationship among biological factors (see Chapter 3, "Biology"), psychological factors, and sociological factors (including familial influences) affecting PTSD development and symptom maintenance. Yehuda and LeDoux (2007) argued that "research must focus on identifying pre- and posttraumatic risk factors that explain the development of the disorder and the failure to reinstate physiological homeostasis" (p. 19). They reviewed research from twin studies that suggest shared genetic risk factors for exposure to interpersonal violence and development of PTSD. Yehuda et al. (2008) argued that epigenetic factors may be important because the risk of PTSD in offspring is related to maternal PTSD or to maternal and paternal PTSD, but not to paternal PTSD alone.

Impact of PTSD on the Community and Health Care System

People with PTSD are seen in all health care settings. Knowledge of PTSD (i.e., the ability to recognize and/or treat symptoms) can enhance the quality of care provided by general health practitioners, given the frequency with which patients with PTSD present in non–mental health settings and the high levels of functional and medical problems associated with the disorder. In a review, Seedat et al. (2006) reported that patients with PTSD have more impairments in quality of life than do general-public patients with other chronic physical conditions (e.g., diabetes, multiple sclerosis) or patients with anxiety disorders. PTSD ranks second only to depression in terms of the quality-of-life decrements associated with mental disorders.

The impact of PTSD is also seen in veteran and active-duty military populations, including veterans from World War II, Korea, Vietnam, the Gulf War, and the wars in Iraq and Afghanistan (Magruder and Yeager 2009; Magruder et al. 2005). For example, service members returning from Iraq reported a fourfold increase in concerns about interpersonal conflict (Milliken et al. 2007). Returning service members from Iraq or Afghanistan who screened positive for mental health concerns had higher rates of attrition from the military (Hoge et al. 2006). Returnees who screened positive for PTSD also had higher rates of sick call visits, somatic complaints, physical symptoms, and missed workdays, as well as overall lower general health (Hoge et al. 2007). Hoge et al. (2008) concluded that PTSD, and not mild traumatic brain injury, accounted for poor general health, missed workdays, medical visits, and a high number of somatic and postconcussive symptoms (except for headache). In community (Zvolensky et al. 2008) and military/veteran samples (Smith et al. 2008), PTSD was associated with increased risks of smoking, even during a self-guided quit attempt (Zvolensky et al. 2008.

PTSD is also associated with educational failure, work impairment (an estimated $3 billion loss in productivity in the United States), unemployment, and marital instability (Kessler 2000). It is even associated with increased mortality (Boscarino 2008) and suicide (McFarlane 2004), although this finding is not generally supported or included in large-scale studies of population health (e.g., Kinder et al. 2008; Michaud et al. 2006).

Freed et al. (2009) summarized the preference-based metrics (a special class of health-related quality-of-life measures used in cost-effectiveness and disease burden analyses) for PTSD, and found that the decrements associated with PTSD are comparable to those of major depression. Severe PTSD is only a slightly more desirable health condition than pretransplant congestive heart failure (van Hout et al. 1993). When combined with measures of disease pervasiveness (i.e., incidence) and persistence (i.e., course of illness), PTSD ranks within the top 20 most burdensome diseases in the United States (Michaud et al. 2006).

The effects of PTSD go far beyond symptom distress. PTSD enervates families, clinics, health care systems, and communities. Only through large-scale epidemiological studies could this information have been gleaned, and these studies on the aftermath of PTSD provide a glib picture. However, the question remains: What can epidemiology tell us about how to clinically manage PTSD?

Applying Epidemiological Knowledge to the Clinical Management of PTSD

We see this chapter as most relevant from three clinical perspectives (see Table 2–9): those of the mental health care provider, the primary care provider, and the health care administrator. PTSD is treatable (arguably to varying degrees of effectiveness) and perhaps preventable (Adler et al. 2007), although more research exists on the efficacy of PTSD treatment than on prevention efforts. A full review of the efficacy literature is beyond the scope of this chapter, but

Table 2–9. Epidemiological contributions by clinical perspective

Epidemiological contribution	Mental health care provider	Primary care provider	Health care administrator
Tailor treatment	X	X	
Screening and assessment	X	X	X
Prevention	X	X	X
Resource allocation			X
Disaster preparation	X	X	X
Community support			X
Clinical decision making	X	X	

several recent reviews determined that psychotherapeutic (Bisson et al. 2007; Bradley et al. 2005) and pharmacological (Davidson 2006; Ipser et al. 2006) interventions for PTSD can be effective. The effectiveness of varying types of therapy or drug treatments depends on the type of intervention and samples studied. In general, treatments were less effective for combat trauma (Bisson et al. 2007; Bradley et al. 2005; Ipser et al. 2006) than for noncombat trauma.

Mental Health Care Provider

Of most obvious relevance to the clinical management of PTSD is the mental health care provider. Beyond just implementing efficacious treatments, the mental health care provider must be aware of the complexities of diagnosing and treating PTSD. Although most individuals who are exposed to trauma do not develop PTSD, some individuals have chronic and unremitting PTSD symptoms for decades. Numerous correlates of PTSD development and maintenance are modifiable with support and treatment. For example, Kleim et al. (2007) found that mental defeat and rumination about prior problems with anxiety or depression were good predictors of PTSD. Clinicians trained in cognitive-behavioral therapy can readily identify and restructure irrational thoughts, thereby potentially improving symptoms. Other researchers argue that "ongoing stressors play a central role in explaining the trajectory" of PTSD and that interventions designed to reduce ongoing adversity may attenuate the consequences of trauma (Galea et al. 2008). In working with children and adolescents, clinicians should be adept at handling family issues, such as parental support, family conflict, overprotectiveness, and parenting practices, all of which may be determinants of PTSD symptom severity (Bokszczanin 2008; Gewirtz et al. 2008).

Primary Care Provider

Primary care is often the first entry point into the health care system by PTSD patients. Primary care providers are tasked not only with treating the patient's chief complaint but also with screening for other treatable problems. Primary care providers can use brief PTSD screens (e.g., Gore et al. 2008; Prins et al. 2004) to identify PTSD symptoms. Primary care providers can also offer pharmacological treatment for PTSD symptoms. The primary care provider's capacity to identify and treat PTSD benefits both the individual patient and the health care system, especially if patients are reluctant to see a mental health specialist (Hoge et al. 2004) or can be treated without seeing a mental health specialist. However, without accurate knowledge of PTSD prevalence in a clinic (prevalence of PTSD in primary care clinics ranges from 6% to 36%, as reported by Gore et al. 2008), primary care providers may overlook this common problem. Conversely, they may assume a PTSD diagnosis, especially when patients report symptoms, such as peritraumatic dissociation, that are unusual in primary care settings. Accurate recognition can lead to appropriate treatment, especially given that patients with PTSD are heavy users of the health care system, and primary care providers generally underdiagnose rather than overdiagnose PTSD (Magruder et al. 2005).

Health Care Administrator

Epidemiological data can help health care systems better predict what resources will be needed to best provide care. For example, in areas prone to natural disasters, a health care administrator may consider an emphasis on community outreach and connectedness to community resources. Abramson et al. (2008) found that factors such as informal social support networks were associated with better mental health status. Health care administrators must also be aware of potential biases of screening tools, given that appropriate cutoff scores may be population dependent. The choice of a cutoff score to determine population prevalence greatly influences results (Terhakopian et al.

2008). Finally, cost-effectiveness and disease burden metrics can help evaluate the real-time health of a population via direct comparisons of medical and mental health conditions.

Conclusion

In this chapter, we by no means provide an exhaustive summary of all that epidemiology can offer to the clinical management of PTSD. Rather, we offer an introduction to the utility of epidemiological principles and knowledge. We did not describe at least a few other factors that are relevant to the population-level understanding of PTSD because epidemiology of PTSD is a large topic, and volumes may be dedicated to each of these in turn. For example, we give a cursory description of resilience factors, which by some are seen as the opposite of risk factors along a single dimension (e.g., low IQ is associated with a high risk of PTSD, and high IQ is associated with a lower risk of PTSD). However, risk and resilience factors may not be unidimensional, and they actually interact with one another by offsetting the impact of each (e.g., good coping may offset the increased risk of PTSD because of low IQ [Yehuda and Flory 2007]). We also say very little about the discordance between science and law, both of which define who has symptoms of posttraumatic stress (Mendelson 1995), and little about current research to identify latent class variables of PTSD (Breslau et al. 2005). Although these topics are important in their own right, they likely are not as useful to the clinical management of PTSD as they are to understanding policy implications and nosological and classification issues.

Epidemiology provides a population-level perspective on issues relevant to improving prevention, identification, and treatment of PTSD. Clinicians, clinic and hospital administrators, and health policy makers must make decisions in the face of competing demands. The following are examples of decisions: How should a primary care provider prioritize patient concerns of traumatic exposure when the patient is also reporting other concerns and appointment times are limited? What problems are frequently presented in a clinic, and are staff members appropriately trained to handle those problems? Following a disaster, what factors may impact a decision to extend mental health services to survivors and rescue workers? All these questions rely on epidemiological studies for answers. Through epidemiology, researchers, health care policy makers, and clinicians gain valuable information regarding the frequency of traumatic exposure, the likelihood of developing PTSD, the expected course of the disorder, and the impact of mitigating factors.

Key Clinical Points

- The epidemiology of PTSD provides 1) evidence of disease rates, risk factors, and correlates; 2) normative screening data; 3) real-world support for interventions to assist the health care practitioner; and 4) rates of detection and treatment and patterns of medical utilization in those with the disease.
- Recently traumatized individuals are several times more likely to present for medical care than for mental health care.
- Rates of traumatic exposure are higher than rates of PTSD; thus, clinicians should be cautious about presuming a diagnosis of PTSD based solely on exposure.
- Several factors, including trauma type, affect rates of PTSD.
- DSM-IV-TR Criterion A2 (the experience of intense fear, helplessness, or horror) is a weak predictor of PTSD, but the *absence* of Criterion A2 is a strong indicator of *no* PTSD (except in highly trained individuals such as military personnel).
- Proximity to a disaster, degree of injury, threat to life, fatalities, and property damage correlate to rates of PTSD.
- The time to onset of PTSD after a traumatic event varies greatly.
- There is a high comorbidity of PTSD and other mental health problems.
- Research suggests that traumatic exposure has a cumulative effect, particularly in women.
- PTSD ranks second only to depression in terms of quality-of-life decrements associated with a mental health disorder.

References

Abramson D, Stehling-Ariza T, Garfield R, et al: Prevalence and predictors of mental health distress post-Katrina: findings from the Gulf Coast Child and Family Health Study. Disaster Med Public Health Prep 2:77–86, 2008

Adler AB, Castro CA, McGurk D: U.S. Army Medical Research Unit—Europe Research Report 2007-001. Heidelberg, Germany, USAMRU-E, 2007

Adler AB, Wright KM, Bliese PD, et al: A2 diagnostic criterion for combat-related posttraumatic stress disorder. J Trauma Stress 21:301–308, 2008

American Psychiatric Association: Diagnostic and Statistical Manual of Mental Disorders, 3rd Edition. Washington, DC, American Psychiatric Association, 1980

American Psychiatric Association: Diagnostic and Statistical Manual of Mental Disorders, 3rd Edition, Revised. Washington, DC, American Psychiatric Association, 1987

American Psychiatric Association: Diagnostic and Statistical Manual of Mental Disorders, 4th Edition, Text Revision. Washington, DC, American Psychiatric Association, 2000

Bills CB, Levy NA, Sharma V, et al: Mental health of workers and volunteers responding to events of 9/11: review of the literature. Mt Sinai J Med 75:115–127, 2008

Bisson JI, Ehlers A, Matthews R, et al: Psychological treatments for chronic posttraumatic stress disorder: systematic review and meta-analysis. Br J Psychiatry 190:97–104, 2007

Bodkin JA, Pope HG, Detke MJ, et al: Is PTSD caused by traumatic stress? J Anxiety Disord 21:176–182, 2007

Bokszczanin A: Parental support, family conflict, and overprotectiveness: predicting PTSD symptom levels of adolescents 28 months after a natural disaster. Anxiety Stress Coping 21:325–335, 2008

Boscarino JA: Psychobiologic predictors of disease mortality after psychological trauma: implications for research and clinical surveillance. J Nerv Ment Dis 196:100–107, 2008

Bradley R, Greene J, Russ E, et al: A multidimensional meta-analysis of psychotherapy for PTSD. Am J Psychiatry 162:214–227, 2005

Breslau N: Epidemiologic studies of trauma, posttraumatic stress disorder, and other psychiatric disorders. Can J Psychiatry 47:923–929, 2002

Breslau N, Anthony JC: Gender differences in the sensitivity to posttraumatic stress disorder: an epidemiological study of urban young adults. J Abnorm Psychol 116:607–611, 2007

Breslau N, Kessler RC: The stressor criterion in DSM-IV posttraumatic stress disorder: an empirical investigation. Biol Psychiatry 50:699–704, 2001

Breslau N, Davis GC, Andreski P, et al: Traumatic events and posttraumatic stress disorder in an urban population of young adults. Arch Gen Psychiatry 48:216–222, 1991

Breslau N, Kessler RC, Chilcoat HD, et al: Trauma and posttraumatic stress disorder in the community: the 1996 Detroit Area Survey of Trauma. Arch Gen Psychiatry 55:626–632, 1998

Breslau N, Reboussin BA, Anthony JC, et al: The structure of posttraumatic stress disorder: latent class analysis in 2 community samples. Arch Gen Psychiatry 62:1343–1351, 2005

Brewin CR: What is it that a neurobiological model of PTSD must explain? Prog Brain Res 167:217–228, 2008

Bronner MB, Knoester H, Bos AP, et al: Posttraumatic stress disorder (PTSD) in children after paediatric intensive care treatment compared to children who survived a major fire disaster. Child Adolesc Psychiatry Ment Health 2:9, 2008

Carty J, O'Donnell ML, Creamer M: Delayed-onset PTSD: a prospective study of injury survivors. J Affect Disord 90:257–261, 2006

Copeland WE, Keeler G, Angold A, et al: Traumatic events and posttraumatic stress in childhood. Arch Gen Psychiatry 64:577–584, 2007

Creamer M, Burgess P, McFarlane AC: Post-traumatic stress disorder: findings from the Australian National Survey of Mental Health and Well-being. Psychol Med 31:1237–1247, 2001

Davidson JR: Pharmacologic treatment of acute and chronic stress following trauma: 2006. J Clin Psychiatry 67 (suppl 2):34–39, 2006

Davidson JR, Foa EB: Diagnostic issues in posttraumatic stress disorder: considerations for the DSM-IV. J Abnorm Psychol 100:346–355, 1991

Davidson JR, Stein DJ, Shalev AY, et al: Posttraumatic stress disorder: acquisition, recognition, course, and treatment. J Neuropsychiatry Clin Neurosci 16:135–147, 2004

Davydow DS, Gifford JM, Desai SV, et al: Posttraumatic stress disorder in general intensive care unit survivors: a systematic review. Gen Hosp Psychiatry 30:421–434, 2008

DeViva JC, Bloem WD: Symptom exaggeration and compensation seeking among combat veterans with posttraumatic stress disorder. J Trauma Stress 16:503–507, 2003

Deykin EY, Keane TM, Kaloupek D, et al: Posttraumatic stress disorder and the use of health services. Psychosom Med 63:835–841, 2001

Freed MC, Goldberg RK, Gore KL, et al: Estimating the disease burden of combat-related posttraumatic stress disorder in United States veterans and military service members, in Handbook of Disease Burdens and Quality of Life Measures. Edited by Preedy VR, Watson RR. New York, Springer-Verlag, 2009, pp 1527–1548

Friedman MJ: Posttraumatic stress disorder among military returnees from Afghanistan and Iraq. Am J Psychiatry 163:586–593, 2006

Galea S, Tracy M, Norris F, et al: Financial and social circumstances and the incidence and course of PTSD in Mississippi during the first two years after Hurricane Katrina. J Trauma Stress 21:357–368, 2008

Gewirtz A, Forgatch M, Wieling E: Parenting practices as potential mechanisms for child adjustment following mass trauma. J Marital Fam Ther 34:177–192, 2008

Gore KL, Engel CC, Freed MC, et al: Test of a single-item posttraumatic stress disorder screener in a military primary care setting. Gen Hosp Psychiatry 30:391–397, 2008

Grieger TA, Cozza SJ, Ursano RJ, et al: Posttraumatic stress disorder and depression in battle-injured soldiers. Am J Psychiatry 163:1777–1783; quiz 1860, 2006

Harris IA, Young JM, Rae H, et al: Predictors of post-traumatic stress disorder following major trauma. ANZ J Surg 78:583–587, 2008

Hepp U, Gamma A, Milos G, et al: Prevalence of exposure to potentially traumatic events and PTSD. The Zurich Cohort Study. Eur Arch Psychiatry Clin Neurosci 256:151–158, 2006

Hoge CW, Castro CA, Messer SC, et al: Combat duty in Iraq and Afghanistan, mental health problems, and barriers to care. N Engl J Med 351:13–22, 2004

Hoge CW, Auchterlonie JL, Milliken CS: Mental health problems, use of mental health services, and attrition from military service after returning from deployment to Iraq or Afghanistan. JAMA 295:1023–1032, 2006

Hoge CW, Terhakopian A, Castro CA, et al: Association of posttraumatic stress disorder with somatic symptoms, health care visits, and absenteeism among Iraq war veterans. Am J Psychiatry 164:150–153, 2007

Hoge CW, McGurk D, Thomas JL, et al: Mild traumatic brain injury in U.S. soldiers returning from Iraq. N Engl J Med 358:453–463, 2008

Institute of Medicine, Subcommittee on Posttraumatic Stress Disorder of the Committee on Gulf War and Health: Posttraumatic Stress Disorder: Diagnosis and Assessment. Washington, DC, National Academies Press, 2006

Ipser J, Seedat S, Stein DJ: Pharmacotherapy for post-traumatic stress disorder—a systematic review and meta-analysis. S Afr Med J 96:1088–1096, 2006

Jones E, Wessely S: A paradigm shift in the conceptualization of psychological trauma in the 20th century. J Anxiety Disord 21:164–175, 2007

Keane TM, Marshall AD, Taft CT: Posttraumatic stress disorder: etiology, epidemiology, and treatment outcome. Annu Rev Clin Psychol 2:161–197, 2006

Kessler RC: Posttraumatic stress disorder: the burden to the individual and to society. J Clin Psychiatry 61 (suppl 5):4–14, 2000

Kessler RC, Sonnega A, Bromet E, et al: Posttraumatic stress disorder in the National Comorbidity Survey. Arch Gen Psychiatry 52:1048–1060, 1995

Kessler RC, Sonnega A, Bromet E, et al: Epidemiological risk factors for trauma and PTSD, in Risk Factors for Posttraumatic Stress Disorder. Edited by Yehuda R. Washington, DC, American Psychiatric Press, 1999, pp 23–60

Kessler RC, Chiu WT, Demler O, et al: Prevalence, severity, and comorbidity of 12-month DSM-IV disorders in the National Comorbidity Survey Replication. Arch Gen Psychiatry 62:617–627, 2005

Kimerling R, Calhoun KS: Somatic symptoms, social support, and treatment seeking among sexual assault victims. J Consult Clin Psychol 62:333–340, 1994

Kinder LS, Bradley KA, Katon WJ, et al: Depression, posttraumatic stress disorder, and mortality. Psychosom Med 70:20–26, 2008

King NS: PTSD and traumatic brain injury: folklore and fact? Brain Inj 22:1–5, 2008

Kleim B, Ehlers A, Glucksman E: Early predictors of chronic post-traumatic stress disorder in assault survivors. Psychol Med 37:1457–1467, 2007

Koenen KC, Moffitt TE, Caspi A, et al: The developmental mental-disorder histories of adults with posttraumatic stress disorder: a prospective longitudinal birth cohort study. J Abnorm Psychol 117:460–466, 2008

Magruder KM, Yeager DE: The prevalence of PTSD across war eras and the effect of deployment on PTSD: a systematic review and meta-analysis. Psychiatric Annals 39:778–788, 2009

Magruder KM, Frueh BC, Knapp RG, et al: Prevalence of posttraumatic stress disorder in Veterans Affairs primary care clinics. Gen Hosp Psychiatry 27:169–179, 2005

McFarlane A: The contribution of epidemiology to the study of traumatic stress. Soc Psychiatry Psychiatr Epidemiol 39:874–882, 2004

McNally RJ: Progress and controversy in the study of posttraumatic stress disorder. Annu Rev Psychol 54:229–252, 2003

Mendelson D: Legal and medical aspects of liability for negligently occasioned nervous shock: a current perspective. J Psychosom Res 39:721–735, 1995

Michaud CM, McKenna MT, Begg S, et al: The burden of disease and injury in the United States 1996. Popul Health Metr 4:11, 2006

Milliken CS, Auchterlonie JL, Hoge CW: Longitudinal assessment of mental health problems among active and reserve component soldiers returning from the Iraq war. JAMA 298:2141–2148, 2007

Mol SS, Arntz A, Metsemakers JF, et al: Symptoms of post-traumatic stress disorder after non-traumatic events: evidence from an open population study. Br J Psychiatry 186:494–499, 2005

Neria Y, Nandi A, Galea S: Post-traumatic stress disorder following disasters: a systematic review. Psychol Med 38:467–480, 2008

Prins A, Ouimette P, Kimerling R, et al: The Primary Care PTSD screen (PC–PTSD): development and operating characteristics. Primary Care Psychiatry 9:9–14, 2004

Schnurr PP, Friedman MJ, Sengupta A, et al: PTSD and utilization of medical treatment services among male Vietnam veterans. J Nerv Ment Dis 188:496–504, 2000

Schnurr PP, Lunney CA, Sengupta A, et al: A descriptive analysis of PTSD chronicity in Vietnam veterans. J Trauma Stress 16:545–553, 2003

Schnurr PP, Hayes AF, Lunney CA, et al: Longitudinal analysis of the relationship between symptoms and quality of life in veterans treated for posttraumatic stress disorder. J Consult Clin Psychol 74:707–713, 2006

Seedat S, Lochner C, Vythilingum B, et al: Disability and quality of life in posttraumatic stress disorder: impact of drug treatment. Pharmacoeconomics 24:989–998, 2006

Smith TC, Ryan MA, Wingard DL, et al: New onset and persistent symptoms of posttraumatic stress disorder self reported after deployment and combat exposures: prospective population based U.S. military cohort study. BMJ 336:366–371, 2008

Spinazzola J, Blaustein M, van der Kolk BA: Posttraumatic stress disorder treatment outcome research: the study of unrepresentative samples? J Trauma Stress 18:425–436, 2005

Stein MB, McQuaid JR, Pedrelli P, et al: Posttraumatic stress disorder in the primary care medical setting. Gen Hosp Psychiatry 22:261–269, 2000

Terhakopian A, Sinaii N, Engel CC, et al: Estimating population prevalence of posttraumatic stress disorder: an example using the PTSD checklist. J Trauma Stress 21:290–300, 2008

Ursano RJ, Santiago P, Hasan N: PTSD and traumatic stress: gender, ethnicity and other problems of knowing and care. Presentation at the National Institutes of Health conference Trauma Spectrum Disorders: The Role of Gender, Race and Other Socioeconomic Factors, Bethesda, MD, October 2008

van der Velden PG, Wittmann L: The independent predictive value of peritraumatic dissociation for PTSD symptomatology after type I trauma: a systematic review of prospective studies. Clin Psychol Rev 28:1009–1020, 2008

van Hout BA, Wielink G, Bonsel GJ, et al: Effects of ACE inhibitors on heart failure in the Netherlands: a pharmacoeconomic model. Pharmacoeconomics 3:387–397, 1993

Wang PS, Berglund P, Olfson M, et al: Failure and delay in initial treatment contact after first onset of mental disorders in the National Comorbidity Survey Replication. Arch Gen Psychiatry 62:603–613, 2005

Weathers FW, Keane TM: The Criterion A problem revisited: controversies and challenges in defining and measuring psychological trauma. J Trauma Stress 20:107–121, 2007

West C, Bernard B, Mueller C, et al: Mental health outcomes in police personnel after Hurricane Katrina. J Occup Environ Med 50:689–695, 2008

Yeager DE, Magruder KM, Knapp RG, et al: Performance characteristics of the posttraumatic stress disorder checklist and SPAN in Veterans Affairs primary care settings. Gen Hosp Psychiatry 29:294–301, 2007

Yehuda R, Flory JD: Differentiating biological correlates of risk, PTSD, and resilience following trauma exposure. J Trauma Stress 20:435–447, 2007

Yehuda R, LeDoux J: Response variation following trauma: a translational neuroscience approach to understanding PTSD. Neuron 56:19–32, 2007

Yehuda R, Bell A, Bierer LM, et al: Maternal, not paternal, PTSD is related to increased risk for PTSD in offspring of Holocaust survivors. J Psychiatr Res 42:1104–1111, 2008

Zatzick DF, Galea S: An epidemiologic approach to the development of early trauma focused intervention. J Trauma Stress 20:401–412, 2007

Zvolensky MJ, Gibson LE, Vujanovic AA, et al: Impact of posttraumatic stress disorder on early smoking lapse and relapse during a self-guided quit attempt among community-recruited daily smokers. Nicotine Tob Res 10:1415–1427, 2008

3

Biology

Espen Walderhaug, Ph.D.
John H. Krystal, M.D.
Alexander Neumeister, M.D.

The definition of posttraumatic stress disorder (PTSD) in the *Diagnostic and Statistical Manual of Mental Disorders*, 4th Edition, Text Revision (DSM-IV-TR; American Psychiatric Association 2000), links a specific syndrome, characterized mainly by symptoms of reexperiencing, avoidance, and hyperarousal, with catastrophic and traumatic events distinguished from ordinary stressful life events. Epidemiological surveys in the United States have documented the

This work was supported by a grant from the Department of Veterans Affairs to the VA National Center for PTSD and VA Alcohol Research Center, as well as by grants 5 AA 14906 04 and 2P50-AA012870-07 (Dr. Krystal). Dr. Krystal is a paid scientific consultant in the area of PTSD to Eli Lilly and Co. Dr. Walderhaug is supported by a postdoctoral fellowship grant from the Research Council of Norway, Division for Science.

probability of developing PTSD following traumatic exposure at approximately 10% (Breslau et al. 1998; Kessler et al. 1995); women are more likely than men to develop PTSD once trauma occurs (Breslau et al. 1999; Norris 1992; Stein et al. 1997b, 2000). The increased morbidity (Hoge et al. 2007; Kubzansky et al. 2007), disability (Schnurr et al. 2006; Zatzick et al. 1997), and mortality (Boscarino 2006) associated with PTSD illustrate the need to develop more informative models to test pathophysiological and treatment hypotheses. Current prevention and treatment strategies for PTSD can be improved, and additional research is needed to investigate basic mechanisms underlying PTSD with the goal of alleviating the devastating impact on public health.

The Interactive Role of Heritability and Environment in the Etiology of PTSD

Converging evidence from family, twin, and molecular genetic studies supports the role of genetic influences in the etiology of PTSD. Family studies indicate an increased risk for PTSD in first-degree relatives of patients with PTSD (Sack et al. 1995). Ongoing research efforts aim to separate environmental from genetic causes; that is, the succession of PTSD from parent to child could be caused by a parent's altering a child's avoidance behavior through poor adjustment to trauma, or the parent could have passed on genetic vulnerabilities to the development of PTSD (Koenen et al. 2008). Twin studies can disentangle and investigate these factors, and have greatly increased understanding of the genetic etiology of PTSD. Twin studies have found genetic influence in three areas: the risk of trauma exposure, the development of PTSD, and the existence of comorbidity (Nugent et al. 2008). Moderators of the disease process in PTSD appear to include a heritable component as well as the individual's environment and coping style.

Although family and twin studies are important in establishing heritability, they cannot identify individual genes that might moderate the PTSD risk. Molecular genetic studies look at the structure and function of genes, as well as how genes are transferred from generation to generation. In contrast to family and twin studies, molecular genetic studies have the potential to identify markers of vulnerability and resilience.

Molecular genetics has established two research strategies: linkage studies and association studies. A linkage study looks for genetic markers that run in a family. Ideally, candidate genes should first appear in linkage studies, where the entire genome of individuals is examined in large family studies to identify genetic markers continuously passed on together with a given disease process, such as PTSD (Broekman et al. 2007). This approach is difficult in PTSD research, because the diagnostic prerequisite is exposure to a potentially traumatic event. This environmental condition for PTSD constitutes a variable that limits the number of eligible participants in a family and makes linkage studies in PTSD difficult.

In contrast, association studies investigate possible connections between genetic variants (polymorphisms) and underlying traits (endophenotypes), such as biochemical, endocrine, neuroanatomical, cognitive, and psychiatric characteristics of an illness, in this case PTSD. To date, only a limited number of genetic studies related to PTSD are available, but the results from these studies indicate a genetic influence on the function of neurochemical systems suspected to be important for PTSD, including brain dopamine and serotonergic systems. Ongoing research aims to identify the genetic influences of the functioning of other neurobiological systems in PTSD, including the hypothalamic-pituitary-adrenal (HPA) axis, γ-aminobutyric acid (GABA), apolipoprotein E, brain-derived neurotrophic factor, and neuropeptide Y (NPY) systems (Broekman et al. 2007).

A potentially important approach to better understanding gene by environment interactions is an exemplary study conducted by Kilpatrick et al. (2007) to test if a polymorphism in the serotonin transporter gene promotor region (5-HTTLPR) moderates risk of developing PTSD after a natural disaster. Kilpatrick and colleagues found the low expression or short (*s*) variant of 5-HTTLPR increased the risk of posthurricane PTSD, but only under the conditions of high hurricane exposure and low social support. As future studies identify more candidate genes, researchers may come to better understand the interactions between genetic vulnerability and traumatic exposure.

Evidence has been found to suggest that the sex of participants should be considered to more fully understand the effects of genes in the pathology of PTSD. Sjöberg et al. (2006) looked at a polymorphism in 5-HTTLPR in 200 adolescent boys and girls to see how environment, sex, and genotype might predict depression. Although measures for PTSD were not included, the findings are highly relevant to the study of PTSD because 5-HTTLPR is one of the most promising candidate genes in PTSD, particularly given its high comorbidity with depression and the emerging evidence of a sex difference in PTSD. Sjöberg et al. (2006) found that homozygous carriers of the short (*s*) 5-HTTLPR allele were more vulnerable to different environmental stressors than heterozygous carriers or carriers of the long (*l*) allele, irrespective of gender. Girls carrying the *s*/*s* allele were more significantly affected by traumatic conflict within the family and developed depressive symptoms in response to high family conflict. In contrast, boys carrying the *s*/*s* allele were more significantly affected by the type of residence in which they lived than by traumatic conflict within the family. Boys carrying the *s*/*s* allele responded to living in public housing, rather than in their own house, with a decrease in depressive symptoms. The unexpected reduction of depressive symptoms in the boys carrying the *s*/*s* allele can be explained by a symptom shift toward other kinds of psychopathological behavior and might reflect a true sex difference in the depressive phenotype (Rihmer et al. 1998; Sjöberg et al. 2006). A recent study using tryptophan depletion to transiently lower brain serotonin function supports such hypotheses. The authors reported that men (but not women) became more impulsive, whereas women (but not men) showed mood reduction in response to tryptophan depletion (Walderhaug et al. 2007). Evidence explaining the sex difference observed in prevalence and clinical presentation of mood and impulse control disorders would help further the understanding and treatment of PTSD.

Influence of Gender in PTSD

Emerging evidence suggests sex differences in both prevalence and duration of PTSD. Women have a higher prevalence of PTSD compared with men regardless of age (Cuffe et al. 1998; Kessler et al. 1995). Furthermore, women typically experience PTSD symptoms for longer periods than men. Breslau (2002) found that the median time to PTSD remission was 12 months in men versus 48 months in women. Notably, evidence indicates that even though women are more likely to meet criteria for PTSD, they are less likely to experience traumatic events in general (Tolin and Foa 2006). The type of trauma may explain some of this discrepancy. Sexual assault is one of the most severe traumatic experiences and has a significantly higher incidence in women. This greater lifetime exposure to sexual assault among women may explain the higher prevalence of PTSD in women despite the lower overall exposure to traumatic events. This notion, however, did not stand up to a "within-trauma type" analysis revealing women to be more likely than men to experience PTSD following exposure to accidents, nonsexual assaults, witnessing death/injury, disaster, fire, and war. Another study found women to be more than twice as likely to develop PTSD following a traumatic event, irrespective of the precipitating trauma, other traumatic experiences, poverty, or history of affective disorders (Breslau et al. 1999). These findings suggest that the greater prevalence of PTSD in women cannot be completely explained by type of trauma (Koenen et al. 2008); however, not all studies have found an increased vulnerability for PTSD in women. In a population-based survey of 30,000 Gulf War era veterans, exposure to either of two kinds of severe trauma—sexual assault or combat—was associated with comparable risk for PTSD in men and women (Kang et al. 2005). Overall, it remains unclear whether there is a "true" gender effect that moderates PTSD risk or instead the increased PTSD risk in women is explained by environmental factors such as the type of trauma.

Neuroendocrine and Neurochemical Aspects of PTSD

PTSD may be related to disturbances in the synthesis, release, or metabolism of a combination of hormones and neurotransmitters. The HPA axis has received considerable attention in PTSD and other stress-related disorders. The HPA axis is an important system in stress response that provides for coordination of energy regulation, immune defenses, brain information processing, and behavioral response.

Cortisol

Cortisol is the primary stress hormone and has numerous effects on the body. One such effect is an increased sensitivity of the thalamus to incoming stimuli (Weiss 2007). Cortisol release increases under stress, resulting in the reduction of many metabolic, neuronal defensive, and immune reactions, as well as an increase in the amount of energy available for responding to the immediate stressor. The concentration of cortisol in patients with PTSD varies across studies, with reports of low (Bremner et al. 2003a; Yehuda et al. 1990), high

(Maes et al. 1998), or normal (Shalev et al. 2008) basal cortisol concentration when compared with that of normal controls. The general assumption that cortisol levels are low in patients with PTSD was disproved in a recent meta-analysis across 37 studies (Meewisse et al. 2007). Nevertheless, there remains support for low cortisol levels in patients with PTSD under certain conditions, based on the type of control group and the specific subpopulation. Statistically significantly lower cortisol levels were found in people with PTSD when compared with nonexposed controls, but not when compared with trauma-exposed controls. Subgroup analysis further revealed lower cortisol in women and abused victims—that is, the populations most at risk for developing PTSD. Finally, cortisol levels were significantly lower in the PTSD groups compared with the control groups when the cortisol samples were collected in the afternoon, but not when collected in the morning (Meewisse et al. 2007). Figure 3–1 gives a graphical presentation of the 37 main articles published on PTSD and cortisol between 1980 and 2005. The results from these studies vary on either side of the dotted line representing "no difference" in cortisol levels between PTSD and control groups.

Thus far, research has shown lower levels of cortisol in PTSD patients compared with controls only under certain conditions. Cortisol levels depend on age, gender, body weight, and metabolism of the participant; type and chronicity of stressor; comorbid depression or other psychopathology; substance abuse; time since the traumatic event; and time in the circadian rhythm during which cortisol is collected for assessment (Pervanidou 2008). Studies reporting on cortisol levels in subjects homogeneous with respect to the above variables or controlling for these variables in statistical analyses have generally been more likely to observe significant differences in cortisol related to PTSD (Yehuda et al. 2006). Studies alleging a link between endocrine "vulnerability factors" and PTSD often lack predictive power, and such models have very little specificity and sensitivity as indicators of the disorder (Shalev et al. 2008). Biological alterations associated with PTSD may be correlates of other pathophysiological processes, or may represent compensatory mechanisms of adaptation rather than constituting a core pathophysiological process. The scientific literature thus far has not suggested an endocrine pathology in PTSD, and in general cortisol levels are reported to be within normal limits for individuals with PTSD (Yehuda 2006).

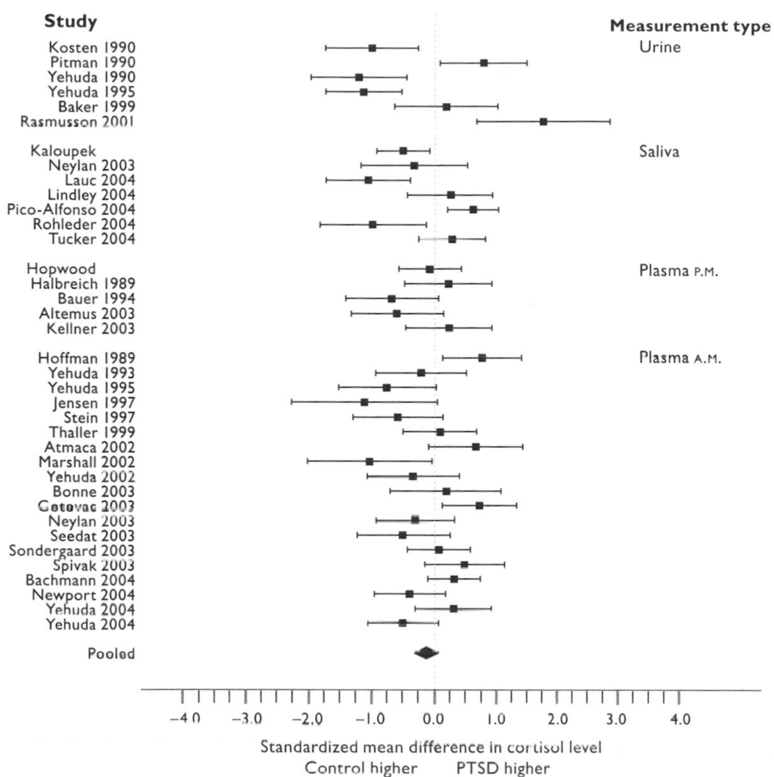

Figure 3–1. Standardized mean difference (with 95% confidence interval) in cortisol levels between people with posttraumatic stress disorder and control subjects (37 studies).

Studies are grouped according to type of measurement and identified by first-named author.

Source. Reprinted from Meewisse M-L, Reitsma JB, De Vries G-J, et al.: "Cortisol and Post-traumatic Stress Disorder in Adults: Systematic Review and Meta-Analysis." *British Journal of Psychiatry* 191:387–392, 2007, p. 389. Copyright 2007 The Royal College of Psychiatrists. Used with permission.

The secretion of cortisol is regulated via an HPA feedback loop. Corticotropin-releasing hormone (CRH) has a regulatory effect on cortisol secretion and serves as a neurotransmitter coordinating stress-induced neural responses in the brain. CRH receptors (CRH1, CRH2) are distributed throughout the brain (Lightman and Young 1988) and have been investigated for possible treatment development. An open-label study of a CRH1 antagonist for the treatment of depression showed promise (Zobel et al. 2000), but the only sufficiently powered and adequately dosed comparator substance and placebo-controlled study failed to demonstrate clinical antidepressant effects (Binneman et al. 2008). This negative finding dampens enthusiasm for using CRH1 antagonists in patients with PTSD, although clinical trials in PTSD have not yet been completed and are currently ongoing.

Norepinephrine

Noradrenergic and serotonergic transmitter systems have both been implicated in core symptoms of PTSD (Southwick et al. 1997a). The noradrenergic systems in patients with PTSD have been found to be hyperresponsive to stressful stimuli (Southwick et al. 1997a). Such hyperresponsiveness would be consistent with the behavioral sensitization model of PTSD, proposing that biochemical, physiological, and behavioral responses to stressors increase over time (Southwick et al. 1997b). With chronic traumatic stress, the norepinephrine system becomes sensitized from repeated activation (Bremner et al. 1996). Although the findings are inconsistent, the levels of norepinephrine and noradrenergic activity (both centrally and peripherally) seem to be significantly higher in patients with PTSD than in control groups. Sensitization of noradrenergic systems may contribute to the arousal symptoms in PTSD, including hypervigilance, exaggerated startle response, anxiety, irritability, and insomnia and nightmares (Southwick et al. 1995). Neurobiological studies also have shown noradrenergic stress system involvement in enhanced encoding of emotional memories and fear conditioning (Elzinga and Bremner 2002). This involvement suggests a role for norepinephrine in PTSD symptoms such as reexperiencing, intrusive memories, and flashbacks. Yohimbine, an alpha-2 adrenergic receptor antagonist that increases neuronal norepinephrine release, was used by Southwick et al. (1993) as a pharmacological challenge to test noradrenergic reactivity. In this study, men, but not women, with PTSD given yohimbine had significant increases in core PTSD symptoms such as flashbacks, intrusive traumatic thoughts, emotional numbing, and grief compared with a healthy male control group. A large body of data from a range of research areas has provided compelling evidence for exaggerated noradrenergic activity in patients with PTSD. This exaggerated activity is generally observed in response to stressors but not under baseline or resting conditions (Southwick et al. 1999).

Neuropeptide Y (NPY)

NPY, a neurotransmitter colocalized with norepinephrine, may play an important role in the stress response system (Heilig and Widerlov 1990). Acute stress exposure appears to elicit increased NPY and norepinephrine release (C.A. Morgan et al. 2002), whereas prolonged trauma exposure is associated with reduced baseline NPY levels (C.A. Morgan et al. 2003). At the synaptic level, NPY has been shown to inhibit the release of norepinephrine (Colmers and Bleakman 1994). Reduced NPY levels translate to a reduced capacity to restrain the noradrenergic system, resulting in an exaggerated release of norepinephrine. This may contribute to hypersensitive reactions to stressors (Southwick et al. 1999). Future yohimbine challenge studies will hopefully determine whether variability in the stress-induced release of NPY, rather than variability in baseline levels of NPY, can differentiate between PTSD and trauma-exposed control groups, and whether stress-induced NPY release plays a role in the development of maladaptive responses to stress. Greater levels of NPY release are associated with less psychological distress (C.A. Morgan et al. 2002); therefore, plasma NPY levels may represent a biological correlate of resilience to or recovery from trauma (Yehuda et al. 2006).

Serotonin

Serotonin, 5-hydroxytryptamine (5-HT), has been associated with a wide variety of physiological or behavioral functions, including affect, aggression, cognition, appetite, nausea, endocrine function, gastrointestinal function, motor function, perception, sensory function, sex, sleep, and vascular function (Bloom 1995). Many drugs currently used for the treatment of psychiatric disorders are thought to act, at least partially, through serotonergic mechanisms. Serotonin plays an important role in the regulation of the prefrontal cortex, amygdala, and hippocampus, each of which has been implicated in the pathophysiology of PTSD (Southwick et al. 2005). Increasing evidence indicates abnormalities in serotonergic function in patients with PTSD. Perhaps the strongest clinical evidence of serotonin's role in PTSD comes from pharmacological treatment studies. Selective serotonin reuptake inhibitors (SSRIs) block reuptake of serotonin from the synapses and make more serotonin available throughout the brain. The Australian guidelines for the treatment of adults with PTSD reviewed 31 pharmacological treatment studies and concluded, "Where medication is considered for the treatment of PTSD in adults, SSRI antidepressants should be the first choice" (Forbes et al. 2007, p. 644). Pharmacological challenge studies have shown meta-chlorophenylpiperazine, a serotonergic agonist, to cause anxiety and flashbacks in a subgroup of patients with PTSD (Southwick et al. 1997a). Davis et al. (1999) used the serotonin-releasing agent and reuptake inhibitor D-fenfluramine in patients with PTSD and demonstrated a significantly lower prolactin response compared with control subjects, suggesting central serotonergic dysfunction in PTSD. Additionally, the low expression variant of the serotonin transporter gene appears to predispose individuals to posthurricane PTSD, given high hurricane exposure and low social support (Kilpatrick et al. 2007), further supporting the role of serotonin in PTSD.

Neuroimaging Studies in PTSD

Functional Neurocircuitry of Fear and Anxiety

Much of the sensory information of fear- and anxiety-inducing stimuli is first processed in the sensory cortex prior to transfer to subcortical structures, which are more involved in affective, behavioral, and somatic responses. The amygdala has strong projections to most areas of the striatum, including the nucleus accumbens, olfactory tubercle, and parts of the caudate and putamen. The portion of the striatum that is innervated by the amygdala also receives efferents from the orbitofrontal cortex and the ventral tegmental area. The dense innervation of the striatum and prefrontal cortex by the amygdala indicates that the amygdala can powerfully regulate both of these systems (McDonald 1991a, 1991b).

Of note, the thalamus sends sensory information directly to the amygdala and hypothalamus. The amygdala is involved in memory processing of particularly emotionally arousing events (McGaugh 2000). Lesions of the amygdala block the enhancing effects of emotional arousal on memory consolidation (Roozendaal 2000) and impair fear conditioning in human subjects. Data support a crucial role for the amygdala in the transmission and interpretation of fear- and anxiety-inducing sensory information because it receives afferents from thalamic and cortical exteroceptive systems, as well as from subcortical visceral afferent pathways (Amaral et al. 1992). The neuronal interactions between the amygdala and the cortical regions, such as the orbitofrontal cortex, enable the individual to initiate adaptive behaviors to threat based on the nature of the threat and prior experience. The interactions between the amygdala and the extrapyramidal motor system may be imperative for generating motor responses to threatening stimuli, especially those related to prior adverse experiences. Current research indicates that the production of emotions may be more dependent on a neural network consisting of cortical and limbic regions than on the activity of one single region (Anand et al. 2005).

Abnormalities in the Hippocampus in PTSD

Bremner et al. (1995) reported a small but significant decrease (8%) of the right hippocampal body in patients with combat-related PTSD, which was subsequently confirmed by three studies from two independent groups (Bremner et al. 1995; Gurvits et al. 1996; Stein et al. 1997a). The decrease in hippocampal volume was seen in patients with PTSD related to either combat or childhood sexual and/or physical abuse. Individuals with early childhood abuse and current major depressive disorder showed an 18% reduction in left hippocampal volume when compared with patients with major depressive disorder without childhood abuse, after controlling for age, race, education, whole-brain volume, alcohol use, and PTSD (Bremner et al. 2003b). Notably, the volume reduction was confined to the posterior hippocampus, which may be relevant for the pathophysiology of PTSD in light of the association between the posterior hippocampus and processing, storage, and retrieval of spatiotemporal information. Other studies failed to find a reduction in hippocampal volume in Holocaust victims (Golier et al. 2000), combat veterans (Schuff et al. 1997), or women with PTSD secondary to domestic violence. Longitudinal magnetic resonance imaging (MRI) studies in adult subjects with PTSD immediately and 6 months after a motor vehicle accident (Bonne et al. 2001) and a 2-year study in children with sexual and/or physical abuse–related PTSD (De Bellis et al. 2001) did not find reductions in hippocampal volume. The largest volumetric study to date, performed in 44 abused children with PTSD and 61 healthy children, found a significant decrease in intracranial volume and corpus callosal volume but not hippocampal volume (De Bellis et al. 1999). A post hoc analysis in patients with alcohol dependence showed that the volume of the hippocampus in women with alcohol dependence and PTSD was similar to that of women with alcohol dependence without PTSD (Agartz et al. 1999).

Several factors could explain the contradictory findings in hippocampal volume studies in PTSD. Trauma variables may play a factor, including differences in type of trauma, duration and frequency of trauma, severity of trauma, and the timing of trauma during one's development. Differences in the prevalence of comorbid disorders, such as major depression and substance problems, could also explain the variance in hippocampal volume. Exposure to antidepressants may enhance dendritic branching (Duman et al. 1999, 2000) and contribute to differences in hippocampal volume in humans. A recent hippocampal volume study in people with major depression, however, suggests that maintenance antidepressant treatment may be necessary to prevent hippocampal volume loss (Neumeister et al. 2005).

Future studies in patients with PTSD should take into account possible factors for heterogeneity in biological markers and study more homogeneous groups of traumatized patients, with comparison to control subjects exposed to similar trauma without current PTSD. An excellent example for this type of study is by Gilbertson et al. (2002), who studied homozygote twins discordant for trauma exposure. In this study, disorder severity in PTSD patients exposed to trauma was negatively correlated with hippocampal volume of both the patient and the patient's trauma-unexposed identical twin. Furthermore, twin pairs with severe PTSD (both trauma-exposed and unexposed twin) had significantly smaller hippocampi than non-PTSD pairs. These data suggest that smaller hippocampal volume may be a vulnerability marker for PTSD rather than a consequence of exposure to trauma.

Abnormalities in the Amygdala and Prefrontal Cortex in PTSD

Although the role of the amygdala in fear conditioning has been repeatedly demonstrated in preclinical studies, few human studies have demonstrated amygdala activation during acquisition and extinction phases of fear conditioning (LaBar et al. 1998). Studies of amygdala activation in PTSD show mixed results and are confounded by variation across studies of the behavioral paradigms of symptom provocation. Right amygdala activation was reported in combat-related PTSD when patients and control subjects were exposed to traumatic imagery and combat pictures (Rauch et al. 1996; Shin et al. 1997), whereas the left amygdala was activated in response to combat sounds (Liberzon et al. 1999). However, other studies that used similar paradigms were unable to replicate the finding of greater amygdala activation in patients with PTSD than in those without (Bremner et al. 1999).

A functional MRI (fMRI) study by Rauch et al. (2000) extended the masked-faces paradigm to patients with PTSD. This study was an important step toward an understanding of how the amygdala responds to emotionally valenced stimuli. Specifically, activity within the amygdala increased in response to pictures of fearful versus neutral versus happy faces. With use of the masked-face paradigm, the automaticity of the amygdala response is highlighted, because activation of other brain regions outside the amygdala is minimized. In particular, non–masked face paradigms lead to amygdala and medial frontal activation, which is important for understanding the circuit involved in processing emotional information. Nonetheless, the non–masked face paradigm does not tell us about amygdala function itself. Using a modified approach by exposing individuals to pictures of fearful versus neutral or happy faces presented below the level of awareness, Whalen et al. (1998) demonstrated activation of the amygdala. In contrast, overt presentation of emotional faces resulted in significant medial frontal activation (Morris et al. 1998; Whalen et al. 1998). Rauch et al. (2000) found exaggerated amygdala responses to mask-fearful versus mask-happy faces in patients with PTSD compared with combat-exposed veterans without PTSD, suggesting that these patients exhibit exaggerated amygdala activation to general threat related stimuli presented at the subliminal level. Studies with similar symptom-provocation designs, but using fMRI techniques in larger samples of patients and controls, may provide definitive answers with respect to the role of the amygdala in PTSD symptoms.

Abnormalities in the functioning of medial prefrontal cortex subregions in patients with PTSD have been shown in positron emission tomography (PET) and single-photon emission computed tomography (SPECT) studies using personalized scripts, combat slides, or sounds (Damsa et al. 2009). The prefrontal cortex is reciprocally connected to the amygdala and inhibits acquisition of the fear response and promotes extinction of behavioral response to fear-conditioned stimuli that are no longer reinforced (M.A. Morgan and LeDoux 1995; Quirk et al. 2000). Various subregions of the medial prefrontal cortex mediate different responses. Lesions of the ventral medial prefrontal cortex or the orbital cortex prolong the extinction phase (M.A. Morgan et al. 1993), whereas lesions of the dorsal medial prefrontal cortex (anterior cingulate) facilitate the fear response during acquisition and extinction phases of fear conditioning, resulting in a generalized increase in fear response (M.A. Morgan and LeDoux 1995). Suppression of neuronal firing in the subgenual prefrontal cortical equivalent in the rat model (prelimbic cortex) is inversely correlated with an increase in amygdala neuronal activity (Garcia et al. 1999). Based on lesion studies, one can hypothesize that dysfunction in the medial prefrontal cortex can result in a disinhibition of amygdala activity. This disinhibition, in turn, promotes acquisition of a fear response to traumatic stimuli and will result in a failure to extinguish the fear response even after the traumatic stimulation has ceased.

Receptor Imaging Studies in PTSD

Relatively few studies have addressed abnormalities of receptors and transporters that play key roles in the regulation of neurochemical functions in PTSD. Of particular relevance to the pathophysiology of PTSD are benzodiazepine receptors and serotonin (5-HT) systems.

A neuroimaging study assessing benzodiazepine receptor binding using SPECT and the radiotracer [^{123}I]iomazenil showed reduced benzodiazepine receptor binding potential in the medial prefrontal cortex in patients with combat-related PTSD relative to controls. Such studies argue for the role of benzodiazepine receptor dysfunction in the pathogenesis of PTSD (Bremner et al. 2000).

Altered benzodiazepine receptor number or function may relate to alterations in serotonergic receptor expression. Several studies have suggested close interactions between serotonergic and GABAergic systems. Mice lacking the 5-HT$_{1A}$ receptor displayed marked anxiety (Heisler et al. 1998; Parks et al. 1998; Ramboz et al. 1998), and animals exposed to stress exhibited downregulation of 5-HT$_{1A}$ receptors (McKittrick et al. 1995). Subordinate rats in a dominance hierarchy showed reduced 5-HT_{1A} receptor levels and severe anxiety (McKittrick et al. 1995). Sibille et al. (2000) found that 5-HT_{1A} receptor knock-out mice had 1) a reduction in the alpha-1 and alpha-2 subunits of the $GABA_A$ receptor function, 2) reduced binding of both benzodiazepine and nonbenzodiazepine $GABA_A$ receptor-ligand, and 3) benzodiazepine-resistant anxiety. These studies suggest pathogenesis from a 5-HT_{1A} receptor deficit, resulting in dysfunction within GABAergic systems and increased levels of anxiety.

A logical next step in the evaluation of brain systems potentially involved in the pathophysiology of PTSD was to determine 5-HT_{1A} receptor expression in patients with PTSD versus controls. Bonne et al. (2005) acquired PET images of 5-HT_{1A} receptor binding using PET imaging of 12 unmedicated PTSD subjects and 11 healthy nontrauma controls using $[^{18}F]$fluorocarbonyl-WAY-100635, a highly selective 5-HT_{1A} receptor radioligand. Unexpectedly, they found no difference in 5-HT_{1A} receptor expression between the groups. This result suggests no direct role for the 5-HT_{1A} receptor in the pathophysiology of PTSD; however, it does not exclude the relevance of 5-HT_{1A} receptors in mediating the effects of SSRIs in PTSD treatment by involving other transmitter systems and neurotrophic systems.

Future Directions of Neuroimaging Research in PTSD

Despite the limited number of neuroimaging studies in PTSD, these studies have predominantly shown a difference between PTSD patients and control groups in the hippocampus, amygdala, and prefrontal cortex. These results are essential for an understanding of structural and functional abnormalities associated with PTSD and serve as a basis to better understand the effects of treatment in PTSD. To date, only a very small number of studies have addressed the impact of treatment on brain function using neuroimaging. For example, cognitive-behavioral therapy (CBT) with in vivo exposure has been shown to be an effective treatment for PTSD (Forbes et al. 2007). The effects of CBT on brain function, however, are not yet fully understood and represent a gap in understanding. Imaging techniques are powerful tools to look at changes in the brain following treatment interventions, and an increasing number of studies are using these tools. A recent fMRI study recorded brain activity before and after CBT in a small sample of individuals with non–combat-related PTSD (Farrow et al. 2005). Interestingly, CBT induced brain cortical activity associated with symptom improvement in brain regions found to be less active at baseline in patients with PTSD. In a SPECT study assessing cerebral blood flow at baseline and postintervention, Peres et al. (2007) compared PTSD subjects randomly assigned to either exposure-based CBT with cognitive restructuring (n=16) or a waiting list (n=11). Increased cerebral blood flow as an equivalent of increased activation in the left hippocampus, left prefrontal cortex, parietal lobes, and thalamus during memory retrieval after CBT was associated with symptom improvement. Another SPECT study found lower activation in right middle frontal gyrus in PTSD outpatients treated with brief eclectic psychotherapy (n=10) compared with a randomized waiting list control group (n=10) during trauma imagery (Lindauer et al. 2008). These initial encouraging, but somewhat controversial, results indicate a need for adequately powered, well-designed imaging studies elucidating the impact of PTSD treatment on neurobiology.

Conclusion

Genetic, neuroimaging, and neurochemical approaches are combined to provide an integrated biotype of PTSD. Studies investigating the association between heredity, rearing, neurobiological function, and stress response are an exceptional example of highly perceptive research and reveal nature-nurture interaction. The magnitude of data collected on PTSD since it was incorporated into psychiatric nosology in 1980 is a tribute to the importance and appeal of this disorder in the eyes of the mental health and neuroscience communities.

Key Clinical Points

- First-degree relatives of individuals with PTSD are at an increased risk of developing the disorder.
- Twin studies have found genetic influence on the risk of trauma exposure, the development of PTSD, and the existence of comorbidity.
- Emerging evidence suggests that women experience both a higher prevalence and a longer duration of PTSD, though whether this dif-

ference is truly a gender difference or the result of environmental factors remains unclear.

- Cortisol is known to be involved in the pathophysiological process of PTSD, but the exact effects and impact on clinical treatments have yet to be fully elucidated.
- Noradrenergic hyperresponsiveness and neuropeptide Y appear to play significant roles in PTSD for individuals with hyperarousal symptoms and may be clinically important avenues for future therapies.
- SSRIs and treatment via the serotonergic system is a key aspect of current therapies. The relevance of other neurobiological systems to treatment development is currently under investigation.
- Neuroimaging studies have shown that PTSD may be associated with abnormalities including decreased hippocampal volume, abnormal amygdala activity, and abnormal medial prefrontal cortex functioning, although such findings have been inconclusive.

References

Agartz I, Momenan R, Rawlings RR, et al: Hippocampal volume in patients with alcohol dependence. Arch Gen Psychiatry 56:356–363, 1999

Amaral DG, Price JL, Pitanken A, et al: Anatomical organization of the primate amygdala complex, in The Amygdala: Neurobiological Aspects of Emotion, Memory, and Mental Dysfunction. Edited by Aggleton JP. New York, Wiley-Liss, 1992, pp 1–66

American Psychiatric Association: Diagnostic and Statistical Manual of Mental Disorders, 4th Edition, Text Revision. Washington, DC, American Psychiatric Association, 2000

Anand A, Li Y, Wang Y, et al: Activity and connectivity of brain mood regulating circuit in depression: a functional magnetic resonance study. Biol Psychiatry 57:1079–1088, 2005

Binneman B, Feltner D, Kolluri S, et al: A 6-week randomized, placebo-controlled trial of CP-316,311 (a selective CRH1 antagonist) in the treatment of major depression. Am J Psychiatry 165:617–620, 2008

Bloom FE: Introduction to preclinical neuropsychopharmacology, in Neuropsychopharmacology: The Fourth Generation of Progress: An Official Publication of the American College of Neuropsychopharmacology. Edited by Bloom FE, Kupfer DJ. New York, Raven, 1995, pp 407–471

Bonne O, Brandes D, Gilboa A, et al: Longitudinal MRI study of hippocampal volume in trauma survivors with PTSD. Am J Psychiatry 158:1248–1251, 2001

Bonne O, Bain E, Neumeister A, et al: No change in serotonin type 1A receptor binding in patients with posttraumatic stress disorder. Am J Psychiatry 162:383–385, 2005

Boscarino JA: Posttraumatic stress disorder and mortality among U.S. Army veterans 30 years after military service. Ann Epidemiol 16:248–256, 2006

Bremner JD, Randall P, Scott TM, et al: MRI-based measurement of hippocampal volume in patients with combat-related posttraumatic stress disorder. Am J Psychiatry 152:973–981, 1995

Bremner JD, Krystal JH, Charney DS, et al: Neural mechanisms in dissociative amnesia for childhood abuse: relevance to the current controversy surrounding the "false memory syndrome." Am J Psychiatry 153:71–82, 1996

Bremner JD, Staib LH, Kaloupek D, et al: Neural correlates of exposure to traumatic pictures and sound in Vietnam combat veterans with and without posttraumatic stress disorder: a positron emission tomography study. Biol Psychiatry 45:806–816, 1999

Bremner JD, Innis RB, Southwick SM, et al: Decreased benzodiazepine receptor binding in prefrontal cortex in combat-related posttraumatic stress disorder. Am J Psychiatry 157:1120–1126, 2000

Bremner JD, Vythilingam M, Anderson G, et al: Assessment of the hypothalamic-pituitary-adrenal axis over a 24-hour diurnal period and in response to neuroendocrine challenges in women with and without childhood sexual abuse and posttraumatic stress disorder. Biol Psychiatry 54:710–718, 2003a

Bremner JD, Vythilingam M, Vermetten E, et al: MRI and PET study of deficits in hippocampal structure and function in women with childhood sexual abuse and posttraumatic stress disorder. Am J Psychiatry 160:924–932, 2003b

Breslau N: Epidemiologic studies of trauma, posttraumatic stress disorder, and other psychiatric disorders. Can J Psychiatry 47:923–929, 2002

Breslau N, Kessler RC, Chilcoat HD, et al: Trauma and posttraumatic stress disorder in the community: the 1996 Detroit Area Survey of Trauma. Arch Gen Psychiatry 55:626–632, 1998

Breslau N, Chilcoat HD, Kessler RC, et al: Vulnerability to assaultive violence: further specification of the sex difference in post-traumatic stress disorder. Psychol Med 29:813–821, 1999

Broekman BFP, Olff M, Boer F: The genetic background to PTSD. Neurosci Biobehav Rev 31:348–362, 2007

Colmers WF, Bleakman D: Effects of neuropeptide Y on the electrical properties of neurons. Trends Neurosci 17:373–379, 1994

Cuffe SP, Addy CL, Garrison CZ, et al: Prevalence of PTSD in a community sample of older adolescents. J Am Acad Child Adolesc Psychiatry 37:147–154, 1998

Damsa C, Kosel M, Moussally J: Current status of brain imaging in anxiety disorders. Curr Opin Psychiatry 22:96–110, 2009

Davis LL, Clark DM, Kramer GL, et al: D-fenfluramine challenge in posttraumatic stress disorder. Biol Psychiatry 45:928–930, 1999

De Bellis MD, Keshavan MS, Clark DB, et al: A.E. Bennett Research Award. Developmental traumatology. Part II: Brain development. Biol Psychiatry 45:1271–1284, 1999

De Bellis MD, Hall J, Boring AM, et al: A pilot longitudinal study of hippocampal volumes in pediatric maltreatment-related posttraumatic stress disorder. Biol Psychiatry 50:305–309, 2001

Duman RS, Malberg J, Thome J: Neural plasticity to stress and antidepressant treatment. Biol Psychiatry 46:1181–1191, 1999

Duman RS, Malberg J, Nakagawa S, et al: Neuronal plasticity and survival in mood disorders. Biol Psychiatry 48:732–739, 2000

Elzinga BM, Bremner JD: Are the neural substrates of memory the final common pathway in posttraumatic stress disorder (PTSD)? J Affect Disord 70:1–17, 2002

Farrow TFD, Hunter MD, Wilkinson ID, et al: Quantifiable change in functional brain response to empathic and forgivability judgments with resolution of posttraumatic stress disorder. Psychiatry Res 140:45–53, 2005

Forbes D, Creamer M, Phelps A, et al: Australian guidelines for the treatment of adults with acute stress disorder and post-traumatic stress disorder. Aust N Z J Psychiatry 41:637–648, 2007

Garcia R, Vouimba RM, Baudry M, et al: The amygdala modulates prefrontal cortex activity relative to conditioned fear. Nature 402:294–296, 1999

Gilbertson MW, Shenton ME, Ciszewski A, et al: Smaller hippocampal volume predicts pathologic vulnerability to psychological trauma. Nat Neurosci 5:1242–1247, 2002

Golier J, Yehuda R, Grossman R, et al: Hippocampal volume and memory performance in Holocaust survivors with and without PTSD. Paper presented at the annual meeting of the American College of Neuropsychopharmacology, San Juan, Puerto Rico, December 2000

Gurvits TV, Shenton ME, Hokama H, et al: Magnetic resonance imaging study of hippocampal volume in chronic, combat-related posttraumatic stress disorder. Biol Psychiatry 40:1091–1099, 1996

Heilig M, Widerlov E: Neuropeptide Y: an overview of central distribution, functional aspects, and possible involvement in neuropsychiatric illnesses. Acta Psychiatr Scand 82:95–114, 1990

Heisler LK, Chu HM, Brennan TJ, et al: Elevated anxiety and antidepressant-like responses in serotonin 5-HT1A receptor mutant mice. Proc Natl Acad Sci USA 95:15049–15054, 1998

Hoge CW, Terhakopian A, Castro CA, et al: Association of posttraumatic stress disorder with somatic symptoms, health care visits, and absenteeism among Iraq war veterans. Am J Psychiatry 164:150–153, 2007

Kang H, Dalager N, Mahan C, et al: The role of sexual assault on the risk of PTSD among Gulf War veterans. Ann Epidemiol 15:191–195, 2005

Kessler RC, Sonnega A, Bromet E, et al: Posttraumatic stress disorder in the National Comorbidity Survey. Arch Gen Psychiatry 52:1048–1060, 1995

Kilpatrick DG, Koenen KC, Ruggiero KJ, et al: The serotonin transporter genotype and social support and moderation of posttraumatic stress disorder and depression in hurricane-exposed adults. Am J Psychiatry 164:1693–1699, 2007

Koenen K, Nugent N, Amstadter A: Gene-environment interaction in posttraumatic stress disorder. Eur Arch Psychiatry Clin Neurosci 258:82–96, 2008

Kubzansky LD, Koenen KC, Spiro A 3rd, et al: Prospective study of posttraumatic stress disorder symptoms and coronary heart disease in the Normative Aging Study. Arch Gen Psychiatry 64:109–116, 2007

LaBar KS, Gatenby JC, Gore JC, et al: Human amygdala activation during conditioned fear acquisition and extinction: a mixed-trial fMRI study. Neuron 20:937–945, 1998

Liberzon I, Taylor SF, Amdur R, et al: Brain activation in PTSD in response to trauma-related stimuli. Biol Psychiatry 45:817–826, 1999

Lightman SL, Young WS 3rd: Corticotrophin-releasing factor, vasopressin and pro-opiomelanocortin mRNA responses to stress and opiates in the rat. J Physiol 403:511–523, 1988

Lindauer RJ, Booij J, Habraken JB, et al: Effects of psychotherapy on regional cerebral blood flow during trauma imagery in patients with post-traumatic stress disorder: a randomized clinical trial. Psychol Med 38:543–554, 2008

Maes M, Lin A, Bonaccorso S, et al: Increased 24-hour urinary cortisol excretion in patients with post-traumatic stress disorder and patients with major depression, but not in patients with fibromyalgia. Acta Psychiatr Scand 98:328–335, 1998

McDonald AJ: Organization of amygdaloid projections to the prefrontal cortex and associated striatum in the rat. Neuroscience 44:1–14, 1991a

McDonald AJ: Topographical organization of amygdaloid projections to the caudatoputamen, nucleus accumbens, and related striatal-like areas of the rat brain. Neuroscience 44:15–33, 1991b

McGaugh JL: Memory—a century of consolidation. Science 287:248–251, 2000

McKittrick CR, Blanchard DC, Blanchard RJ, et al: Serotonin receptor binding in a colony model of chronic social stress. Biol Psychiatry 37:383–393, 1995

Meewisse M-L, Reitsma JB, De Vries G-J, et al: Cortisol and post-traumatic stress disorder in adults: systematic review and meta-analysis. Br J Psychiatry 191:387–392, 2007

Morgan CA, Rasmusson AM, Wang S, et al: Neuropeptide-Y, cortisol, and subjective distress in humans exposed to acute stress: replication and extension of previous report. Biol Psychiatry 52:136–142, 2002

Morgan CA, Rasmusson AM, Winters B, et al: Trauma exposure rather than posttraumatic stress disorder is associated with reduced baseline plasma neuropeptide-Y levels. Biol Psychiatry 54:1087–1091, 2003

Morgan MA, LeDoux JE: Differential contribution of dorsal and ventral medial prefrontal cortex to the acquisition and extinction of conditioned fear in rats. Behav Neurosci 109:681–688, 1995

Morgan MA, Romanski LM, LeDoux JE: Extinction of emotional learning: contribution of medial prefrontal cortex. Neurosci Lett 163:109–113, 1993

Morris JS, Friston KJ, Buchel C, et al: A neuromodulatory role for the human amygdala in processing emotional facial expressions. Brain 121:47–57, 1998

Neumeister A, Wood S, Bonne O, et al: Reduced hippocampal volume in unmedicated, remitted patients with major depression versus control subjects. Biol Psychiatry 57:935–937, 2005

Norris FH: Epidemiology of trauma: frequency and impact of different potentially traumatic events on different demographic groups. J Consult Clin Psychol 60:409–418, 1992

Nugent NR, Amstadter AB, Koenen KC, et al: Genetics of post-traumatic stress disorder: informing clinical conceptualizations and promoting future research. Am J Med Genet C Semin Med Genet 148:127–132, 2008

Parks CL, Robinson PS, Sibille E, et al: Increased anxiety of mice lacking the serotonin1A receptor. Proc Natl Acad Sci USA 95:10734–10739, 1998

Peres JF, Newberg AB, Mercante JP, et al: Cerebral blood flow changes during retrieval of traumatic memories before and after psychotherapy: a SPECT study. Psychol Med 37:1481–1491, 2007

Pervanidou P: Biology of post-traumatic stress disorder in childhood and adolescence. J Neuroendocrinol 20:632–638, 2008

Quirk GJ, Russo GK, Barron JL, et al: The role of ventromedial prefrontal cortex in the recovery of extinguished fear. J Neurosci 20:6225–6231, 2000

Ramboz S, Oosting R, Amara DA, et al: Serotonin receptor 1A knockout: an animal model of anxiety-related disorder. Proc Natl Acad Sci USA 95:14476–14481, 1998

Rauch SL, van der Kolk BA, Fisler RE, et al: A symptom provocation study of posttraumatic stress disorder using positron emission tomography and script-driven imagery. Arch Gen Psychiatry 53:380–387, 1996

Rauch SL, Whalen PJ, Shin LM, et al: Exaggerated amygdala response to masked facial stimuli in posttraumatic stress disorder: a functional MRI study. Biol Psychiatry 47:769–776, 2000

Rihmer Z, Pestality P, Pihlgren H, et al: "Anxiety/aggression-driven depression" and "male depressive syndrome": are they the same? Psychiatry Res 77:209–210, 1998

Roozendaal B: 1999 Curt P. Richter award. Glucocorticoids and the regulation of memory consolidation. Psychoneuroendocrinology 25:213–238, 2000

Sack WH, Clarke GN, Seeley J: Posttraumatic stress disorder across two generations of Cambodian refugees. J Am Acad Child Adolesc Psychiatry 34:1160–1166, 1995

Schnurr PP, Hayes AF, Lunney CA, et al: Longitudinal analysis of the relationship between symptoms and quality of life in veterans treated for posttraumatic stress disorder. J Consult Clin Psychol 74:707–713, 2006

Schuff N, Marmar CR, Weiss DS, et al: Reduced hippocampal volume and n-acetyl aspartate in posttraumatic stress disorder. Ann N Y Acad Sci 821:516–520, 1997

Shalev AY, Videlock EJ, Peleg T, et al: Stress hormones and post-traumatic stress disorder in civilian trauma victims: a longitudinal study. Part I: HPA axis responses. Int J Neuropsychopharmacol 11:365–372, 2008

Shin LM, Kosslyn SM, McNally RJ, et al: Visual imagery and perception in posttraumatic stress disorder. A positron emission tomographic investigation. Arch Gen Psychiatry 54:233–241, 1997

Sibille E, Pavlides C, Benke D, et al: Genetic inactivation of the serotonin(1A) receptor in mice results in downregulation of major GABA(A) receptor alpha subunits, reduction of GABA(A) receptor binding, and benzodiazepine-resistant anxiety. J Neurosci 20:2758–2765, 2000

Sjöberg RL, Nilsson KW, Niklas N, et al: Development of depression: sex and the interaction between environment and a promoter polymorphism of the serotonin transporter gene. Int J Neuropsychopharmacol 9:443–449, 2006

Southwick SM, Krystal JH, Morgan CA, et al: Abnormal noradrenergic function in posttraumatic stress disorder. Arch Gen Psychiatry 50:266–274, 1993

Southwick SM, Yehuda R, Morgan CA 3rd: Clinical studies of neurotransmitter alterations in post-traumatic stress disorder, in Neurobiological and Clinical Consequences of Stress: From Normal Adaptation to Post-Traumatic Stress Disorder. Edited by Friedman MJ, Charney DS, Deutch AY. New York, Lippincott-Raven, 1995, pp 335–349

Southwick SM, Krystal JH, Bremner JD, et al: Noradrenergic and serotonergic function in posttraumatic stress disorder. Arch Gen Psychiatry 54:749–758, 1997a

Southwick SM, Morgan CA 3rd, Bremner AD, et al: Noradrenergic alterations in posttraumatic stress disorder. Ann NY Acad Sci 821:125–141, 1997b

Southwick SM, Bremner JD, Rasmusson A, et al: Role of norepinephrine in the pathophysiology and treatment of posttraumatic stress disorder. Biol Psychiatry 46:1192–1204, 1999

Southwick SM, Rasmusson A, Barron J, et al: Neurobiological and neurocognitive alterations in PTSD, in Neuropsychology of PTSD. Edited by Vasterling JJ, Brewin CR. New York, Guilford, 2005, pp 27–58

Stein MB, Koverola C, Hanna C, et al: Hippocampal volume in women victimized by childhood sexual abuse. Psychol Med 27:951–959, 1997a

Stein MB, Walker JR, Hazen AL, et al: Full and partial posttraumatic stress disorder: findings from a community survey. Am J Psychiatry 154:1114–1119, 1997b

Stein MB, Walker JR, Forde DR: Gender differences in susceptibility to posttraumatic stress disorder. Behav Res Ther 38:619–628, 2000

Tolin DF, Foa EB: Sex differences in trauma and posttraumatic stress disorder: a quantitative review of 25 years of research. Psychol Bull 132:959–992, 2006

Walderhaug E, Magnusson A, Neumeister A, et al: Interactive effects of sex and 5-HTTLPR on mood and impulsivity during tryptophan depletion in healthy people. Biol Psychiatry 62:593–599, 2007

Weiss SJ: Neurobiological alterations associated with traumatic stress. Perspect Psychiatr Care 43:114–122, 2007

Whalen PJ, Rauch SL, Etcoff NL, et al: Masked presentations of emotional facial expressions modulate amygdala activity without explicit knowledge. J Neurosci 18:411–418, 1998

Yehuda R: Advances in understanding neuroendocrine alterations in PTSD and their therapeutic implications. Ann NY Acad Sci 1071:137–166, 2006

Yehuda R, Southwick SM, Nussbaum G, et al: Low urinary cortisol excretion in patients with posttraumatic stress disorder. J Nerv Ment Dis 178:366–369, 1990

Yehuda R, Brand S, Yang R-K: Plasma neuropeptide Y concentrations in combat exposed veterans: relationship to trauma exposure, recovery from PTSD, and coping. Biol Psychiatry 59:660–663, 2006

Zatzick DF, Marmar CR, Weiss DS, et al: Posttraumatic stress disorder and functioning and quality of life outcomes in a nationally representative sample of male Vietnam veterans. Am J Psychiatry 154:1690–1695, 1997

Zobel AW, Nickel T, Künzel HE, et al: Effects of the high-affinity corticotropin-releasing hormone receptor 1 antagonist R121919 in major depression: the first 20 patients treated. J Psychiatr Res 34:171–181, 2000

4

Assessment and Diagnosis

Douglas C. Johnson, Ph.D.
Murray B. Stein, M.D., M.P.H.

Our aim in this chapter is to provide researchers and clinicians alike with essential information for conducting comprehensive assessment of posttraumatic stress disorder (PTSD). We begin by outlining diagnostic guidelines and identifying some of the challenges to accurate assessment of PTSD. A brief background of the development of symptom classification and a summary comparison of diagnostic criteria in the American Psychiatric Association's *Diagnostic and Statistical Manual of Mental Disorders* (DSM) and the World Health Organization's *International Statistical Classification of Diseases and Related Health Problems* (ICD) systems are also provided. We then discuss emerging evidence regarding the factor structure of PTSD symptoms, as well as how this factor structure differs from current symptom clusters specified in DSM-IV (American Psychiatric Association 1994). Next, we touch on implications that emerging, evidence-based factor structures may have for treatment. This is followed by an outline of unique threats to valid and reliable diagnosis of PTSD.

Brief descriptions of psychometric properties for some recommended measures for assessing PTSD are provided. The assessment section focuses primarily on clinician-administered and self-report measures. Because discussion of promising cognitive, neuroanatomical, and biological correlates of PTSD is well beyond the scope of this chapter, we refer readers interested in those approaches to other chapters within this manual. The chapter concludes with differential diagnosis, followed by key clinical points for assessing PTSD in clinical, research, and forensic settings.

General Considerations

Perhaps no mental health diagnosis has received more attention in the twenty-first century than PTSD. Moreover, since the publication of DSM-IV, few disorders have been the subject of more controversy. PTSD is often the focus of scrutiny in personal injury litigation, compensation and pension examinations within the Veterans Administration, and fitness-for-duty determinations in military and law enforcement settings.

Controversy surrounding PTSD is due in part to challenges involving reliable and valid assessment. These challenges stem from the fact that PTSD has only recently entered into psychiatric nosology. PTSD was introduced in DSM-III (American Psychiatric Association 1980); the diagnostic criteria were changed substantially in DSM-IV (American Psychiatric Association 1994), which invited further scrutiny. DSM-IV introduced a subjective criterion (Criterion A2) requiring the clinician to determine whether an individual's response to trauma involves fear, helplessness, or horror; this change continues to be a source of controversy. Additionally, for some patients and clinicians alike, experience of a life-changing traumatic event is tantamount to a diagnosis of PTSD. Although such a conceptualization of PTSD is understandable from an empathetic viewpoint, it is contrary to the required evidence base and diagnostic guidelines. Further complicating reliable and valid diagnosis is that assessment of PTSD in clinical and research settings often relies exclusively on patient self-report of symptoms. This is not to suggest that self-report measures of PTSD offer little utility. On the contrary, several self-report instruments reviewed in this chapter offer excellent reliability and validity, and are useful for diagnosis and treatment outcome tracking. The concern with self-report instruments is that they are valuable but insufficient diagnostic tools when used exclusively.

When optimized via a structured format and further informed by collateral reports, the clinical interview remains the most reliable form of PTSD assessment. That being said, multiple clinicians are likely to have different opinions about a patient's psychiatric diagnosis, and even the most careful and comprehensive assessment has limitations. However, methods and metrics exist that when used in combination, minimize threats to valid and reliable assessment of PTSD. In this regard, assessment is predicated on identifying the challenges to PTSD diagnosis, and then addressing those challenges with the best clinical assessment tools available. The potential for error is inherent in all mental health assessments—clinical judgment and instrument error are intrinsic to the assessment process—but there are diagnostic challenges unique to PTSD, beginning with the diagnostic criteria.

PTSD Diagnostic Criteria

DSM-IV diagnostic criteria for PTSD (reprinted from DSM-IV-TR; American Psychiatric Association 2000) are presented in Table 4–1. Diagnosis of PTSD requires exposure to a life-threatening trauma (Criterion A1), and a response to that trauma that includes fear, helplessness, or horror (Criterion A2). PTSD is further characterized by the development of symptoms that fall into three groups: reexperiencing (Criterion B), avoidance and emotional numbing (Criterion C), and hyperarousal (Criterion D). An individual must experience a combination of at least one reexperiencing symptom, three avoidance symptoms, and two hyperarousal symptoms for more than 1 month to meet diagnostic criteria. Furthermore, the individual must demonstrate some degree of impairment in social or occupational functioning related to these symptoms.

As noted, DSM-IV introduced changes to Criterion A that continue to engender controversy. Diagnostic confusion regarding Criterion A revolves around the combination of its objective and subjective dimensions. It is a diagnostic point of emphasis that Criterion A requires meeting *both* Criteria A1 and A2. Criterion A1 states that the individual must have "experienced, wit-

Table 4–1. DSM-IV-TR diagnostic criteria for PTSD

A. The person has been exposed to a traumatic event in which both of the following were present:

(1) the person experienced, witnessed, or was confronted with an event or events that involved actual or threatened death or serious injury, or a threat to the physical integrity of self or others

(2) the person's response involved intense fear, helplessness, or horror. **Note:** In children, this may be expressed instead by disorganized or agitated behavior.

B. The traumatic event is persistently reexperienced in one (or more) of the following ways:

(1) recurrent and intrusive distressing recollections of the event, including images, thoughts, or perceptions. **Note:** In young children, repetitive play may occur in which themes or aspects of the trauma are expressed.

(2) recurrent distressing dreams of the event. **Note:** In children, there may be frightening dreams without recognizable content.

(3) acting or feeling as if the traumatic event were recurring (includes a sense of reliving the experience, illusions, hallucinations, and dissociative flashback episodes, including those that occur on awakening or when intoxicated). **Note:** In young children, trauma-specific reenactment may occur.

(4) intense psychological distress at exposure to internal or external cues that symbolize or resemble an aspect of the traumatic event

(5) physiological reactivity on exposure to internal or external cues that symbolize or resemble an aspect of the traumatic event

C. Persistent avoidance of stimuli associated with the trauma and numbing of general responsiveness (not present before the trauma), as indicated by three (or more) of the following:

(1) efforts to avoid thoughts, feelings, or conversations associated with the trauma

(2) efforts to avoid activities, places, or people that arouse recollections of the trauma

(3) inability to recall an important aspect of the trauma

(4) markedly diminished interest or participation in significant activities

(5) feeling of detachment or estrangement from others

Table 4–1. DSM-IV-TR diagnostic criteria for PTSD *(continued)*

(6) restricted range of affect (e.g., unable to have loving feelings)

(7) sense of a foreshortened future (e.g., does not expect to have a career, marriage, children, or a normal life span)

D. Persistent symptoms of increased arousal (not present before the trauma), as indicated by two (or more) of the following:

(1) difficulty falling or staying asleep

(2) irritability or outbursts of anger

(3) difficulty concentrating

(4) hypervigilance

(5) exaggerated startle response

E. Duration of the disturbance (symptoms in Criteria B, C, and D) is more than 1 month.

F. The disturbance causes clinically significant distress or impairment in social, occupational, or other important areas of functioning.

Specify if:

Acute: if duration of symptoms is less than 3 months
Chronic: if duration of symptoms is 3 months or more

Specify if:

With Delayed Onset: if onset of symptoms is at least 6 months after the stressor

Source. Reprinted from *Diagnostic and Statistical Manual of Mental Disorders,* 4th Edition, Text Revision. Washington, DC, American Psychiatric Association, 2000. Copyright 2000, American Psychiatric Association. Used with permission.

nessed, or [been] confronted with an event or events that involved actual or threatened death or serious injury, or a threat to the physical integrity of self or others." Thus, Criterion A1 appears to be more objective in that it requires that the event be life threatening or present a risk of serious injury. For example, a combat zone is generally accepted as an environment in which there are routine threats, whether perceived or not, to life, to physical integrity, or of serious injury. Conversely, job loss and divorce, although life changing and occasionally perceived as traumatic, are not objectively life-threatening events.

Criterion A1, however, does have its problems. Whereas some events are unequivocally considered life threatening (e.g., being robbed at gunpoint), many events are not as clear-cut (e.g., being beaten up in a bar fight), with the likelihood of threat to life very much in the eye of the beholder. Moreover, controversy exists about whether an individual needs to directly experience the threat (e.g., the gun is pointed at his head) or can experience it indirectly (e.g., a gun is pointed at someone else who is nearby) or even vicariously (e.g., if he had entered the room a few minutes earlier, he might have been shot at). In combination with Criterion A2, which relies on the patient's response to the trauma, the possibility exists for any event (including nontraumatic events) to qualify as traumatic per se, as long as the individual perceives it with "fear, helplessness, or horror."

The applicability of Criterion A2 to military personnel in combat situations has recently been questioned. The challenges to its applicability arise from the notion that many professional warriors, as well as many first responders and emergency medical service personnel, make confronting death and other potentially traumatic events their life's vocation. These individuals may not typically respond to events meeting Criterion A1 with fear, helplessness, or horror, and therefore may fail to meet Criterion A2. Reasons for their not meeting Criterion A2 remain speculative, and factors that contribute to the absence of fear in these situations have been part of the discussion regarding psychological resilience (e.g., Maddi 2007; Southwick et al. 2005). However, what is often overlooked is that depending on the definition of *resilience,* many of these individuals may experience symptoms of PTSD but miss being diagnosed because they fail to endorse Criterion A2. Indeed, the absence of so-called fear, helplessness, or horror during a response to potentially traumatic events does not preclude significant PTSD symptom severity. In an assessment of military personnel exposed to combat in Iraq, 79% did not endorse Criterion A2 (Adler et al. 2008). Furthermore, 18% of those without an A2 response met diagnostic criteria for PTSD symptom clusters B, C, and D, and nearly 8% endorsed impaired functioning and emotional distress. Moreover, the overwhelming majority (61%) of those service members who did not endorse Criterion A2 stated that their response was one of fulfilling an "occupational" duty. Other frequently endorsed responses to combat trauma included "anger," "anxiety," "dissociation," and being "sad." These results suggest that strict application of Criterion A2 when evaluating subjective

Table 4–2. Threats to reliable and valid PTSD assessment

Diagnostic standards: ICD-10 vs. DSM-IV
Factor structure: theoretical vs. empirical
Symptom heterogeneity
Variable course
Symptom overlap and comorbidity
Malingering and response bias

Note. DSM-IV = *Diagnostic and Statistical Manual of Mental Disorders*, 4th Edition (American Psychiatric Association 1994); ICD-10 = *International Statistical Classification of Diseases and Related Health Problems*, 10th Revision (World Health Organization 1992).

responses to trauma may result in underdiagnosis and a failure to refer many who are symptomatic and in need of treatment.

Threats to Reliability and Validity

Table 4–2 highlights the threats to reliable and valid diagnosis of PTSD.

DSM-IV Versus ICD-10

Research evaluating meaningful differences between DSM-IV and ICD-10 is limited, and comparison of diagnostic symptom criteria for PTSD is even rarer. Peters et al. (1999) found that DSM-IV and ICD-10 criteria for PTSD are characterized by distinctions that do make for slight differences diagnostically. An outline of these differences is presented in Table 4–3. Findings indicate that ICD-10 criteria are a slighter lower diagnostic threshold. Of individuals who met DSM-IV criteria for PTSD, 85% also met ICD-10 criteria; however, of individuals who met ICD-10 criteria, only 37% met diagnosis according to DSM-IV. Criterion C (avoidance and numbing) and Criterion E (social and occupational impairment) accounted for the majority of variance between the two classification systems.

Factor Structure of PTSD

It is worth noting that the diagnostic criteria for PTSD introduced in DSM-III, and modified through DSM-IV, were not empirically derived, but rather were

Table 4–3. Comparison between ICD-10 and DSM-IV-TR diagnostic criteria for PTSD

ICD-10	DSM-IV
A. Exposure to stressor	A1. Exposure to stressor A2. Emotional reaction to stressor
B. Persistent remembering of the stressor in one of the following: intrusive flashbacks, vivid memories or recurring dreams, experiencing distress when reminded of the stressor	B. One or more of the following: B1. Recurrent and intrusive recollections B2. Recurrent distressing dreams B3. Acting or feeling as though event were recurring B4. Psychological distress when exposed to reminders B5. Physiological reactivity when exposed to reminders
C. Requires only one symptom of actual or preferred avoidance	C. Three or more of the following: C1. Avoidance of thoughts, feelings, or conversations associated with the stressor C2. Avoidance of activities, places, or people that arouse recollections of the stressor C3. Inability to recall important aspect of stressor C4. Diminished interest or participation in significant activities C5. Detachment from others C6. Restricted affect C7. Sense of foreshortened future

Table 4–3. Comparison between ICD-10 and DSM-IV-TR diagnostic criteria for PTSD *(continued)*

ICD-10	DSM-IV
D. Either D1 or D2: D1. Inability to recall D2. Two or more of the following: A. Sleep problems B. Irritability C. Concentration problems D. Hypervigilance E. Exaggerated startle response	D. Two or more of the following: D1. Sleep problems D2. Irritability D3. Concentration problems D4. Hypervigilance D5. Exaggerated startle response
E. Onset of symptoms within 6 months of the stressor	E. Duration of disturbance of at least 1 month
	F. Distress or impairment in areas of functioning

Note. DSM-IV=*Diagnostic and Statistical Manual of Mental Disorders*, 4th Edition (American Psychiatric Association 1994); ICD-10=*International Statistical Classification of Diseases and Related Health Problems*, 10th Revision (World Health Organization 1992).

Source. Adapted from Peters L, Slade T, Andrews G: "A Comparison of ICD10 and DSM-IV Criteria for Posttraumatic Stress Disorder. *Journal of Traumatic Stress* 12:335–343, 1999.

the products of expert consensus. This is not to suggest that diagnostic criteria derived from this method are somehow invalid. In fact, over the last 20 years, a substantial literature supports the notion that the constellation of symptoms specific to PTSD is characteristic of a maladaptive response to trauma. However, data seem to indicate that all three symptom clusters are not equally predictive of PTSD. For example, assessment of survivors of the 1994 Oklahoma City bombing highlights the role of Criterion C (avoidance and emotional numbing) in predicting PTSD diagnosis. In the subsample of individuals who had Criterion C symptoms (i.e., by endorsing three out of seven symptoms), 76% went on to later be diagnosed with PTSD (North et al. 1999). In contrast, in the subsample of survivors who met Criterion B or D, approximately 49% went on to meet full diagnostic criteria for PTSD. Criterion C was also the strongest predictor of those who would not develop PTSD. Of those who did not meet Criterion C, less than 3% were later diagnosed with PTSD; in contrast, of those who did not meet criteria for reexperiencing or hyperarousal symptoms, approximately 75% went on to a positive diagnosis of PTSD.

Emerging evidence for the factor structure of PTSD has also engendered closer examination of diagnostic criteria. Instead of a three-factor model represented by Criteria B, C, and D, confirmatory factor analytic studies of trauma survivors support single-factor, two-factor, or four-factor models of PTSD. For example, in a study of Vietnam combat veterans, factor analysis suggested that avoidance and emotional numbing symptoms, although combined in DSM-IV under PTSD diagnostic Criterion C, were actually distinct factors (King et al. 1998). Another model, the four-factor dysphoria model, has demonstrated validity in samples of Persian Gulf War veterans (Simms et al. 2002) and in samples of veterans from Operations Enduring Freedom and Iraqi Freedom (R.H. Pietrzak, D.C. Johnson, M.B. Goldstein, et al., "Confirmatory Factor Analysis of the PTSD Checklist-Military Version in Veterans of Operations Enduring and Iraqi Freedom," manuscript submitted for publication, 2010). The four-factor dysphoria model comprises reexperiencing, avoidance and emotional numbing, dysphoria, and hyperarousal. Table 4–4 outlines symptom composition of each factor.

The value of the four-factor dysphoria model is the potential for informing treatment and assessing treatment progress. Evidence from assessment of individuals with experience in Operations Enduring Freedom and Iraqi Freedom suggests that the dysphoria factor is most strongly associated with comorbid

Table 4–4. Four-factor dysphoria model of PTSD

Reexperiencing
B1. Repeated, disturbing memories
B2. Repeated, disturbing dreams
B3. Reliving (flashbacks)
B4. Emotionally upset at reminders
B5. Physical reactions to reminders
Avoidance and emotional numbing
C1. Avoiding thinking or talking about event
C2. Avoiding activities or situations that remind
Dysphoria
C3. Inability to recall aspects of trauma
C4. Loss of interest
C5. Detachment
C6. Restricted affect
C7. Sense of foreshortened future
D1. Sleep disturbance
D2. Irritability
D3. Difficulty concentrating
Hyperarousal
D4. Hypervigilance
D5. Exaggerated startle response

depression, psychosocial functioning, and psychological resilience (Pietrzak et al., "Confirmary Factor Analysis," 2010). From a treatment perspective, early therapeutic progress might be gained more readily when interventions target dysphoria factor symptoms. Given the strong correlation that dysphoria factor symptoms have with depression and psychosocial impairment, early symptom reduction may facilitate improvement in conditions that frequently co-occur with PTSD (e.g., alcohol abuse, major depressive disorder). Additionally, early targeting of dysphoria factor symptoms may be less threatening to patients who are unlikely to adhere to fear conditioning and exposure-based treatments. Therapeutic interventions that target dysphoria factor symptoms can focus on sleep (D1), emotion regulation (C6 and D2), or cognitive remediation (D3) without broaching the topic of trauma memories and exposure. Moreover, because dysphoria factor symptoms appear to be more strongly correlated with resilience and psychosocial impairment, early symptom reduction may bolster resilience and improve social support networks that make adherence to empirically validated exposure-based treatments more likely.

Symptom Heterogeneity

PTSD can also be difficult to assess reliably due to a large degree of symptom variability. To meet DSM-IV diagnostic criteria, an individual must endorse or experience one of five reexperiencing symptoms, three of seven avoidance symptoms, and two of five hyperarousal symptoms. Thus, there are 1,750 different combinations of PTSD symptoms that meet diagnostic criteria. Such heterogeneity of symptoms makes it unlikely that any two cases of PTSD will look exactly the same. Further complicating assessment and treatment is that even those individuals who do not meet full diagnostic criteria for PTSD often suffer significant social and occupational impairment. These observations have led some investigators to propose that a truncated, simplified set of diagnostic criteria be applied, incorporating symptoms that are commonly associated with impairment following trauma exposure (Norman et al. 2007).

Variable Course

Comprehensive assessment of PTSD must also take into consideration variability in the course of symptom presentation. Some individuals have delayed onset—that is, they manifest symptoms of PTSD beginning several months, or in rarer cases years, after exposure to trauma. Moreover, symptom intensity can wax and wane over the course of several months. For clinicians attempting to accurately screen for the presence of PTSD symptoms, the variable course of PTSD symptoms can be problematic.

The variable course of PTSD symptoms has been a critical issue in attempts to screen large numbers of combat veterans returning from Afghanistan and Iraq. In the early years of these military operations, it was common for military treatment facilities to screen personnel for PTSD immediately upon return from deployment as part of a standard health reassessment. However, mental health assessments within days or weeks of returning from combat deployment were yielding unanticipated low rates of PTSD symptoms (e.g., <5%).

Much speculation continues about why PTSD screening that takes place soon after return from deployment yields lower rates of symptoms; however, there is little disagreement that longitudinal assessment following trauma exposure optimizes the potential for accurate classification of PTSD. In a study of active-duty hospitalized military personnel, symptoms of PTSD were assessed at 1 month, 4 months, and 7 months after battlefield injury. The rates of probable PTSD at the 1-month assessment were 4.2%, whereas rates at the 4-month and 7-month marks were 12.2% and 12.0%, respectively (Grieger et al. 2006). Moreover, nearly 80% of those individuals who screened positive for probable PTSD at the 7-month mark did not report the presence of significant symptoms at the 1-month assessment. As a result of these and other similar findings, the U.S. Department of Defense has implemented mandatory serial screening for symptoms of combat stress at 1 month, 3 months, and 6 months following return from deployment.

Symptom Overlap

PTSD shares several symptoms with substance abuse disorders, panic disorder, adjustment disorder, obsessive-compulsive disorder (OCD), and major depressive disorder. Moreover, several of these shared symptoms are often easily recognizable in other disorders, and this overlap may challenge accurate diagnosis. For example, PTSD symptoms of anger, irritability, sleep disturbances, and sense of a foreshortened future are also often present in major depressive disorder. There is also significant overlap of symptoms between PTSD and mild traumatic brain injury (mTBI; Table 4–7). In a study of 2,525 U.S. Army infantry soldiers, 4.9% reported loss of consciousness (LOC) while deployed in support of Operation Iraqi Freedom (OIF). Of those soldiers reporting history of LOC, 43.9% met criteria for PTSD. Furthermore, the association between mTBI and poorer general health was completely mediated by PTSD and depressive symptoms (Hoge et al. 2008). This result suggests that in many cases, social, occupational, and physical impairment following head trauma may best be explained as complex PTSD sequelae rather than mTBI.

Malingering

Malingering is a threat to valid and reliable assessment of PTSD. DSM-IV-TR indicates that differential diagnosis of PTSD should involve an evaluation to rule out malingering. That this diagnostic imperative is explicitly expressed for assessing PTSD, but not for assessing mood disorders or other anxiety disorders, underscores the need for comprehensive assessment to include an evaluation of malingering.

In general, PTSD can be malingered in two ways: 1) malingered memory for the event, which includes intentional inaccuracies about the nature of the trauma (i.e., Criterion A1) and exaggeration of the response to the trauma (i.e., Criterion A2); and 2) feigned symptom severity (e.g., frequency or intensity). With respect to memory for the Criterion A event, it is a misconception that inconsistency of memory suggests deception or fabrication. Schacter (1999) referred to memory as having "fragile power." That is, humans have an impressive capacity for remembering the gist of events, yet the ability to recall detail accurately is less impressive and highly vulnerable to numerous types of information processing errors. Assessment of memory for PTSD Criterion A events can often reveal seemingly contradictory results. Survivors of life-threatening trauma may be unable to recall some details (e.g., posttraumatic amnesia) while also being unable to forget other details (e.g., intrusive memories). The PTSD literature sometimes refers to this phenomenon as "islands of memory," in that portions of memory are distinct and salient, but are disconnected and form a fragmented whole. It is also worth noting that memory, including memory for traumatic events, is dynamic. Remembering one portion of an experience often activates memories for associated aspects of the event that may not have previously been remembered. For example, the victim of a sexual assault may not remember the type of car in which her attacker drove away. However, efforts to retrieve memories about other details of her trauma, such as time of day, location, or facial features, may activate a network of other memories associated (e.g., semantically, sensorially) with the entire trauma. Accordingly, variability in recall for traumatic events does not necessarily suggest malingering.

To date, there is no commonly used test specific to malingering PTSD. Excellent instruments that assess nonspecific symptom exaggeration include the Miller Forensic Assessment of Symptoms Test (M-FAST; Miller 2005) and the Victoria Symptom Validity Checklist (VSVT; Slick et al. 1997), but these do not specifically address PTSD symptoms. Other tests, such as the Test of Memory Malingering (TOMM; Tombaugh 1996) identify poor effort on tests of neurocognitive functioning. However, such tests do not assess malingering specific to PTSD-related cognitive impairments or symptoms.

Assessment of PTSD

Self-Report Measures

PTSD Checklist

The PTSD Checklist (PCL; Weathers et al. 1991) is one of the most widely used self-report measures for PTSD. The original PCL comprised items corresponding to DSM-III diagnostic criteria for PTSD, and was validated in combat veterans from the Vietnam and Persian Gulf Wars. Since then, the PCL has been modified to correspond to DSM-IV diagnostic criteria, and a substantial literature exists outlining its reliability, validity, and utility for assessing symptoms in a variety of populations. Additionally, three alternate versions of the PCL have been created: a military version (PCL-M), a civilian version (PCL-C), and a stressor-specific version designed for serial assessment on a weekly basis (PCL-S; Weathers and Ford 1996).

The PCL consists of 17 items, scored on a 5-point Likert scale (1 = *not at all;* 5 = *extremely)*, that directly assess PTSD Criteria B, C, and D from DSM-IV. Scores range from 17 to 85, and represent frequency of PTSD symptoms. Various scoring conventions and cutoffs have been examined. In general, a PCL total score of 50 and a symptom score of 3 or higher are recommended as diagnostic cutoffs for military personnel. For civilians, recommended PCL total cutoff scores range from 44 to as low as 30 in some primary care settings. Regarding symptom change, the PCL tends to underrate improvement and is less diagnostically accurate in cases at or near diagnostic threshold when compared to the Clinician-Administered PTSD Scale (Forbes et al. 2001).

Abbreviated versions of the PCL may be preferred in settings where time and resources for more comprehensive psychiatric screening are limited (e.g., combat theater and deployment health clinics, civilian primary care clinics). Two-item and six-item versions of the PCL have demonstrated acceptable diagnostic reliability and validity as screening instruments (Lang and Stein 2005). These shorter versions appear in Table 4–5.

Davidson Trauma Scale

The Davidson Trauma Scale (DTS; Davidson et al. 1997) assesses the frequency and severity of PTSD symptoms among individuals with a history of trauma exposure. Like the PCL, the DTS comprises 17 items corresponding to DSM-IV diagnostic criteria. However, the DTS differs from the PCL in

Table 4–5. Two- and six-item versions of PTSD Checklist (PCL)

Below is a list of problems and complaints that veterans sometimes have in response to stressful military experience. Please read each one carefully, then circle one of the numbers to the right [5-point Likert scale, not shown here] *to indicate how much you have been bothered by that problem in the past month.*

Two-item PCL

1 Repeated, disturbing memories, thoughts, or images of a stressful experience from the past?

2 Feeling very upset when something reminded you of a stressful experience from the past?

Cutoff score = 4
Sensitivity 0.96, specificity 0.58

Six-item PCL

1 Repeated, disturbing memories, thoughts, or images of a stressful experience from the past?

2 Feeling very upset when something reminded you of a stressful experience from the past?

3 Avoiding activities or situations because they reminded you of a stressful experience from the past?

4 Feeling distant or cut off from other people?

5 Feeling irritable or having angry outbursts?

6 Having difficulty concentrating?

Cutoff score = 14
Sensitivity 0.92, specificity 0.72

Source. Lang and Stein 2005.

that the DTS assesses symptom frequency and symptom severity as separate factors. Whereas the PCL records only one response to "how much you have been bothered" by each symptom, the DTS provides a 5-point Likert scale for frequency (0 = *not at all;* 4 = *every day*) and another for intensity (0 = *not at all;* 4 = *extremely distressing*) for each symptom. The scale has good internal consistency and test-retest reliability. Additionally, the DTS correlates with clinician-administered and self-report measures of PTSD, as well as with symptoms of general psychological distress.

Deployment Risk and Resilience Inventory

The Deployment Risk and Resilience Inventory (DRRI; King et al. 2003) is a collection of measures designed to assess before- and after-deployment factors associated with behavioral health outcomes. Factors include training and preparation, unit cohesion, social support, and combat exposure. In an effort to improve upon scales oriented to Vietnam-era combat (e.g., Combat Experiences Scale; Keane et al. 1989), measures within the DRRI were developed specifically to assess "stereotypical combat experiences" of Persian Gulf War veterans. Initial validation of the DRRI conducted with veterans from Persian Gulf I (King et al. 2006) indicated adequate to good psychometric properties for DRRI scales. See Table 4–6 for specific scales relevant to assessment of combat stress and exposure.

Following scale development in Persian Gulf War samples, the DRRI has also been validated in a sample of Operation Iraqi Freedom (OIF) veterans (Vogt et al. 2008). Reliability and validity of the DRRI was assessed in a sample of 640 active-duty military service members deployed to Iraq from 2003 to 2006. Data for the DRRI were collected as part of a larger study that assessed soldiers before and after deployment in support of OIF (Neurocognitive Deployment Health Study; Brailey et al. 2007). Internal consistency of the DRRI in the OIF sample was comparable to results obtained in the Gulf War I sample 15 years earlier. Cronbach's alphas ranged from 0.77 to 0.90 for combat exposure–related scales. Combat exposure–related scales demonstrated good convergent validity in comparisons between frontline combat personnel and those assigned to support/logistics. Moreover, these scales revealed a significant dose-response relationship between degree of exposure and several behavioral health symptoms, including posttraumatic stress, depression, physical health, and cognitive functioning (Vogt et al. 2008).

Perceived Stress Scale

The Perceived Stress Scale (PSS; Cohen et al. 1983) is one of the most widely used self-report measures of subjective perceptions of stress. The PSS is available in 4-item, 10-item, and 14-item versions, all of which demonstrate adequate psychometric properties. Instructions ask the respondent about "feelings and thoughts during the last month." Each item is scored on a 5-point Likert scale, with items measuring the perceived frequency of "unpredictable, uncontrollable, and overloaded stress." The following are examples

Table 4–6. Deployment Risk and Resilience Inventory subscales relevant to assessment of combat stress

Subscale	Measures	No. of items	Sample items
Perceived Threat	Fear for one's safety in the war zone	15	"I thought I would never survive." "I felt that I was in great danger of being killed or wounded."
Combat Experiences	Exposure to stereotypical warfare	15	"I or members of my unit were attacked by terrorists or civilians." "My unit engaged in battle in which it suffered casualties."
Aftermath of Battle	Exposure to consequences of combat	15	"I was exposed to the sight, sound, or smell of dying men and women." "I saw allies after they had been severely wounded or disfigured in combat."
NBC Exposures	Exposure to nuclear, biological, and chemical agents	20	"While deployed I was exposed to depleted uranium in munitions." "I took pyridostigmine or NAPPs."

Note. NAPP = nerve agent pyridostigmine pretreatment; NBC = nuclear, biological, and chemical.

of item content: "How often have you felt that you were on top of things?" "How often have you felt that you were unable to control the important things in your life?" and "How often have you felt confident about your ability to handle your personal problems?" Normative data were obtained from 2,387 U.S. respondents to a 1983 Harris Poll (Cohen and Williamson 1988). Higher scores on the PSS are indicative of a higher frequency of perceived stressors. Results of studies utilizing the PSS indicate that higher levels of perceived stress are associated with a host of poor behavioral health outcomes that include difficulty with smoking cessation, higher incidence of depressive symptoms, and weakened immune response.

Posttraumatic Cognitions Inventory

The Posttraumatic Cognitions Inventory (PTCI; Foa et al. 1999) is a 33-item measure of the thoughts and beliefs an individual has about potentially traumatic events. Each item is scored on a 7-point Likert scale ranging from 1 (*totally agree*) to 7 (*totally disagree*). Item development leveraged theory from Aaron Beck's cognitive triad, and psychometric analysis supports a three-factor model of trauma-related cognitions: 1) negative cognitions about self, 2) negative cognitions about the world, and 3) self-blame (Foa et al. 1999). Validation of the PTCI revealed significant positive correlation with trait anxiety (i.e., State-Trait Anxiety Inventory), as well as with depressive symptoms (Beck Depression Inventory). PTCI items include "My life has been destroyed by the trauma," "I can't stop bad things from happening to me," and "If I think about the event now, I will not be able to handle it." Because such statements are often the focus of restructuring and altering perspective in the course of cognitive-behavioral therapy, the PTCI can be a valuable tool for tracking treatment outcome.

Trauma Symptom Inventory

The Trauma Symptom Inventory (TSI; Briere 1995) is a 100-item evaluation of acute and chronic symptomatology from a wide variety of traumas, including rape, combat experiences, major accidents, natural disasters, and childhood abuse. The TSI comprises three validity scales and 10 clinical scales that assess a wide range of psychological impacts. These include not only symptoms typically associated with PTSD or acute stress disorder, but also those intrapersonal and interpersonal difficulties often associated with more chronic psychological trauma (e.g., dissociation, lack of social support, tension reduction behavior). The TSI does not generate DSM-IV diagnoses; instead, it is intended to evaluate the relative level of various forms of posttraumatic distress (Briere 1995).

Clinician-Administered Scales

Structured Clinical Interview for DSM Disorders

The Structured Clinical Interview for DSM-IV-TR Axis I Disorders, Research Version, Patient Edition (SCID-I/P; First et al. 2002) is a clinician-based structured interview designed to comprehensively assess the majority of Axis I disorders. The PTSD portion of the SCID is found in Module F, Anxiety Disorders. The SCID covers each of the 17 DSM-IV symptoms for PTSD, and clinicians rate symptoms along a 3-point scale ranging from 1 (*symptom not present*) to 3 (*symptom present*). A dichotomous (yes/no) rating is made by the clinician after determining if each of three symptom criteria (i.e., reexperiencing, avoidance, hyperarousal) has been met. Several versions of the SCID are available for use dependent on the setting (e.g., research, clinical, and nonpatient populations). The SCID is also available in several different languages.

Mini-International Neuropsychiatric Interview

The Mini-International Neuropsychiatric Interview (MINI; Sheehan et al. 1998) is a brief structured interview. Similar to the SCID, the MINI was designed to assess major Axis I disorders according to DSM-IV criteria. The primary strengths of the MINI are its ease of administration and brief administration time. The mean time for administering the entire MINI is 18.7±11.6 minutes. The PTSD module of the MINI (Module I) is a total of six questions, each with dichotomous (yes/no) response options. Questions I1 and I2 assess PTSD Criteria A1 and A2, respectively. Question I3 assesses the presence of reexperiencing symptoms. Questions I4 and I5 evaluate symptoms of avoidance and emotional numbing (Criterion C) and hyperarousal (Criterion D). The final question of the PTSD module addresses social and occupational functioning.

Essential to the MINI's brief administration time is the MINI Screen. The MINI Screen is a 20-question interview intended to help select which modules of the subsequent MINI should be fully administered. Three items in the MINI Screen are associated with Module I (PTSD). A positive ("yes") response to any of these three items directs the interviewer to administer the entire PTSD module. Psychometric evaluations of the MINI indicate strong diagnostic reliability and validity in comparison with the SCID and the Composite International Diagnostic Interview (CIDI). The MINI is one of the most widely used clinical assessment instruments in the world, and is available in multiple languages. A MINI Tracking version is also available, which measures symptoms along a continuum and is useful for measuring treatment outcome (Sheehan et al. 1998).

Clinician-Administered PTSD Scale

The Clinician-Administered PTSD Scale (CAPS; Weathers 1996) is a structured clinical interview measuring the frequency and intensity of the 17 DSM-IV symptoms of PTSD and eight associated symptoms. The CAPS also contains five global rating questions regarding the impact of symptoms on social and occupational functioning, improvement since previous assessment, and overall validity and severity of reported symptoms (Blake et al. 1990). The CAPS is often considered the "gold standard" in assessment of PTSD, and a literature comprising more than 200 published studies supports its diagnostic reliability and validity (for review, see Weathers et al. 2001).

One advantage of the CAPS over other structured clinical interviews, such as the SCID, is that CAPS scoring goes beyond dichotomous (yes/no) ratings. The clinician uses a 5-point Likert scale to rate each PTSD symptom assessed via the CAPS along two dimensions: 1) symptom frequency (0 = *never;* 4 = *daily or almost every day*) and 2) symptom intensity (0 = *none;* 4 = *extreme, incapacitating distress*). The CAPS total score is the sum of the frequency and intensity scores for each of the 17 PTSD symptoms. CAPS total scores range from 0 to 136, and several scoring conventions have been evaluated (e.g., Weathers et al. 1999). The lowest score that may be used to make a diagnosis of PTSD is 24; however, this is the extreme liberal end of diagnostic threshold and is very rarely used. Sensitivity and specificity of PTSD diagnoses are optimized by using a CAPS total score cutoff in the range of 60–70. A CAPS cutoff score of 65 is recommended by the National Center for PTSD (Weathers 1999) for forensic evaluations.

Anxiety Disorders Interview Schedule for DSM-IV

Developed by DiNardo et al. (1994), the Anxiety Disorders Interview Schedule for DSM-IV (ADIS) is a structured clinical interview designed to assess patients for current episodes of anxiety disorders. The strength of the ADIS is that it allows for assessment of symptoms, including frequency and intensity, along a continuum that facilitates robust evaluation of subthreshold diagnoses. The ADIS is also an excellent tool for differential diagnosis. For example, panic attacks are common to panic disorder, social phobia, and specific phobias, in addition to PTSD. Similarly, intrusive, unwanted thoughts are characteristic of PTSD as well as obsessive-compulsive disorder. Because the ADIS assesses associated symptoms of anxiety in greater detail, it is also particularly well suited for evaluating disorders that are highly comorbid with PTSD (e.g., depression, substance abuse). Additional features of the ADIS include a diagnostic timeline, a section for DSM-IV multiaxial assessment, and designation of primary and secondary diagnoses. Psychometric data for the PTSD module of the ADIS indicate strong reliability and validity in a military sample (sensitivity 1.00; specificity 0.91), whereas clinician agreement was less reliable in civilian community mental health samples (e.g., kappa=0.55).

Morel Emotional Numbing Test (MENT)

As mentioned, there is an absence of well-validated tests that specifically assess malingering of PTSD symptoms. However, one promising test developed to address this gap is the Morel Emotional Numbing Test (MENT; Morel 1998). The MENT is a 60-item forced-choice recognition test. Administration involves displaying a series of easily recognizable facial expressions (e.g., sad, angry, happy, fearful). The respondent is instructed to correctly identify the emotion associated with each facial expression. Just prior to administration, the respondent is read an instruction set, which includes a statement that individuals with PTSD often have difficulty identifying facial expressions (i.e., an intentional misinterpretation of the PTSD symptom "emotional numbing). However, similar to neuropsychological tests that indirectly measure effort, the faces presented during the MENT should be recognizable to anyone with intact visual functioning. Respondents are additionally aided by the fact that the MENT is a recognition test that presents the correct answer along with only one foil.

Validity of the MENT as a tool for assessing malingering in PTSD is supported by several published studies that highlight its sensitivity and specificity for differentiating malingerers from those who truly have PTSD. For example, in a study that included a sample of compensation-seeking combat veterans, the hit rate (i.e., the ratio of true malingerers minus false-positives) was 95.6% (Morel 1998). Subsequent evaluations of the MENT indicated that it performs comparably to well-established instruments commonly used in neuropsychology to identify insufficient effort and endorsement of improbable, low-frequency items (e.g., Messer and Fremouw 2007; Morel 2007). Additionally, a 2008 meta-analysis of five studies that used the MENT (Morel and Shepherd 2008) showed consistently larger mean error rates by malingerers than by credible respondents. The mean number of errors on the MENT by malingerers ranged from 22.9 to 8.4, whereas errors by credible respondents ranged from 6.8 to 1.1.

Differential Diagnosis of PTSD

PTSD is not an especially difficult clinical diagnosis to make, but clinicians should maintain an index of suspicion and a habit of inquiring about potentially traumatic events. Because many patients will not spontaneously report traumatic experiences to a treating clinician, direct inquiry is often required. A case in point is the reporting of experiences of childhood maltreatment, wherein individuals may not endorse abuse unless the questions are behaviorally specific (Thombs et al. 2006). It is strongly recommended, so as to avoid missing cases of PTSD, that clinicians routinely inquire about a range of potentially traumatic experiences (e.g., exposure to intimate partner violence; serious physical injury from any source; combat exposure) in a patient's initial evaluation and revisit this area of inquiry in subsequent sessions when the index of suspicion is raised by particular symptoms (e.g., insomnia) or the failure to respond to treatment as expected. See Table 4–7 for some keys to accurate and reliable assessment of PTSD.

Adjustment Disorder

For a patient who has experienced a "stressful" event but lacks traumatic exposure of sufficient severity (Criterion A1), a diagnosis of adjustment disorder may apply. According to the definition of adjustment disorder, once the stressor has remitted, the symptoms should not persist beyond 6 months. However, if the stressor (e.g., marital discord) fails to remit and the symptoms persist beyond 6 months, other diagnoses (e.g., major depression) should also be considered. If symptoms do persist, the clinician should revisit whether

Table 4–7. Keys to accurate and reliable assessment of PTSD

Carefully establish that both the trauma and the response meet diagnostic criteria.
Ask about "shock," "anxiety," or "stress" if there is no endorsement of "fear, helplessness, or horror."
Establish that specific symptoms are anchored to the trauma (otherwise, they are not symptoms of PTSD).
Do not rely on screeners for diagnosis.
Seek information from a combination of self-report measures, formal testing, collateral sources, and clinician interview.
Obtain specific examples of social and occupational functioning impairments.
Perform serial assessment of symptoms (i.e., track multiple time points).
Utilize psychometrically valid instruments with published cutoff scores.
Screen or formally assess malingering of PTSD symptoms.

Criterion A1 (and Criterion A2) had indeed been met, and reconsider a diagnosis of PTSD.

Acute Stress Disorder

Acute stress disorder, first introduced in DSM-IV, has been a controversial diagnosis and may not persist into DSM-5 (Stein and Bienvenu 2004). Acute stress disorder should pose little difficulty in terms of differential diagnosis with PTSD, given that the former, by definition, is short-lived, enduring for a maximum of 4 weeks following exposure to the stressor. In some instances, acute stress disorder can be construed as a forerunner of PTSD, because the symptoms persist beyond 4 weeks in a proportion of individuals (10%–15%, depending on the nature of the traumatic stressor), at which time a diagnosis of PTSD may supervene. Acute stress disorder, as conceptualized in DSM-IV, emphasizes dissociative symptoms (e.g., feeling dazed or disoriented), which themselves may be confused with symptoms of traumatic brain injury (see "Traumatic Brain Injury" section later in this chapter).

Major Depression

In clinical and epidemiological samples, the majority of patients with PTSD will have comorbid depressive symptoms, with many also meeting diagnostic criteria for major depression. As such, major depression is often not a differential diagnosis, but rather a co-occurring diagnosis. However, some symptoms of major depression and PTSD can be difficult to disaggregate, such as anhedonia in major depressive disorder and emotional numbing (i.e., Criterion C avoidance symptoms) in PTSD. When in doubt, the clinician can make a provisional comorbid diagnosis of major depression, therein pointing to the need for vigilant assessment of suicidality.

Obsessive-Compulsive Disorder

Intrusive thoughts and images and the performance of behaviors intended to avoid the discomfort associated with such cognitions are common to both obsessive-compulsive disorder and PTSD. The disclosure of an inciting traumatic event may be useful in making a diagnosis of PTSD, and the elucidation of the particular thought content (which, in the case of PTSD, will be tied to one or more traumatic events) will aid in differential diagnosis. However, certain forms of trauma exposure (e.g., military conflict) may be associated with behaviors (e.g., checking related to prior military duties) that make differential diagnosis a challenging endeavor (Tuerk et al. 2009).

Psychotic Disorders

It is being increasingly recognized that psychotic disorders such as schizophrenia are associated with early and often pervasive exposure to traumatic events (Conus et al. 2009) and with high rates of PTSD, which often goes unrecognized and untreated in community mental health settings (Mueser et al. 2008). Accordingly, a comorbid diagnosis of PTSD should be strongly considered among patients with psychotic disorders, although the elucidation of a focal traumatic "event" may be difficult, in part because the patient is likely to have experienced many Criterion A events over a lifetime. There is also the possibility of an individual with a principal diagnosis of PTSD experiencing psychotic symptoms, such as the recurring visual hallucination of seeing a prior assailant, or the tendency to extrapolate risk to the point that it can be considered "paranoia." In those cases where the principal diagnosis is PTSD, these psychotic symptoms should be relatively short-lived (although they can be recurrent), and reality testing should be intact (although it may temporarily fail upon reexposure to reminders of the traumatic event). Bizarre delusions or hallucinations and grossly disorganized thought processes are inconsistent with a principal diagnosis of PTSD.

Personality Disorders

Historically, particularly in the military, there may have been a tendency to diagnose "personality disorders"—rather than PTSD—among individuals who developed maladaptive responses to traumatic stress. This predilection to assign a personality disorder rather than PTSD likely reflected a long-standing bias against those persons who experience mental illness. It may also have reflected concerns about malingering and secondary gain, as well as a general unwillingness to acknowledge that severe traumatic stress can cause mental illness that may be compensable. In terms of differential diagnosis, it is important to remember that personality disorder diagnoses are meant to refer to lifelong patterns of maladaptive behaviors and troubled interpersonal interactions. Thus, a history consistent with personality disorder prior to trauma exposure may indicate a preexisting personality disorder, but would not rule out a concurrent diagnosis of PTSD given that preexisting personality disorder (e.g., antisocial personality disorder) is a risk factor for developing PTSD following trauma exposure. Borderline personality disorder is increased among persons with childhood maltreatment and, accordingly, may be seen in conjunction with PTSD, particularly in women. Considering personality disorders to be, in most cases, co-occurring conditions on another diagnostic axis—rather than necessarily differential diagnoses—may be helpful in terms of therapeutic formulation and treatment planning.

Traumatic Brain Injury

Mild traumatic brain injury has been noted to be common among military personnel deployed to the recent conflicts in Afghanistan and Iraq, and to frequently be associated with PTSD (Hoge et al. 2008). This observation has raised questions about the nature of this relationship, and attention has been drawn to the fact that syndromal conceptualizations of sequelae of mild traumatic brain injury (i.e., postconcussive symptoms) and exposure to traumatic events (i.e., PTSD symptoms) overlap substantially (Stein and McAllister 2009). A summary of overlap between symptoms characterizing response to a traumatic stressor and postconcussive symptoms is presented in Table 4–8.

Table 4–8. Diagnostic criteria and associated features of posttraumatic stress disorder and traumatic brain injury

Symptom	PTSD	TBI
Emotional numbing	✓	✓
Reduced awareness	✓	✓
Depersonalization	✓	✓
Derealization	✓	✓
Amnesia	✓	✓
Recurrent images	✓	✓
Nightmares	✓	—
Distress on reminders	✓	—
Avoidance of reminders	✓	—
Social detachment	✓	✓
Diminished interest	✓	✓
Sense of foreshortened future	✓	—
Insomnia	✓	✓
Irritability	✓	✓
Concentration deficits	✓	✓
Hypervigilance	✓	—
Elevated startle response	✓	—

Lack of objective assessment metrics has also created challenges for differential diagnosis, and assessment of PTSD via self-report questionnaires may be especially vulnerable to false-positive diagnosis in individuals with traumatic brain injury. For example, Sumpter and McMillan (2006) compared rates of PTSD diagnosis in patients with traumatic brain injury. When assessed via patient self-report questionnaire, 59% were diagnosed with PTSD; when assessed via structured clinical interview, only 3% were diagnosed with PTSD. The increase in false-positives with self-report questionnaires was ultimately attributed to patient failure to follow instructions, inattention, misinterpretation of symptoms, and symptom overlap. Such a disparity in diagnosis is a caution to clinicians against overreliance on self-report measures, and further underscores the proper place of clinician-administered interviews as the standard in psychodiagnostic assessment of PTSD.

At present, this is a very controversial topic, with experts variously suggesting that mild traumatic brain injury has been grossly underdiagnosed or overdiagnosed among military personnel. Given this controversy, recommendations about concurrent assessment of traumatic brain injury (above and beyond the requisite questioning about change in or loss of consciousness in association with an injury) and its place in differential diagnosis are uncertain.

Key Clinical Points

- The diagnosis of PTSD requires 1) exposure to trauma; 2) a response of fear, helplessness, or horror; and 3) development of symptoms categorized as reexperiencing, avoidance, and hyperarousal.
- Military personnel and other highly trained individuals may not respond to life-threatening situations with fear, helplessness, or horror (DSM Criterion A2).
- Criterion C (avoidance and emotional numbing) appears to be the criterion most predictive of PTSD.
- PTSD can be difficult to assess acutely, owing to the large degree of interindividual symptom variability; longitudinal assessments may provide a more thorough means of evaluating PTSD.
- Self-report measures of PTSD such as the PCL, PTCI, and TSI are validated instruments that provide a variety of information to a clinician in assessing an individual's likelihood of having PTSD.
- Clinician-administered measures of PTSD such as the SCID, MINI, and CAPS provide structured evaluation tools for assessment of PTSD.
- In cases where a "stressful" but not a traumatic experience occurred for an individual, a diagnosis of adjustment disorder may apply.
- Major depressive disorder may be concurrent with a diagnosis of PTSD or may better explain an individual's symptoms and should be considered, given the high comorbidity of these two disorders.

- The presence of a psychotic disorder should not dissuade a provider from exploring the possibility of PTSD as a comorbid diagnosis, given the evidence of early, and often pervasive, traumatic experiences for individuals with psychotic disorders.
- In most cases, providers should consider personality disorders to be co-occurring with PTSD rather than a differential diagnosis.
- Differentiating malingering of PTSD from true PTSD is a difficult and complex task, but instruments such as the Miller Forensic Assessment of Symptoms Test (M-FAST) and the MENT may assist providers in clarifying this diagnostic uncertainty.

References

Adler AB, Wright KM, Bliese PD, et al: A2 diagnostic criterion for combat-related posttraumatic stress disorder. J Trauma Stress 21:301–308, 2008

American Psychiatric Association: Diagnostic and Statistical Manual of Mental Disorders, 3rd Edition. Washington, DC, American Psychiatric Association, 1980

American Psychiatric Association: Diagnostic and Statistical Manual of Mental Disorders, 4th Edition. Washington, DC, American Psychiatric Association, 1994

American Psychiatric Association: Diagnostic and Statistical Manual of Mental Disorders, 4th Edition, Text Revision. Washington, DC, American Psychiatric Association, 2000

Blake DD, Weathers FW, Nagy LM, et al: A clinician rating scale for assessing current and lifetime PTSD: the CAPS-1. Behav Ther 13:187–188, 1990

Brailey K, Vasterling JJ, Proctor SP, et al: PTSD symptoms, life-events, and unit cohesion in US soldiers: baseline findings from the neurocognition deployment health study. J Trauma Stress 20:495–503, 2007

Briere J: Trauma Symptom Inventory Professional Manual. Odessa, FL, Psychological Assessment Resources, 1995

Cohen S, Kamarck T, Mermelstein R: A global measure of perceived stress. J Health Soc Behav 24:386–396, 1983

Cohen S, Williamson G: Perceived stress in a probability sample of the United States, in The Social Psychology of Health: Claremont Symposium on Applied Social Psychology. Edited by Spacapan S, Oskamp S. Newbury Park, CA, Sage, 1988, pp 31–67

Conus P, Cotton S, Schimmelmann BG, et al: Pretreatment and outcome correlates of sexual and physical trauma in an epidemiological cohort of first-episode psychosis patients. Schizophr Bull Apr 21, 2009 [Epub ahead of print]

Davidson JR, Book SW, Colket JT, et al: Assessment of a new self-rating scale for post-traumatic stress disorder. Psychol Med 27:153–160, 1997

DiNardo PA, Brown TA, Barlow DH: Anxiety Disorders Interview Schedule for DSM-IV: Lifetime Version (ADIS-IV-L). San Antonio, TX, Psychological Corporation, 1994

First MB, Spitzer RL, Gibbon M, et al: Structured Clinical Interview for DSM-IV-TR Axis I Disorders, Research Version, Patient Edition (SCID I/P). New York, Biometrics Research, New York State Psychiatric Institute, November 2002

Foa EB, Ehlers A, Clark DM, et al: The Posttraumatic Cognitions Inventory (PTCI): development and validation. Psychol Assess 11:303–314, 1999

Forbes D, Creamer M, Biddle D: The validity of the PTSD Checklist as a measure of symptomatic change in combat-related PTSD. Behav Res Ther 39:977–986, 2001

Grieger TA, Cozza SJ, Ursano RJ, et al: Posttraumatic stress disorder and depression in battle-injured soldiers. Am J Psychiatry 163:1777–1783; quiz 1860, 2006

Hoge CW, McGurk D, Thomas JL, et al: Mild traumatic brain injury in U.S. soldiers returning from Iraq. N Engl J Med 358:453–463, 2008

Keane TM, Fairbank JA, Caddell JM, et al: Clinical evaluation of a measure to assess combat exposure. Psychol Assess 1:53–55, 1989

King DW, Leskin GA, King LA, et al: Confirmatory factor analysis of the Clinician-Administered PTSD Scale: evidence for the dimensionality of posttraumatic stress disorder. Psychol Assess 10:90–96, 1998

King DW, King LA, Vogt DS: Manual for the Deployment Risk and Resilience Inventory (DRRI): A Collection of Measures for Studying Deployment-Related Experiences of Military Veterans. Boston MA, National Center for PTSD, 2003

King L, King D, Vogt D, et al: Deployment Risk and Resilience Inventory: a collection of measures for studying deployment-related experiences of military personnel and veterans. Mil Psychol 18:89–120, 2006

Lang AJ, Stein MB: An abbreviated PTSD checklist for use as a screening instrument in primary care. Behav Res Ther 43:585–594, 2005

Maddi SR: Relevance of hardiness assessment and training to the military context. Mil Psychol 19:61–70, 2007

Messer JM, Fremouw WJ: Detecting malingered posttraumatic stress disorder using the Morel Emotional Numbing Test–Revised (MENT-R) and the Miller Forensic Assessment of Symptoms Test (M-FAST). Journal of Forensic Psychology Practice 7:33–57, 2007

Miller HA: M-FAST: Miller Forensic Assessment of Symptoms Test. Lutz, FL, Psychological Assessment Resources, 2005

Morel KR: Development and preliminary validation of a forced-choice test of response bias for posttraumatic stress disorder. J Pers Assess 70:299–314, 1998

Morel KR, Shepherd BE: Meta-analysis of the Morel Emotional Numbing Test for PTSD: comment on Singh, Avasthi, and Grover. German Journal of Psychiatry 11:128–131, 2008

Mueser KT, Rosenberg SD, Xie H, et al: A randomized controlled trial of cognitive-behavioral treatment for posttraumatic stress disorder in severe mental illness. J Consult Clin Psychol 76:259–271, 2008

Norman SB, Stein MB, Davidson JR: Profiling posttraumatic functional impairment. J Nerv Ment Dis 195:48–53, 2007

North CS, Nixon SJ, Shariat S, et al: Psychiatric disorders among survivors of the Oklahoma City bombing. JAMA 282:755–762, 1999

Peters L, Slade T, Andrews G: A comparison of ICD10 and DSM-IV criteria for posttraumatic stress disorder. J Trauma Stress 12:335–343, 1999

Schacter DL: The seven sins of memory: insights from psychology and cognitive neuroscience. Am Psychol 54:182–203, 1999

Sheehan DV, Lecrubier Y, Sheehan KH, et al: The Mini-International Neuropsychiatric Interview (M.I.N.I.): the development and validation of a structured psychiatric interview for DSM-IV and ICD-10. J Clin Psychiatry 59:22–33, 1998

Simms LJ, Watson D, Doebbeling BN: Confirmatory factor analysis of posttraumatic stress-symptoms in deployed and non-deployed veterans of the Gulf war. J Abnorm Psychol 111:637–647, 2002

Slick DJ, Hopp G, Strauss E, et al: Manual for the Victoria Symptom Validity Test, Odessa, FL, Psychological Assessment Resources, 1997

Southwick SM, Vythilingam M, Charney DS: The psychobiology of depression and resilience to stress: implications for prevention and treatment. Annu Rev Clin Psychol 1:255–291, 2005

Stein MB, Bienvenu OJ: Diagnostic classification of anxiety disorders: DSM-V and beyond, in The Neurobiology of Mental Illness, 3rd Edition. Edited by Charney DS, Nestler EJ. New York, Oxford University Press, 2008, pp 525–534

Stein MB, McAllister TW: Exploring the convergence of posttraumatic stress disorder and mild traumatic brain injury. Am J Psychiatry 166:768–776, 2009

Sumpter RE, McMillan TM: Errors in self-report of post-traumatic stress disorder after severe traumatic brain injury. Brain Inj 20:93–99, 2006

Thombs BD, Bernstein DP, Ziegelstein RC, et al: An evaluation of screening questions for childhood abuse in 2 community samples: implications for clinical practice. Arch Intern Med 166:2020–2026, 2006

Tombaugh TN: TOMM: Test of Memory Malingering. Toronto, ON, Canada, MHS, 1996

Tuerk PW, Grubaugh AL, Hamner MB, et al: Diagnosis and treatment of PTSD-related compulsive checking behaviors in veterans of the Iraq war: the influence of military context on the expression of PTSD symptoms. Am J Psychiatry 166:762–767, 2009

Vogt DS, Proctor SP, King DW, et al: Validation of scales from the Deployment Risk and Resilience Inventory in a sample of Operation Iraqi Freedom veterans. Assessment 15:391–403, 2008

Weathers FW: Psychometric review of Clinician-Administered PTSD Scale (CAPS), in Measurement of Stress, Trauma, and Adaptation. Edited by Stamm BH. Lutherville, MD, Sidran Press, 1996

Weathers FW, Ford J: Psychometric review of PTSD Checklist (PCL-C, PCL-S, PCL-M, PCL-PR), in Measurement of Stress, Trauma, and Adaptation. Edited by Stamm BH. Lutherville, MD, Sidran Press, 1996

Weathers F, Huska J, Keane T: The PTSD Checklist Military Version (PCL-M), Boston, MA, National Center for Posttraumatic Stress Disorder, 1991

Weathers FW, Ruscio AM, Keane TM: Psychometric properties of nine scoring rules for the Clinician-Administered Posttraumatic Stress Disorder Scale. Psychol Assess 11:124–133, 1999

Weathers FW, Keane TM, Davidson JR: Clinician-Administered PTSD Scale: a review of the first ten years of research. Depress Anxiety 13:132–156, 2001

World Health Organization: International Statistical Classification of Diseases and Related Health Problems, 10th Revision. Geneva, World Health Organization, 1992

5

Psychiatric Comorbidities

Carol S. North, M.D., M.P.E.
Alina M. Suris, Ph.D., A.B.P.P.
Sunday Adewuyi, M.B.B.S.

Posttraumatic stress disorder (PTSD) is widely considered the "signature diagnosis" of trauma. Epidemiological studies have confirmed that PTSD is the most prevalent psychiatric disorder in most populations after exposure to trauma (David et al. 1996; Foa et al. 2006; Norris et al. 2002; North et al. 1994, 1999; Raja et al. 2008; Shalev et al. 1998). PTSD, however, is not the only disorder arising after trauma. Research conducted in a variety of populations and settings has shown that PTSD has an abundance of psychiatric comorbidities (Brady et al. 2000; Breslau et al. 1991; Deering et al. 1996; Keane and Kaloupek 1997; Kessler et al. 1995; Koenen et al. 2008; Kulka et al. 1990; J.C. McMillen et al. 2000). Comorbidity is said to be the rule rather than the exception for patients with PTSD (Brady et al. 2000).

The *Diagnostic and Statistical Manual of Mental Disorders*, 4th Edition, Text Revision (DSM-IV-TR; American Psychiatric Association 2000), lists several comorbid psychiatric disorders found in association with PTSD: panic disorder, agoraphobia, social or other phobias, obsessive-compulsive disorder, major depression, somatization disorder, and substance use disorders. Narrowly focused efforts to understand and recognize PTSD may divert attention from the other psychiatric disorders likely to be found in patients following exposure to trauma.

In this chapter, we explore potential mechanisms for the co-occurrence of comorbid psychiatric disorders with PTSD and review existing literature on the types of psychiatric disorders that accompany PTSD in various populations exposed to different types of trauma. After a discussion of the importance and relevance of PTSD comorbidity to clinical practice, we highlight strategies for addressing comorbidity in patients with PTSD.

Theories of Psychiatric Comorbidity With PTSD

Several potential explanations have been advanced for psychiatric comorbidity in patients with PTSD. The following discussion describes the evidence supporting the three main hypothetical causal models (or explanations) for PTSD comorbidity (Brady et al. 2000; Breslau et al. 2000; Keane and Kaloupek 1997; Stewart et al. 1998; Wittmann et al. 2008).

Explanation 1: Diagnostic Artifact

The diagnostic artifact model considers the possibility that observed associations between PTSD and other psychiatric disorders following traumatic events are a function of diagnostic imprecision and overlapping criteria (Davidson and Foa 1991; Green et al. 1985). If PTSD cannot be differentiated from its accompanying comorbidities, this represents a serious challenge to the validity and reliability of PTSD as an independent construct (Breslau and Davis 1987, 1992; Brett et al. 1988; Goldberg et al. 1990; Green et al. 1985; Keane and Wolfe 1990; North et al. 2009; Robins 1990; Solomon and Canino 1990).

A potential contributor to apparent diagnostic overlap is a known tendency for some people to indiscriminately describe many symptoms of various disorders; some individuals habitually overreport or exaggerate symptoms or express high levels of distress (Brady et al. 2000; C. McMillen et al. 2002).

These behaviors are observed in patients with somatization disorder, which by definition presents with a wide array of somatic and neuropsychological symptoms nonspecific to single disorders. Patients with somatization disorder also report many symptoms of psychiatric disorders, including posttraumatic symptoms, thus confounding differential diagnosis. Although somatization disorder is relatively uncommon in general populations, it is surprisingly prevalent in treatment settings (North 2005) and among patients seeking treatment for problems associated with a history of childhood molestation (Modestin et al. 2005; Moreau and Zisook 2002; C. Spitzer et al. 2008).

Stewart et al. (1998) considered the possibility that patients with substance use disorders may misinterpret drug and alcohol withdrawal symptoms as PTSD symptoms (e.g., anxiety and hyperarousal). Confusion between PTSD and withdrawal symptoms may further blur the distinction between PTSD and psychiatric comorbidities.

A potential source of diagnostic overlap is apparent nonspecificity inherent in certain symptoms that recur in diagnostic criteria for more than one disorder. Factor analytic studies have been applied to clarify the structure of PTSD and its naturally occurring boundaries from other disorders by documenting patterns of coherence and separation of symptoms occurring in nature. Factor analysis, however, does not confer diagnostic validity; it is simply an exercise that demonstrates cohesive symptom groups whose members tend to travel together. Factor analytic studies fail to achieve consensus on the structure of PTSD symptom groups. The recommended number of separate symptom clusters varies from two to five or more (Rosen and Lilienfeld 2008), variably arranged. Some factor analysis studies have confirmed the symptom categories as currently constructed in DSM-IV-TR (Cordova et al. 2000; Fawzi et al. 1997; Silver and Iacono 1984). Other studies have provided evidence to support breaking the avoidance/numbing category into two separate groups (Asmundson et al. 2004; McDonald et al. 2009; Palmieri et al. 2007; Sack et al. 1997; Shelby et al. 2005). Yet other studies have identified a two-factor solution regrouping the avoidance and arousal symptoms together and the numbing and intrusion symptoms together (Buckley et al. 1998; Feuer et al. 2005; Taylor et al. 1998). One study observed grouping of PTSD symptom groups with symptoms of other disorders: depressive symptoms grouped with avoidance symptoms, and anxiety symptoms grouped with arousal symptoms (Maes et al. 1998).

In factor analytic studies, as well as other research on PTSD comorbidity, methodological shortcomings undoubtedly contribute to impressions of symptom overlap of other disorders with PTSD. DSM-IV-TR criteria specify that PTSD symptoms must be temporally or contextually related to sufficient exposure to qualify for the diagnosis. Failure to address this temporal or contextual linkage in assessment of PTSD symptoms is destined to yield a nonspecific collection of symptoms that fail to coalesce into the constellations of PTSD symptoms defined by DSM-IV-TR, or even to define any coherent and meaningful syndrome (Bodkin et al. 2007; Breslau et al. 2002; Coyne and Thompson 2007; McHugh and Treisman 2007; Rosen and Taylor 2007; R.L. Spitzer et al. 2007; Yehuda and McFarlane 1995). More careful examination of PTSD symptoms in conformity with the diagnostic criteria will be needed to clarify the cohesiveness and differentiation of PTSD and its symptoms from other disorders. Adherence to specified diagnostic criteria in assessing symptoms is paramount for research into PTSD comorbidity. Not attending to this issue has resulted in inadequate research and limited progress in understanding the potential contribution of symptom overlap in existing criteria to comorbidity in PTSD.

Explanation 2: PTSD Leads to Other Disorders

According to a second theory regarding comorbidity, other disorders arising in the posttrauma setting are considered secondary to PTSD, occurring as a consequence of PTSD rather than independently resulting from the traumatic exposure itself. This model would be best supported if development of other disorders was restricted to exposed individuals with PTSD and did not occur in exposed individuals without PTSD. A finding of frequent occurrence of other disorders in people without PTSD, however, would argue against this causal model.

In a study of 801 community mothers, Breslau et al. (1997) found that trauma exposure not followed by the development of PTSD did not confer risk for first-onset major depression. In that study, risk for major depression was largely confined to those who developed PTSD after exposure, thus representing a diagnosis comorbid with PTSD rather than an independent entity and consistent with the model in which PTSD leads to other disorders. Even though major depression following traumatic exposure is most likely to occur in people who develop PTSD, research has demonstrated that some people do develop major depression in the absence of PTSD, and therefore psychiatric evaluation should not end with assessment of PTSD (Nemeroff et al. 2006; North 2004; North et al. 1999).

In the aftermath of trauma, substance use disorders in particular are assumed to start as a part of escalation of use of a substance initiated for the purpose of relieving unpleasant posttraumatic symptoms. This is the basis of a widely held "self-medication" hypothesis of substance abuse following trauma exposure (Brady et al. 2000; Breslau et al. 2003; Brown and Wolfe 1994; Chilcoat and Breslau 1998a, 1998b; Jacobsen et al. 2001; Khantzian 1985, 1997; Stewart 1996). If substance use disorders arise in this way, then first onset of substance use disorders should regularly occur after traumatic exposures only in highly traumatized individuals with PTSD.

A general population study (Breslau et al. 2003; Chilcoat and Breslau 1998a, 1998b) found that risk for development of drug use disorders following trauma occurred primarily among those with PTSD, whereas trauma exposure without subsequent PTSD did not increase the risk of developing a drug use disorder. The findings were different for alcohol, however; neither exposure to trauma nor development of PTSD was associated with development of alcohol use disorders (Breslau et al. 2003). Using lifetime retrospective data, survival analysis models demonstrated time-dependent cumulative incidence of PTSD and drug use disorders relative to one another, suggesting that PTSD likely led to drug use disorders rather than vice versa (Chilcoat and Breslau 1998a, 1998b). The authors concluded that their findings do not establish causality and do not clarify whether the association between PTSD and development of drug use disorders represents self-medication of posttraumatic symptoms or shared susceptibilities to psychopathology.

This work leaves several issues unresolved. First, the survival analysis did not examine temporal proximity of onset of substance abuse within individuals after exposure to trauma (Chilcoat and Breslau. 1998a). A temporal link between the onsets of substance abuse and PTSD would be important for a causal explanation. Second, the lack of association between the onset of an alcohol use disorder and PTSD (Breslau et al. 2003) is not consistent with a unified self-medication hypothesis frequently invoked to explain the development of a substance use disorder in the wake of trauma. Third, the association of drug use disorders with PTSD was confined only to prescription psychoactive medications and did not include common illicit substances of abuse, such as cocaine and marijuana (Chilcoat and Breslau 1998b). This finding would suggest that the development of drug abuse in association with PTSD may be largely confined to complications arising from potentially abusable psychotropic medications prescribed for PTSD rather than representing a consequence of PTSD itself. In a study by Bremner et al. (1996), Vietnam veterans with PTSD reported that alcohol, marijuana, heroin, and benzodiazepines improved their PTSD symptoms, whereas cocaine worsened hyperarousal symptoms. The latter finding would also seem inconsistent with a self-medication hypothesis for cocaine abuse in association with PTSD. Among those with PTSD, 34% had comorbid cocaine dependence and 6% had cocaine abuse. The PTSD comorbidity rates were similar for sedative dependence and abuse (32% and 9%, respectively) and opiate dependence and abuse (26% and 2%, respectively).

Others have entertained the possibility of a reverse causal directionality, specifically that substance use disorders might heighten vulnerability for PTSD after exposure to trauma (Deering et al. 1996; Stewart et al. 1998). One retrospective study of Vietnam veterans found that alcohol use disorders preceded PTSD by more than 3 years (Davidson et al. 1990).

Efforts to understand the associations of alcohol and other drugs with trauma have been further confused by research inconsistencies; some studies have examined substance *use* and others have examined substance abuse/dependence *disorders*. Substance *use* and substance use *disorders* may have quite different associations with trauma or PTSD and will likely yield different sets of consequences, dictating different treatment needs. For example, although a small but statistically significant increase in the use of substances was documented in the population of Manhattan after the 9/11 terrorist attacks (Vlahov et al. 2002), disaster research has demonstrated that even with an increase in substance use after disaster, this increase does not translate into new substance use *disorders* with any regularity (David et al. 1996; North et al. 2004). Cottler et al. (1992) found that the onset of substance *use* in a general population sample was more likely to precede PTSD than to follow it, contrary to others' findings that drug use *disorders* follow rather than precede PTSD (Breslau et al. 2003; Chilcoat and Breslau 1998a, 1998b).

Finally, if substance use disorders arise as part of a posttraumatic self-medication process, such disorders should arise in association with all types of trauma exposure. However, research on disaster survivors has consistently failed to demonstrate a postdisaster increase in the development of substance use disorders (David et al. 1996; North et al. 1994, 1999, 2002a, 2004, 2008a).

Taken together, the nonassociations of alcohol and recreational drug use disorders with PTSD and trauma in general populations, the nonoccurrence of new substance use disorders after disasters, and the lack of data on the temporal association of development of PTSD and substance use disorders fail to support the self-medication hypothesis of origins of substance use disorders following trauma. One underexplored area within this topic is the likelihood for relapse of existing substance use disorders following trauma.

Explanation 3: Trauma Leads to Multiple Disorders (Shared Vulnerability)

In the shared vulnerability model, exposure to trauma leads not only to PTSD but also to other disorders. This model suggests two possible mechanisms: 1) trauma produces broad psychopathological effects, as evidenced by multiple disorders arising independently in the wake of trauma, and 2) several disorders result from trauma through shared vulnerabilities within individuals prone to psychopathology, as evidenced by a tendency for development of more than one disorder among those who become ill. Disorders with shared vulnerabilities should cluster within individuals; however, if different disorders arise independently from trauma, the pattern of occurrence in the population should be more randomly distributed. Breslau et al. (2000) offered the observation that because only a minority of people exposed to traumatic events develop psychiatric illness afterward, personal vulnerability must play a critical role in determining the likelihood of psychopathology following exposure to trauma.

An obvious candidate for a shared vulnerability factor is preexisting psychopathology. A study by Breslau et al. (2000) of a community sample of 1,007 young adults from a health maintenance organization explored lifetime relationships among preexisting major depression and development of PTSD and major depression after trauma exposure. In this study, history of a depressive disorder at some time before exposure to a traumatic event was associated with a more than threefold risk for PTSD after the traumatic event. Among individuals with no history of major depression prior to traumatic exposure, development of PTSD afterward was also strongly associated with the development of a first major depressive episode. Additionally, people exposed to trauma who did not develop PTSD experienced little more major depression afterward than did unexposed individuals. These findings are consistent with the model of preexisting personal vulnerability to a variety of psychopathology in the wake of trauma rather than a vulnerability to a specific disorder. Numerous studies of disaster survivors have found that preexisting psychopathology strongly predicts PTSD and other psychiatric sequelae of the disaster, and that other postdisaster psychopathology in the absence of PTSD is uncommon (Bromet et al. 1982; Gabriel et al. 2007; J.C. McMillen et al. 2000; Norris et al. 2002; North et al. 1994, 1999, 2004, 2008a; Phifer 1990; Smith et al. 1990).

A complication to these considerations is that exposure to trauma is not as arbitrary as commonly assumed, stated perhaps most succinctly by Breslau et al. (2002, p. 926): "Traumatic events are not random." Trauma exposure is more likely for some groups than others, with multiple occurrences tending to cluster in some individuals (Breslau et al. 1995). Epidemiological research has demonstrated several individual risk factors for trauma exposure: low socioeconomic status, ethnic minority group membership, illicit drug use, personal psychiatric history (childhood conduct problems, substance use disorders, and other major psychiatric illness), family history (substance abuse, antisocial behaviors, and other psychopathology), and personality traits (Brady et al. 2000; Breslau 2002; Breslau et al. 1991, 1995; Cottler et al. 1992; Helzer et al. 1987; McFarlane 1998; Norris 1992; Perkonigg et al. 2000).

Risk for exposure to trauma can therefore be considered a preexisting shared vulnerability factor, given the diagnostic requirement of a traumatic exposure. For example, if alcoholism puts people at risk for having accidents, then selecting a sample from emergency department patients undergoing treatment for accidental injuries will yield a group that is unrepresentative of other populations in terms of the prevalence of alcohol use disorders. Recognition of selection bias in traumatized samples is critical to interpretation of research findings given that these intertwined relationships with preexisting risk factors indelibly confound the occurrence of trauma and its relationship with psychopathology (PTSD and comorbid psychiatric disorders) in most trauma-exposed populations. To the degree that preexisting psychopathology, which confers risk for trauma exposure, increases likelihood of PTSD afterward, it also increases likelihood of other disorders afterward, and comorbidity is to be expected.

In contrast, disasters generally appear to be more "equal-opportunity" events than other kinds of traumatic events more typically associated with individual preexisting selection factors (North 1995, 2007; North et al. 1999), as discussed above. Not all disasters, however, share this characteristic. For example, Midwestern floods and Hurricane Katrina have been found to preferentially expose people with predisaster vulnerability factors (e.g., preexisting alcoholism among flood victims who inhabit flood-prone land because it is affordable, and chronic and persistent psychiatric and medical disabilities among people without resources to evacuate before Hurricane Katrina) (North et al. 2004, 2008b). Aside from these exceptions, other large-scale disasters provide opportunities to examine PTSD comorbidities without the usual confounding of risk factors for trauma and psychopathology afterward. Co-occurrence of disorders within the same disaster-exposed individuals may be expected to occur without confounding effects of elevated rates of preexisting psychopathology.

Summary of Comorbidity Models

These three potential models have been proposed to account for psychiatric comorbidity with PTSD. Evidence to date suggests that psychiatric comorbidity with PTSD cannot simply be dismissed as an artifact of overlapping diagnostic criteria. Much of the work providing the evidence lacks the methodological precision to ensure that PTSD symptoms are specifically associated with the traumatic event, either temporally or in content, as required by DSM-IV-TR. Unless symptom data are collected in conformity with the accepted definition of the disorder, apparent overlap between PTSD and other symptoms may reflect only measurement imprecision and cannot be considered evidence in support of the first model. Regarding the two models involving PTSD causation and shared vulnerability, research has demonstrated that other psychiatric disorders appear to cluster with PTSD within individuals, but available data do not clarify whether this pattern represents shared vulnerability or a causal pathway from PTSD to other disorders. Confounding of outcomes with risk for trauma exposure further impedes untangling of these relationships. It remains to be seen, therefore, how future methodologically adequate research will demonstrate the comorbidity with PTSD to be ultimately explained by any, or a synthesis, of these proposed explanatory models.

Psychiatric Comorbidities in Different PTSD Populations: Review of the Research Literature

An extensive array of trauma research conducted in a variety of populations and settings has consistently demonstrated remarkably high PTSD comorbidity rates. Psychiatric comorbidity has been measured in excess of 80% in studies of combat veterans with PTSD (Deering et al. 1996; Keane and Wolfe 1990; Kulka et al. 1990; Orsillo et al. 1996; Sierles et al. 1986), in 60%–80% of disaster survivors with PTSD (McFarlane and Papay 1992; J.C. McMillen et al. 2000; North et al. 1999), and in 70%–90% of individuals with PTSD in general population studies (Breslau 2001a, 2001b; Kessler et al. 1995; Perkonigg et al. 2000). Although a high prevalence of psychiatric comorbidity appears to be a constant of PTSD regardless of the setting or the population examined, the specific types and relative prevalence of various psychiatric disorders comorbid with PTSD may differ from population to population and by trauma type (Deering et al. 1996; Keane and Kaloupek 1997).

Specific characteristics of PTSD as a psychiatric disorder complicate the understanding not only of the disorder itself but also of comorbidities. The diagnosis of PTSD, unlike most other psychiatric disorders in DSM-IV-TR, is defined in relation to a potential etiological factor—namely, a traumatic event. Most major diagnoses in DSM-IV-TR, such as schizophrenia, bipolar disorder, major depression, and panic disorder, are based on descriptions of symptom clusters and clinical characteristics, with an agnostic stance toward etiology. The more straightforward definitions of these other descriptive finding–based diagnoses promote relatively uncomplicated relationships between disorders and characteristic features.

Because the diagnosis of PTSD as currently defined hinges first on the occurrence of an external event and second on the constellation of symptoms that follow, associations with the defining traumatic event must be entered into any equations predicting the occurrence of PTSD linked to that event (North et al. 2009). Comorbidities in PTSD must be considered within the context of the defining traumatic exposure of PTSD, which—as noted above—differs among populations and trauma types. In the following sections, we consider PTSD comorbidities separately by trauma groups. For reference in reviewing this material, Table 5–1 provides a concise summary of comorbidities most likely to be found in association with PTSD in different populations and general implications of the comorbid disorders for the course and management of the PTSD.

Combat Veterans

Most PTSD comorbidity data come from studies of combat veterans (Deering et al. 1996). In a comprehensive review of the PTSD comorbidity literature,

Deering et al. (1996) observed that comorbidity appears to be more prevalent in combat-related PTSD than in PTSD from noncombat sources. They also noted that specific comorbid disorders occurred with different relative frequencies in combat-related PTSD and in PTSD from other sources of trauma. In particular, the authors pointed out that combat veterans with PTSD appeared to have much higher rates of comorbid substance use disorders than did people with PTSD from other sources of trauma. Deering et al. attributed the high prevalence of PTSD comorbidity in combat veterans to possible cultural factors, chronicity of PTSD, preexisting substance abuse, type of trauma, intensity and duration of trauma exposure, demographics (e.g., gender, age), treatment received, and methodological differences in research.

A review of psychiatric comorbidity with combat-related PTSD by Keane and Kaloupek (1997), however, concluded that psychiatric comorbidity is extensive among Vietnam veterans regardless of whether they were selected for study from treatment or community settings. The psychiatric disorders most often found to be comorbid with PTSD in combat veterans are alcohol use disorders, followed by major depression, other drug abuse, and Cluster B (especially antisocial, but also borderline) personality disorders (Bremner et al. 1996; Deering et al. 1996; Keane and Kaloupek 1997).

Comparing rates of disorders in combat veterans with those in other populations is difficult for several reasons. First, instead of performing full diagnostic assessment, many studies have substituted screening measures not designed to assess established diagnostic criteria. Second, time frames have been inconsistent for diagnoses reported (e.g., current prevalence such as last month or last year, lifetime cumulative prevalence, incidence for new cases only). Third, research has often relied on nonrepresentative samples (especially treatment samples). For example, only 2 of the 19 combat veteran studies included in Deering et al.'s (1996) review of PTSD comorbidity selected veterans from sources outside of psychiatric treatment settings, precluding comparability to other groups. Fourth, combat PTSD is often studied retrospectively over years to decades; PTSD from other sources, such as motor vehicle accidents and disasters, is generally studied in closer temporality with the event (Deering et al. 1996).

Table 5–1. Expected psychiatric comorbidities with PTSD in different traumatized populations

Comorbid disorder	Select populations	General implications for prognosis and treatment
Major depression	General/all; women	More severe PTSD Treatments overlap
Other anxiety disorders	General/all; women	More severe PTSD Treatments overlap
Substance use disorders	General/all; accident and assault survivors; men; disadvantaged populations (disorder is preexisting)	Most are overlooked
Alcohol	Combat veterans; rescue workers; accident and assault survivors; disadvantaged populations; men (disorder is generally preexisting)	Contributes to severity and chronicity of anxiety and depression
Other drugs	Combat veterans; accident and assault survivors; disadvantaged populations; men (disorder is generally preexisting)	Contributes to severity and chronicity of anxiety and depression
Personality disorders (Cluster B)	Varies by type of personality disorder (disorder is preexisting)	Anticipate more difficult treatment
Antisocial	Combat veterans; accident and assault survivors; men (disorder is preexisting)	May be associated with malingering
Conduct disorder	Childhood abuse survivors; men (disorder is preexisting)	Childhood precursor to antisocial personality
Borderline	Patient populations; childhood abuse survivors (disorder is preexisting)	Anticipate a severe, complicated course

Table 5–1. Expected psychiatric comorbidities with PTSD in different traumatized populations *(continued)*

Comorbid disorder	Select populations	General implications for prognosis and treatment
Somatization disorder	Patient populations; childhood abuse survivors; women (disorder is preexisting)	Not the same as malingering Psychiatric symptoms are often part of somatization disorder Anticipate a severe, complicated course
Somatoform symptoms or disorders	Patient populations; childhood abuse survivors; women (disorder is usually preexisting)	Not the same as malingering
Psychosis (e.g., schizophrenia)	Patient populations; populations selected for socioeconomic disadvantage and chronic illness (disorder is preexisting)	Need to stabilize psychosis to enable effective PTSD treatment
Bipolar disorder	Patient populations; populations selected for socioeconomic disadvantage and chronic illness (disorder is preexisting)	Need to stabilize mood disorder to enable effective PTSD treatment

Survivors of Community Accidents, Assaults, and Childhood Abuse

Because the groups are subject to similar, and substantial, selection bias, survivors of community accidents, assaults, and childhood abuse are combined into one section in this chapter. Although some children may be victims of random child abuse (e.g., a child abducted by a sexual predator), many abused children have chaotic, multiproblem families whose members abuse them or subject them to adverse circumstances through neglect or inability to protect them from exposure to dangerous environments (e.g., drug-addicted parents who fail to monitor their children's safety). Associations of these risk factors with child abuse can be expected to yield psychopathology that may be confounded with the effects of the abuse. Because children at risk for abuse on average have dysfunctional family backgrounds with excessive substance abuse, sociopathy, and economic disadvantage (Annerback et al. 2007; Sartor et al. 2008; Sunday et al. 2008; Turner et al. 2007), they can be expected to have an increased likelihood of substance abuse, personality disorders, and economic disadvantage later in their lives, emerging from other elements of their backgrounds, even if they have not been abused.

Authors of studies of individuals abused as children have predictably recorded high rates of substance abuse, delinquency and other conduct problems, borderline personality disorder, and somatoform disorders (De Bellis 2002; Nurcombe 2000). Although one may be tempted to attribute all of these later disorders to the earlier abuse, many of them may represent associations arising from the individuals' original risk factors for child abuse. Nonetheless, PTSD in this population is associated with these comorbidities, which may require different intervention plans than for PTSD in other populations.

The situation is somewhat similar for populations selected for having survived community accidents and assaults. Even though some accidents and assaults may be essentially random occurrences, exposure to accidents and assaults is generally associated with predisposing factors, such as substance abuse, sociopathy, serious mental illness, and economic disadvantage (Dumais et al. 2005). Findings from research on motor vehicle accident victims with PTSD have identified Cluster B personality and substance use disorder comorbidities (Bryant and Harvey 1995; Dumais et al. 2005; Levy et al. 1996). Thus, populations selected for having survived community accidents and assaults can be expected to have distinct preexisting characteristics even before the traumatic event.

Disaster Survivors

As discussed in the earlier section on the shared vulnerability hypothesis, most disasters are relatively nonselective regarding preexisting characteristics of individuals in affected populations. Therefore, one would expect psychiatric comorbidity to reflect less influence from preexisting characteristics in this population. In contrast with comorbidities most typical among veteran populations, the most prevalent comorbidity among disaster survivors is major depression, and substance use disorders are less common (David et al. 1996; Deering et al. 1996; Norris et al. 2002; North 2007; North et al. 1994, 1999; Smith et al. 1990). Alcohol and drug use disorders identified after disasters are almost always preexisting, and the onset of new substance use disorders in the first few months and years after disasters is infrequently observed (David et al. 1996; Norris et al. 2002; North 2007; North et al. 1994, 1999; Smith et al. 1990). Comorbidity with PTSD confers greater severity of illness and effects on the individual's life. Among Oklahoma City bombing survivors, PTSD was found to be associated with difficulties functioning, but psychiatric comorbidities with PTSD after the bombing were associated with even more problems with functioning (North et al. 1999).

Rescue workers responding to disasters represent a special subgroup of disaster-exposed populations. Depending on the timing of their response, they may be directly exposed to the danger or they may be exposed only to the aftermath of a disaster. Few studies of disaster responders have assessed alcohol use disorders, and even fewer have examined predisaster alcohol history.

A systematic study assessing Oklahoma City firefighter responders with structured diagnostic interviews found that the most prevalent diagnosis was not PTSD (13%) but rather alcohol use disorder (24%), and the prevalence of psychiatric comorbidity with PTSD was 54%. In this study, the most common comorbidity with PTSD was alcohol use disorder (North et al. 2002a). Virtually all the firefighters with an alcohol use disorder diagnosis after the bombing had a predisaster history of the disorder, and in fact 47% of the firefighters met lifetime criteria for alcohol abuse or dependence. Curiously, the proportion of firefighters who said they coped by drinking alcohol was not significantly higher (19%) than among directly exposed survivors (16%), who had only a 9% postdisaster prevalence of alcohol use disorder (North et al. 1999, 2002b). Use of alcohol to cope after the bombing was four times as common among firefighters with alcohol use disorders as among those without, and the majority of firefighters with an alcohol use disorder denied that they consumed alcohol as a means of coping with the disaster. These findings suggest that the use of alcohol by these firefighters may have represented rationalization of drinking inherent in the disease of alcoholism more than self-medication of their distress.

Other studies of firefighters not selected for disaster exposure have described similarly high prevalence rates for current alcohol (29%) and substance use (19%) disorders (Boxer and Wild 1993; Wagner et al. 1998). The combined evidence from these studies suggests that alcoholism among firefighters responding to the Oklahoma City bombing may represent a longstanding characteristic of this group rather than a reaction to having participated in a particular disaster response.

General Populations

Research on trauma in general populations involves a mix of subpopulations by trauma type. The most common lifetime traumatic events observed in population studies are accidental injuries (especially motor vehicle accidents), assaults (especially robbery but also sexual and other physical assaults), witnessing others being severely injured or killed, and receiving news of a tragic death or severe injury of a loved one (Breslau et al. 1995, 1998; Norris 1992; Resnick et al. 1993). Lifetime psychiatric comorbidities with lifetime diagnoses of PTSD recorded in these studies are 73% and 79% among women and 88% among men (Breslau et al. 1997; Kessler et al. 1995).

In the National Comorbidity Survey, the most commonly observed lifetime disorders comorbid with a lifetime history of PTSD were major depression, substance use disorders, conduct disorder, and anxiety disorders. Specifically, prevalence rates among men for comorbid disorders were as follows: major depression, 48%; alcohol use disorder, 52%; drug use disorder, 31%; conduct disorder, 43%; and other anxiety disorders, ranging from 7% to 29%. Among women, prevalence rates were as follows: major depression, 49%; alcohol use disorder, 28%; drug use disorder, 27%; conduct disorder, 15%; and other anxiety disorders, ranging from 13% to 29% (Kessler et al. 1995). All these disorders were significantly more prevalent among those with than without a lifetime diagnosis of PTSD (odds ratios mostly ranging between 3 and 6). Therefore, in general populations, the most prevalent comorbidity with PTSD is major depression, followed by substance use disorders (particularly in men).

Specific Comorbidities and Population Characteristics

Specific populations may be expected to show PTSD comorbidities related to characteristics inherent in the population, and specific comorbidities may be found in different trauma-exposed populations. In the general population, women have higher rates of depressive, anxiety (including PTSD), and somatoform disorders than men, and men have higher rates of sociopathy and substance use disorders than women. Therefore, estimates of psychopathology in populations such as military veterans (predominantly male) should consider these gender differences in interpreting rates of specific gender-related psychiatric disorders in comparison with other populations. Samples selected from treatment settings can be expected to have elevated rates of psychopathology, and thus PTSD comorbidities in populations identified from nontreatment settings can be expected to be influenced by this selection bias.

Although the collective findings of studies reviewed in this chapter abundantly demonstrate that comorbidity is to be expected with PTSD, the associated comorbidities are typically confined to certain psychiatric disorders—as noted above, most commonly major depression, substance use disorders, anxiety disorders, and personality disorders. It should be noted that schizophrenia and bipolar disorder are not among the psychiatric disorders reported to begin in the aftermath of trauma. Although psychotic symptoms have been described in association with PTSD, they are largely considered artifacts of problems in research methodology or misinterpretation of PTSD symptoms (Deering et al. 1996; Escobar et al. 1983; Keane and Kaloupek 1997).

Somatoform symptoms have been reported to accompany PTSD among trauma survivors (Andreski et al. 1998; Breslau 2001b; Foa et al. 2006; Ford et al. 2001; McFarlane et al. 1994; Moreau and Zisook 2002; Shalev et al. 1990). Significant associations between PTSD and somatoform disorders have been identified in patient populations (Breslau 2001b; Escalona et al. 2004) and among survivors of childhood abuse (Modestin et al. 2005; Moreau and Zisook 2002; C. Spitzer et al. 2008). In a study of flood survivors, however, examination of the timing of onset of somatoform symptoms revealed that the large majority of these symptoms were preexisting (North et al. 2004). Research has consistently demonstrated that somatization disorder does not newly arise following exposure to disasters (North 2002; North et al. 1994, 1999, 2004; Raja et al. 2008). Somatization disorder is a condition largely or completely confined to women and typically begins in the decade following puberty and by definition cannot begin after age 30. These characteristics of somatization disorder are inconsistent with its occurrence in male combat veterans or onset following trauma in adults, and therefore one would not anticipate new onset of somatization disorder after trauma in these populations.

Despite recognized associations between personality disorders and trauma, personality disorders have received relatively little attention in relation to PTSD (Deering et al. 1996). The personality disorder most commonly reported among combat veterans with PTSD is antisocial personality disorder (Deering et al. 1996; Keane and Kaloupek 1997; Keane and Wolfe 1990; Sierles et al. 1986), though there is evidence for other personality disorders as well (Sunday et al. 2008). Part of the reason for the prevalence of antisocial personality in military veterans may be the predominantly male population of the armed forces. By definition, antisocial personality disorder begins before age 15, and thus the origins of the disorder precede military service. A large study of Vietnam veterans from a military registry (Fontana and Rosenheck 2005) concluded that the major determinant of postmilitary antisocial behavior is premilitary experience rather than traumatic war zone exposure.

Studies of civilians in treatment for PTSD have focused on associations with borderline personality disorder (Golier et al. 2003; Gunderson and Sabo 1993; McLean and Gallop 2003; Yen et al. 2002). Although PTSD is commonly identified in patients with borderline personality disorder (as high as 50% of the time) (Golier et al. 2003; Moreau and Zisook 2002), borderline personality disorder is not often observed in traumatized populations selected for having PTSD in the absence of preexisting risk factors for borderline personality disorder.

Clinical Implications of Psychiatric Comorbidity With PTSD

The remarkable comorbidity of other psychiatric disorders with PTSD detailed throughout this chapter has enormous implications for both practice and research. Clinicians and researchers alike must consider the likelihood of psychiatric comorbidity with PTSD in traumatized populations, as well as the types of psychiatric disorders most likely to be encountered in different groups with different exposures, to fully understand each individual case of PTSD. The clinical significance of psychiatric comorbidity with PTSD is that the accompanying disorders may be as important as PTSD for determining prognosis and treatment (Brady et al. 2000; Koenen et al. 2008). Considerable evidence demonstrates diagnostic comorbidity with PTSD to be a severity marker for illness and disability (Brady et al. 2000; Breslau 2001b; Deering et al. 1996; North 2007; North et al. 1999). Because PTSD is unlikely to be the only psychiatric disorder in trauma settings, clinicians must not stop with assessment of PTSD. When comorbid psychiatric disorders are identified, clinicians can anticipate the PTSD to be typically more severe, chronic, and resistant to treatment (Brady et al. 2000; Breslau 2001b; Breslau et al. 1991; Moreau and Zisook 2002).

Specific comorbid disorders, demonstrated in this chapter as differing by trauma type and selection source, must be considered in developing treatment plans. Treatment of combat veterans may require special attention to substance use disorders, whereas women hospitalized for PTSD related to childhood abuse need additional consideration of somatoform and borderline personality disorders. All traumatized populations, regardless of the source of the trauma, are likely to have comorbid depressive and anxiety disorders in association with PTSD. These comorbidities are a vital consideration to ensure effective treatment planning for all individuals with PTSD (Brady 1977; North 2007; Schafer and Najavits 2007; Stewart et al. 1998; Vieweg et al. 2006).

Key Clinical Points

- A comorbidity should be considered the rule rather than the exception for PTSD. Comorbidities have been reported at rates in excess of 80%.
- Combat-associated trauma appears to be associated with greater prevalence of alcohol abuse/dependence in PTSD compared with other trauma types.
- Understanding an individual's comorbid disorders in conjunction with PTSD will aid in effective treatment planning and implementation.

- For disaster survivors, major depressive disorder is usually the most prevalent comorbidity with PTSD; substance use disorders are usually less common.
- Substance use disorder accompanying PTSD among disaster survivors usually began before the disaster rather than representing new substance abuse problems after the disaster.
- The most common comorbid disorders with PTSD in the general population are major depression, substance use disorders, conduct disorder, and anxiety disorders.
- Men diagnosed with PTSD have higher rates of comorbid substance use compared with women.
- Somatoform disorder is predominantly a preexisting comorbidity and is almost exclusively found in women.
- Evidence indicates that when additional psychiatric disorders accompany PTSD, the PTSD will be more severe and disabling than PTSD without diagnostic comorbidity.

References

American Psychiatric Association: Diagnostic and Statistical Manual of Mental Disorders, 4th Edition, Text Revision. Washington, DC, American Psychiatric Association, 2000

Andreski P, Chilcoat H, Breslau N: Post-traumatic stress disorder and somatization symptoms: a prospective study. Psychiatry Res 79:131–138, 1998

Annerback EM, Lindell C, Svedin CG, et al: Severe child abuse: a study of cases reported to the police. Acta Paediatr 96:1760–1764, 2007

Asmundson GJ, Stapleton JA, Taylor S: Are avoidance and numbing distinct PTSD symptom clusters? J Trauma Stress 17:467–475, 2004

Bodkin JA, Pope HG, Detke MJ, et al: Is PTSD caused by traumatic stress? J Anxiety Disord 21:176–182, 2007

Boxer PA, Wild D: Psychological distress and alcohol use among fire fighters. Scand J Work Environ Health 19:121–125, 1993

Brady KT: Posttraumatic stress disorder and comorbidity: recognizing the many faces of PTSD. J Clin Psychiatry 58 (suppl 9):12–15, 1997

Brady KT, Killeen TK, Brewerton T, et al: Comorbidity of psychiatric disorders and posttraumatic stress disorder. J Clin Psychiatry 61 (suppl 7):22–32, 2000

Bremner JD, Southwick SM, Darnell A, et al: Chronic PTSD in Vietnam combat veterans: course of illness and substance abuse. Am J Psychiatry 153:369–375, 1996

Breslau N: The epidemiology of posttraumatic stress disorder: what is the extent of the problem? J Clin Psychiatry 62:16–22, 2001a

Breslau N: Outcomes of posttraumatic stress disorder. J Clin Psychiatry 62 (suppl 17):55–59, 2001b

Breslau N: Epidemiologic studies of trauma, posttraumatic stress disorder, and other psychiatric disorders. Can J Psychiatry 47:923–929, 2002

Breslau N, Davis GC: Posttraumatic stress disorder: the etiologic specificity of wartime stressors. Am J Psychiatry 144:578–583, 1987

Breslau N, Davis GC: Posttraumatic stress disorder in an urban population of young adults: risk factors for chronicity. Am J Psychiatry 149:671–675, 1992

Breslau N, Davis GC, Andreski P, et al: Traumatic events and posttraumatic stress disorder in an urban population of young adults. Arch Gen Psychiatry 48:216–222, 1991

Breslau N, Davis GC, Andreski P: Risk factors for PTSD-related traumatic events: a prospective analysis. Am J Psychiatry 152:529–535, 1995

Breslau N, Davis GC, Peterson EL, et al: Psychiatric sequelae of posttraumatic stress disorder in women. Arch Gen Psychiatry 54:81–87, 1997

Breslau N, Kessler RC, Chilcoat HD, et al: Trauma and posttraumatic stress disorder in the community: the 1996 Detroit area survey of trauma. Arch Gen Psychiatry 55:626–632, 1998

Breslau N, Davis GC, Peterson EL, et al: A second look at comorbidity in victims of trauma: the posttraumatic stress disorder-major depression connection. Biol Psychiatry 48:902–909, 2000

Breslau N, Chase GA, Anthony JC: The uniqueness of the DSM definition of post-traumatic stress disorder: implications for research. Psychol Med 32:573–576, 2002

Breslau N, Davis GC, Schultz LR: Posttraumatic stress disorder and the incidence of nicotine, alcohol, and other drug disorders in persons who have experienced trauma. Arch Gen Psychiatry 60:289–294, 2003

Brett EA, Spitzer RL, Williams JB: DSM-III-R criteria for posttraumatic stress disorder. Am J Psychiatry 145:1232–1236, 1988

Bromet EJ, Parkinson DK, Schulberg HC: Mental health of residents near the Three Mile Island reactor: a comparative study of selected groups. J Prev Psychiatry 1:225–276, 1982

Brown PJ, Wolfe J: Substance abuse and post-traumatic stress disorder comorbidity. Drug Alcohol Depend 35:51–59, 1994

Bryant RA, Harvey AG: Psychological impairment following motor vehicle accidents. Aust J Public Health 19:185–188, 1995

Buckley TC, Blanchard EB, Hickling EJ: A confirmatory factor analysis of posttraumatic stress symptoms. Behav Res Ther 36:1091–1099, 1998

Chilcoat HD, Breslau N: Investigations of causal pathways between PTSD and drug use disorders. Addict Behav 23:827–840, 1998a

Chilcoat HD, Breslau N: Posttraumatic stress disorder and drug disorders: testing causal pathways. Arch Gen Psychiatry 55:913–917, 1998b

Cordova MJ, Studts JL, Hann DM, et al: Symptom structure of PTSD following breast cancer. J Trauma Stress 13:301–319, 2000

Cottler LB, Compton WM, Mager D, et al: Posttraumatic stress disorder among substance users from the general population. Am J Psychiatry 149:664–670, 1992

Coyne JC, Thompson R: Posttraumatic stress syndromes: useful or negative heuristics? J Anxiety Disord 21:223–229, 2007

David D, Mellman TA, Mendoza LM, et al: Psychiatric morbidity following Hurricane Andrew. J Trauma Stress 9:607–612, 1996

Davidson JR, Foa EB: Diagnostic issues in posttraumatic stress disorder: considerations for the DSM-IV. J Abnorm Psychol 100:346–355, 1991

Davidson JR, Kudler HS, Saunders WB, et al: Symptom and comorbidity patterns in World War II and Vietnam veterans with posttraumatic stress disorder. Compr Psychiatry 31:162–170, 1990

De Bellis MD: Developmental traumatology: a contributory mechanism for alcohol and substance use disorders. Psychoneuroendocrinology 27:155–170, 2002

Deering GG, Glover SG, Ready D, et al: Unique patterns of comorbidity in posttraumatic stress disorder from different sources of trauma. Compr Psychiatry 37:336–346, 1996

Dumais A, Lesage AD, Boyer R, et al: Psychiatric risk factors for motor vehicle fatalities in young men. Can J Psychiatry 50:838–844, 2005

Escalona R, Achilles G, Waitzkin H, et al: PTSD and somatization in women treated at a VA primary care clinic. Psychosomatics 45:291–296, 2004

Escobar JI, Randolph ET, Puente G, et al: Post-traumatic stress disorder in Hispanic Vietnam veterans. Clinical phenomenology and sociocultural characteristics. J Nerv Ment Dis 171:585–596, 1983

Fawzi MC, Pham T, Lin L, et al: The validity of posttraumatic stress disorder among Vietnamese refugees. J Trauma Stress 10:101–108, 1997

Feuer CA, Nishith P, Resick P: Prediction of numbing and effortful avoidance in female rape survivors with chronic PTSD. J Trauma Stress 18:165–170, 2005

Foa EB, Stein DJ, McFarlane AC: Symptomatology and psychopathology of mental health problems after disaster. J Clin Psychiatry 67 (suppl 2):15–25, 2006

Fontana A, Rosenheck R: The role of war-zone trauma and PTSD in the etiology of antisocial behavior. J Nerv Ment Dis 193:203–209, 2005

Ford JD, Campbell KA, Storzbach D, et al: Posttraumatic stress symptomatology is associated with unexplained illness attributed to Persian Gulf War military service. Psychosom Med 63:842–849, 2001

Gabriel R, Ferrando L, Corton ES, et al: Psychopathological consequences after a terrorist attack: an epidemiological study among victims, the general population, and police officers. Eur Psychiatry 22:339–346, 2007

Goldberg J, True WR, Eisen SA, et al: A twin study of the effects of the Vietnam War on posttraumatic stress disorder. JAMA 263:1227–1232, 1990

Golier JA, Yehuda R, Bierer LM, et al: The relationship of borderline personality disorder to posttraumatic stress disorder and traumatic events. Am J Psychiatry 160:2018–2024, 2003

Green BL, Lindy JD, Grace MC: Posttraumatic stress disorder: toward DSM-IV. J Nerv Ment Dis 173:406–411, 1985

Gunderson JG, Sabo AN: The phenomenological and conceptual interface between borderline personality disorder and PTSD. Am J Psychiatry 150:19–27, 1993

Helzer JE, Robins LN, McEvoy L: Post-traumatic stress disorder in the general population. Findings of the Epidemiologic Catchment Area survey. N Engl J Med 317:1630–1634, 1987

Jacobsen LK, Southwick SM, Kosten TR: Substance use disorders in patients with posttraumatic stress disorder: a review of the literature. Am J Psychiatry 158:1184–1190, 2001

Keane TM, Kaloupek DG: Comorbid psychiatric disorders in PTSD. Implications for research. Ann N Y Acad Sci 821:24–34, 1997

Keane TM, Wolfe J: Comorbidity in post-traumatic stress disorder: an analysis of community and clinical studies. J Appl Soc Psychol 20:1776–1778, 1990

Kessler RC, Sonnega A, Bromet E, et al: Posttraumatic stress disorder in the National Comorbidity Survey. Arch Gen Psychiatry 52:1048–1060, 1995

Khantzian EJ: The self-medication hypothesis of addictive disorders: focus on heroin and cocaine dependence. Am J Psychiatry 142:1259–1264, 1985

Khantzian EJ: The self-medication hypothesis of substance use disorders: a reconsideration and recent applications. Harv Rev Psychiatry 4:231–244, 1997

Koenen KC, Moffitt TE, Caspi A, et al: The developmental mental-disorder histories of adults with posttraumatic stress disorder: a prospective longitudinal birth cohort study. J Abnorm Psychol 117:460–466, 2008

Kulka RA, Schlenger WE, Fairbank JA, et al: Trauma and the Vietnam War Generation: Report of Findings From the National Vietnam Veterans Readjustment Study. New York, Brunner/Mazel, 1990

Levy RS, Hebert CK, Munn BG, et al: Drug and alcohol use in orthopedic trauma patients: a prospective study. J Orthop Trauma 10:21–27, 1996

Maes M, Delmeire L, Schotte C, et al: The two-factorial symptom structure of post-traumatic stress disorder: depression-avoidance and arousal-anxiety. Psychiatry Res 81:195–210, 1998

McDonald SD, Beckham JC, Morey RA, et al: The validity and diagnostic efficiency of the Davidson Trauma Scale in military veterans who have served since September 11th, 2001. J Anxiety Disord 23:247–255, 2009

McFarlane AC: Epidemiological evidence about the relationship between PTSD and alcohol abuse: the nature of the association. Addict Behav 23:813–825, 1998

McFarlane AC, Papay P: Multiple diagnoses in posttraumatic stress disorder in the victims of a natural disaster. J Nerv Ment Dis 180:498–504, 1992

McFarlane AC, Atchison M, Rafalowicz E, et al: Physical symptoms in post-traumatic stress disorder. J Psychosom Res 38:715–726, 1994

McHugh PR, Treisman G: PTSD: a problematic diagnostic category. J Anxiety Disord 21:211–222, 2007

McLean LM, Gallop R: Implications of childhood sexual abuse for adult borderline personality disorder and complex posttraumatic stress disorder. Am J Psychiatry 160:369–371, 2003

McMillen C, North C, Mosley M, et al: Untangling the psychiatric comorbidity of posttraumatic stress disorder in a sample of flood survivors. Compr Psychiatry 43:478–485, 2002

McMillen JC, North CS, Smith EM: What parts of PTSD are normal: intrusion, avoidance, or arousal? Data from the Northridge, California, earthquake. J Trauma Stress 13:57–75, 2000

Modestin J, Furrer R, Malti T: Different traumatic experiences are associated with different pathologies. Psychiatr Q 76:19–32, 2005

Moreau C, Zisook S: Rationale for a posttraumatic stress spectrum disorder. Psychiatr Clin North Am 25:775–790, 2002

Nemeroff CB, Bremner JD, Foa EB, et al: Posttraumatic stress disorder: a state-of-the-science review. J Psychiatr Res 40:1–21, 2006

Norris FH: Epidemiology of trauma: frequency and impact of different potentially traumatic events on different demographic groups. J Consult Clin Psychol 60:409–418, 1992

Norris FH, Friedman MJ, Watson PJ, et al: 60,000 disaster victims speak: Part I. An empirical review of the empirical literature, 1981–2001. Psychiatry 65:207–239, 2002

North CS: Human response to violent trauma. Baillière's Clinical Psychiatry 1:225–245, 1995

North CS: Somatization in survivors of catastrophic trauma: a methodological review. Environ Health Perspect 110:637–640, 2002

North CS: Psychiatric effects of disasters and terrorism: empirical basis from study of the Oklahoma City bombing, in Fear and Anxiety: The Benefits of Translational Research. Edited by Gorman JM. Washington, DC, American Psychiatric Publishing, 2004, pp 105–117

North CS: Somatoform disorders, in Adult Psychiatry. Edited by Rubin EH, Zorumski CF. Malden, MA, Blackwell, 2005, pp 261–274

North CS: Epidemiology of disaster mental health response, in Textbook of Disaster Psychiatry. Edited by Ursano RJ, Fullerton CS, Weisaeth L, et al. New York, Cambridge University Press, 2007, pp 29–46

North CS, Smith EM, Spitznagel EL: Posttraumatic stress disorder in survivors of a mass shooting. Am J Psychiatry 151:82–88, 1994

North CS, Nixon SJ, Shariat S, et al: Psychiatric disorders among survivors of the Oklahoma City bombing. JAMA 282:755–762, 1999

North CS, McMillen JC, Pfefferbaum B, et al: Coping, functioning, and adjustment of rescue workers after the Oklahoma City bombing. J Trauma Stress 15:171–175, 2002a

North CS, Tivis L, McMillen JC, et al: Psychiatric disorders in rescue workers after the Oklahoma City bombing. Am J Psychiatry 159:857–859, 2002b

North CS, Kawasaki A, Spitznagel EL, et al: The course of PTSD, major depression, substance abuse, and somatization after a natural disaster. J Nerv Ment Dis 192:823–829, 2004

North CS, Hong BA, Suris A, et al: Distinguishing distress and psychopathology among survivors of the Oakland/Berkeley firestorm. Psychiatry 71:35–45, 2008a

North CS, King RV, Fowler RL, et al: Psychiatric disorders among transported hurricane evacuees: acute-phase findings in a large receiving shelter site. Psychiatr Ann 38:104–113, 2008b

North CS, Suris AM, Davis M, et al: Toward validation of the diagnosis of posttraumatic stress disorder. Am J Psychiatry 166:1–8, 2009

Nurcombe B: Child sexual abuse I: psychopathology. Aust N Z J Psychiatry 34:85–91, 2000

Orsillo SM, Weathers FW, Litz BT, et al: Current and lifetime psychiatric disorders among veterans with war zone-related posttraumatic stress disorder. J Nerv Ment Dis 184:307–313, 1996

Palmieri PA, Weathers FW, Difede J, et al: Confirmatory factor analysis of the PTSD Checklist and the Clinician-Administered PTSD Scale in disaster workers exposed to the World Trade Center Ground Zero. J Abnorm Psychol 116:329–341, 2007

Perkonigg A, Kessler RC, Storz S, et al: Traumatic events and post-traumatic stress disorder in the community: prevalence, risk factors and comorbidity. Acta Psychiatr Scand 101:46–59, 2000

Phifer JF: Psychological distress and somatic symptoms after natural disaster: differential vulnerability among older adults. Psychol Aging 5:412–420, 1990

Raja M, Onofri A, Azzoni A, et al: Post-traumatic stress disorder among people exposed to the Ventotene street disaster in Rome. Clin Pract Epidemiol Ment Health 4:5, 2008

Resnick HS, Kilpatrick DG, Dansky BS, et al: Prevalence of civilian trauma and posttraumatic stress disorder in a representative national sample of women. J Consult Clin Psychol 61:984–991, 1993

Robins LN: Steps toward evaluating post-traumatic stress reaction as a psychiatric disorder. J Appl Soc Psychol 20:1674–1677, 1990

Rosen GM, Lilienfeld SO: Posttraumatic stress disorder: an empirical evaluation of core assumptions. Clin Psychol Rev 28:837–868, 2008

Rosen GM, Taylor S: Pseudo-PTSD. J Anxiety Disord 21:201–210, 2007

Sack WH, Seeley JR, Clarke GN: Does PTSD transcend cultural barriers? A study from the Khmer Adolescent Refugee Project. J Am Acad Child Adolesc Psychiatry 36:49–54, 1997

Sartor CE, Agrawal A, McCutcheon VV, et al: Disentangling the complex association between childhood sexual abuse and alcohol-related problems: a review of methodological issues and approaches. J Stud Alcohol Drugs 69:718–727, 2008

Schafer I, Najavits LM: Clinical challenges in the treatment of patients with posttraumatic stress disorder and substance abuse. Curr Opin Psychiatry 20:614–618, 2007

Shalev A, Bleich A, Ursano RJ: Posttraumatic stress disorder: somatic comorbidity and effort tolerance. Psychosomatics 31:191–203, 1990

Shalev AY, Freedman S, Peri T, et al: Prospective study of posttraumatic stress disorder and depression following trauma. Am J Psychiatry 155:630–637, 1998

Shelby RA, Golden-Kreutz DM, Andersen BL: Mismatch of posttraumatic stress disorder (PTSD) symptoms and DSM-IV symptom clusters in a cancer sample: exploratory factor analysis of the PTSD Checklist-Civilian Version. J Trauma Stress 18:347–357, 2005

Sierles FS, Chen J-J, Messing ML, et al: Concurrent psychiatric illness in non-Hispanic outpatients diagnosed as having posttraumatic stress disorder. J Nerv Ment Dis 174:171–173, 1986

Silver SM, Iacono CU: Factor-analytic support for DSM-III's post-traumatic stress disorder for Vietnam veterans. J Clin Psychol 40:5–14, 1984

Smith EM, North CS, McCool RE, et al: Acute postdisaster psychiatric disorders: identification of persons at risk. Am J Psychiatry 147:202–206, 1990

Solomon SD, Canino GJ: Appropriateness of DSM-III-R criteria for post-traumatic stress disorder. Compr Psychiatry 31:227–237, 1990

Spitzer C, Barnow S, Gau K, et al: Childhood maltreatment in patients with somatization disorder. Aust N Z J Psychiatry 42:335–341, 2008

Spitzer RL, First MB, Wakefield JC: Saving PTSD from itself in DSM-V. J Anxiety Disord 21:233–241, 2007

Stewart SH: Alcohol abuse in individuals exposed to trauma: a critical review. Psychol Bull 120:83–112, 1996

Stewart SH, Pihl RO, Conrod PJ, et al: Functional associations among trauma, PTSD, and substance-related disorders. Addict Behav 23:797–812, 1998

Sunday S, Labruna V, Kaplan S, et al: Physical abuse during adolescence: gender differences in the adolescents' perceptions of family functioning and parenting. Child Abuse Negl 32:5–18, 2008

Taylor S, Kuch K, Koch WJ, et al: The structure of posttraumatic stress symptoms. J Abnorm Psychol 107:154–160, 1998

Turner HA, Finkelhor D, Ormrod R: Family structure variations in patterns and predictors of child victimization. Am J Orthopsychiatry 77:282–295, 2007

Vieweg WV, Julius DA, Fernandez A, et al: Posttraumatic stress disorder: clinical features, pathophysiology, and treatment. Am J Med 119:383–390, 2006

Vlahov D, Galea S, Resnick H, et al: Increased use of cigarettes, alcohol, and marijuana among Manhattan, New York, residents after the September 11th terrorist attacks. Am J Epidemiol 155:988–996, 2002

Wagner D, Heinrichs M, Ehlert U: Prevalence of symptoms of posttraumatic stress disorder in German professional firefighters. Am J Psychiatry 155:1727–1732, 1998

Wittmann L, Moergeli H, Martin-Soelch C, et al: Comorbidity in posttraumatic stress disorder: a structural equation modelling approach. Compr Psychiatry 49:430–440, 2008

Yehuda R, McFarlane AC: Conflict between current knowledge about posttraumatic stress disorder and its original conceptual basis. Am J Psychiatry 152:1705–1713, 1995

Yen S, Shea MT, Battle CL, et al: Traumatic exposure and posttraumatic stress disorder in borderline, schizotypal, avoidant, and obsessive-compulsive personality disorders: findings from the Collaborative Longitudinal Personality Disorders Study. J Nerv Ment Dis 190:510–518, 2002

PART II

Therapeutics and Management

6

Pharmacotherapy

Matthew J. Friedman, M.D., Ph.D.

Effective medications for posttraumatic stress disorder (PTSD) are currently available. Two selective serotonin reuptake inhibitors (SSRIs), sertraline and paroxetine, have been approved by the U.S. Food and Drug Administration (FDA) for treatment of PTSD and are considered first-line treatments for PTSD by many clinical practice guidelines. In addition, in multisite clinical trials, the SSRI fluoxetine and the serotonin-norepinephrine reuptake inhibitor (SNRI) venlafaxine have produced significant improvement, compared with placebo. Other medications, reviewed in this chapter, have also shown promise in single-site trials and are currently being tested in large-scale multisite investigations.

Although cognitive-behavioral therapy (CBT), especially prolonged exposure and cognitive processing therapy, has consistently outperformed pharmacotherapy with regard to efficacy (see Foa et al. 2009), medication remains an important clinical option for a number of reasons. First, medications are effective. Second, medications are often useful for treating comorbid depression and other anxiety disorders that often accompany PTSD. Third, medications are generally accepted by patients, especially those receiving integrated primary and behavioral care in primary care settings. Finally, medications may be readily obtained from any prescribing clinician, whereas qualified CBT therapists may be hard to find because only 10%–20% of practicing psychotherapists are qualified to provide such treatment (Rosen et al. 2004).

To readers familiar with the many alterations in neurocircuitry and neurobiological systems associated with PTSD (Neumeister et al. 2007), the superiority of CBT may be surprising. Several explanations are possible. First, most randomized controlled trials (RCTs) have focused on SSRIs, which target only the serotonergic system. Although SSRIs are effective for a variety of affective and anxiety disorders, their efficacy in PTSD (see the section on SSRIs below) may be much less specific than the efficacy of CBT. Second, medications affecting key systems altered in PTSD (e.g., adrenergic, dopaminergic, γ-aminobutyric acid [GABA]–ergic, glutamatergic, and hypothalamic-pituitary-adrenocortical [HPA] mechanisms) have received relatively little attention. Given the emerging understanding of the pathophysiology of PTSD, it is entirely possible that medications modulating these systems will eventually prove more effective than SSRIs. Third, medications currently under development may prove to have greater efficacy and specificity, especially corticotropin-releasing factor (CRF) antagonists and neuropeptide Y enhancers. Finally, the best treatment for PTSD may prove to be a combination of CBT and medication, as in ongoing trials of CBT enhancement with the glutamatergic agent D-cycloserine, as well as CBT augmentation for partial responders to sertraline (Rothbaum et al. 2006, 2008).

In this chapter, we consider all the major classes of medication that have been investigated in clinical trials with PTSD patients. The greatest emphasis is placed on results from RCTs, where the strongest evidence can be found. Because the preponderance of RCTs have tested SSRIs and SNRIs, we also consider findings from less rigorous studies to provide a comprehensive overview of results using other medications. We also consider the few studies in which medications were administered acutely posttrauma to prevent the development of PTSD. Indications and contraindications for PTSD medications are summarized in Table 6–1.

Antidepressants

Selective Serotonin Reuptake Inhibitors

SSRIs are currently the medication of choice for use with PTSD patients. As stated previously, two SSRIs, sertraline and paroxetine, have received FDA approval for PTSD treatment based on industry-sponsored multisite RCTs (Brady et al. 2000; Davidson et al. 2001b; Marshall et al. 2001; Tucker et al. 2001). Additionally, when sertraline treatment was extended from 12 to 36 weeks, 55% of nonresponding or partially responding patients converted to medication responders (Londborg et al. 2001). Notably, however, a large RCT conducted with Vietnam veteran chronic PTSD patients receiving sertraline treatment in Veterans Affairs (VA) settings had negative results (Friedman et al. 2007). As in depression and other anxiety disorders, discontinuation of SSRI treatment results in increased clinical relapse and return of PTSD symptoms (Davidson et al. 2001a; Martényi et al. 2002a; Rapaport et al. 2002).

RCTs with fluoxetine (Martényi et al. 2002b; van der Kolk et al. 1994) and open-label studies with fluvoxamine and citalopram (see Friedman et al. 2007 for references) indicate that these SSRIs are also effective agents. SSRIs have been shown to reduce PTSD reexperiencing, avoidance/numbing, and hyperarousal symptoms, and also appear to promote rapid improvement in quality of life that is sustained during treatment (Rapaport et al. 2002).

Other Serotonergic Antidepressants

Nefazodone and trazodone are two antidepressants that enhance serotonergic activity through a dual mechanism combining SSRI action with postsynaptic 5-hydroxytryptamine (serotonin) type 2 (5-HT_2) receptor blockade. An RCT showed nefazodone to be as effective as sertraline (Saygin et al. 2002). Similar positive results have been obtained in open-label nefazodone trials (see Friedman et al. 2007 for references); however, nongeneric nefazodone has been withdrawn from the U.S. market because of liver toxicity. Trazodone as monotherapy has limited efficacy. Because of its sedating effects and synergistic serotonergic action, however, trazodone is often used in conjunction with SSRIs.

Tricyclic Antidepressants

Tricyclic antidepressants (TCAs) are older antidepressants that block presynaptic reuptake of norepinephrine, serotonin, or both, depending on the med-

Table 6–1. Medications for PTSD: indications and contraindications

Class	Medication	Strength of evidence[a]	Daily dose (mg)	Indications	Contraindications
SSRIs	Paroxetine[b]	A	10–60	Reduce B, C, and D symptoms[c]	May produce insomnia, restlessness, nausea, decreased appetite, daytime sedation, nervousness, anxiety
	Sertraline[b]	A	50–200	Produce clinical global improvement	May produce sexual dysfunction, decreased libido, delayed orgasm or anorgasmia
	Fluoxetine	A	20–80	Effective treatment for depression, panic disorder, social phobia, obsessive-compulsive disorder	Clinically significant interactions for people prescribed MAOIs
	Citalopram	F	20–60	Reduce associated symptoms (rage, aggression, impulsivity, suicidal thoughts)	Significant interactions with hepatic enzymes produce other drug interactions
	Fluvoxamine	B	50–300		
Other serotonergic antidepressants	Nefazodone	A	200–600	Superior to placebo in male combat veterans Effective antidepressant	Reports of hepatotoxicity associated with nefazodone treatment
	Trazodone	C	50–600	Trazodone has limited efficacy by itself but is synergistic with SSRIs and may reduce SSRI-induced insomnia Effective antidepressant	May be too sedating; rare priapism

Table 6–1. Medications for PTSD: indications and contraindications *(continued)*

Class	Medication	Strength of evidence[a]	Daily dose (mg)	Indications	Contraindications
Other serotonergic agents	Cyproheptadine	A	4–24	Not recommended Makes PTSD symptoms worse	Drowsiness, weight gain
	Buspirone	F	15–60	Little evidence of efficacy	Few side effects Rare dizziness, headache, nausea
Other second-generation antidepressants	Venlafaxine	A	75–225	Effective antidepressant	May exacerbate hypertension; patients to follow a strict dietary regimen
	Mirtazapine	A	15–45	Efficacy in PTSD has been demonstrated Effective antidepressant	May produce somnolence, increased appetite, weight gain
	Bupropion	A	200–450	Efficacy in PTSD has not been shown Effective antidepressant	May exacerbate seizure disorder

Table 6–1. Medications for PTSD: indications and contraindications *(continued)*

Class	Medication	Strength of evidence[a]	Daily dose (mg)	Indications	Contraindications
MAOIs	Phenelzine	A	15–90	Reduces B symptoms[c] Produces global improvement Effective agent for depression, panic, social phobia Efficacy in PTSD has not been demonstrated for other MAOIs	Risk of hypertensive crisis necessitates strict dietary regimen Contraindicated in combination with most other antidepressants, CNS stimulants, and decongestants Contraindicated in patients with alcohol or substance abuse or dependence May produce insomnia, hypotension, anticholinergic effects, and severe liver toxicity
TCAs	Imipramine Amitriptyline	A A	150–300 150–300	Reduce B symptoms[c] Produce global improvement Effective antidepressant and antipanic agents Imipramine prevented onset of PTSD in pediatric burn patients	Anticholinergic side effects (dry mouth, rapid pulse, blurred vision, constipation) May produce ventricular arrhythmias May produce orthostatic hypotension, sedation, arousal

Table 6–1. Medications for PTSD: indications and contraindications *(continued)*

Class	Medication	Strength of evidence[a]	Daily dose (mg)	Indications	Contraindications
	Desipramine	A	100–300	Desipramine ineffective in PTSD in one randomized clinical trial	Same as for imipramine and amitriptyline
				Other TCAs have not been tested in PTSD	
Antiadrenergic agents	Prazosin	A	6–10	Marked efficacy for PTSD nightmares and insomnia	May be more effective for PTSD in divided doses
	Propranolol	B	40–160	Some effectiveness against B and D symptoms[c]	May produce hypotension, bradycardia
				Reduced physiological reactivity but not PTSD when given acutely	May produce depressive symptoms, hypotension, bradycardia, bronchospasm
	Guanfacine	A	1–3	Ineffective in RCT, but positive results in open trials	May produce hypotension, bradycardia
Glucocorticoids	Hydrocortisone	A	5–30	Prevents later development of PTSD in septic shock and post–cardiac surgery patients	Immunosuppression, osteopenia, hyperglycemia, hypertension

Table 6–1. Medications for PTSD: indications and contraindications *(continued)*

Class	Medication	Strength of evidence[a]	Daily dose (mg)	Indications	Contraindications
Anticonvulsant/ mood stabilizer agents					Gastrointestinal problems, sedation, tremor, thrombocytopenia
	Valproate	A	750–1,750	Ineffective in large RCT Effective in bipolar affective disorder	Teratogenic—should not be used in pregnancy
	Tiagabine	A	4–12	Ineffective in large randomized trial	Dizziness, somnolence, tremor, seizures
	Carbamazepine	B	400–1,600	Reduces B and D symptoms[c] Effective in bipolar affective disorder Possibly effective in reducing impulsive, aggressive, violent behavior	Neurological symptoms, ataxia, drowsiness, low sodium, leukopenia
	Gabapentin[d]	F	300–3,600	Small trials suggest favorable effects	Sedation, ataxia
	Lamotrigine	A/B	50–400	Modestly favorable results in small RCT	Stevens-Johnson syndrome, skin rash, fatigue

Table 6–1. Medications for PTSD: indications and contraindications *(continued)*

Class	Medication	Strength of evidence[a]	Daily dose (mg)	Indications	Contraindications
	Topiramate[d]	B	200–400	Efficacy not demonstrated in PTSD	Glaucoma, sedation, dizziness, ataxia
Glutamatergic agent (partial NMDA agonist)	D-cycloserine	F	250–1,000	Reduction in PTSD severity when combined with prolonged exposure therapy Improved cognition Promising RCTs currently in progress	Somnolence, headache, tremor, dysarthria, vertigo, confusion, nervousness, irritability, psychotic reactions, hyperreflexia, seizures Despite above side effects, has been used safely for tuberculosis for many years
Benzodiazepines	Alprazolam Clonazepam	A B	0.5–6 1–8	Not recommended Do not reduce core B and C symptoms[c] Effective only for general anxiety and insomnia Other benzodiazepines have not been tested in PTSD	Sedation, memory impairment, ataxia Not recommended for patients with past or present alcohol/drug abuse/dependency because of risk for dependence May exacerbate depressive symptoms Aprazolam may produce rebound anxiety

Table 6–1. Medications for PTSD: indications and contraindications *(continued)*

Class	Medication	Strength of evidence[a]	Daily dose (mg)	Indications	Contraindications
Conventional antipsychotics	Thioridazine	F	20–800	Not recommended	Sedation, orthostatic hypotension, anticholinergic effects, extrapyramidal effects, tardive dyskinesia, neuroleptic malignant syndrome, endocrinopathies, ECG abnormalities, blood dyscrasias, hepatotoxicity
	Chlorpromazine	F	30–800		
	Haloperidol	F	1–20		
Atypical antipsychotics	Risperidone	A	4–16	Preliminary data suggest effectiveness against PTSD symptom clusters and aggression May have a role as augmentation treatment for partial responders to other agents	Weight gain with all agents Risk of Type II diabetes with olanzapine
	Olanzapine	A	5–20		
	Quetiapine	B	50–750		

Table 6–1. Medications for PTSD: indications and contraindications *(continued)*

Note. CNS=central nervous system; ECG=electrocardiogram; MAOI=monoamine oxidase inhibitor; NMDA=*N*-methyl-D-aspartate; RCT=randomized controlled trial; SSRI=selective serotonin reuptake inhibitor; TCA=tricyclic antidepressant.

[a]*Strength of evidence:*

Level A=randomized clinical trials

Level B=well-designed clinical studies without randomization or placebo comparison

Level C=service and naturalistic clinical studies, combined with clinical observations that are sufficiently compelling to warrant use of this drug

Level F=a few observations that have not been subjected to clinical or empirical test

[b]U.S. Food and Drug Administration approval for PTSD treatment.

[c]B symptoms: intrusive recollections; C symptoms: avoidant/numbing; D symptoms: hyperarousal.

[d]The only data are from small trials and case reports.

Source. Adapted from Friedman et al. 2009.

ication. As antidepressants, TCAs are no less effective than SSRIs, but they have complicated side-effect profiles that make them more difficult to manage than SSRIs. RCTs with imipramine (Kosten et al. 1991) and amitriptyline (Davidson et al. 1990), but not those with desipramine (Reist et al. 1989), have demonstrated symptom reduction in patients with PTSD.

No new PTSD clinical trials have been done with TCAs during the past 10 years. This is not only because SSRIs and other new antidepressants have more benign side-effect profiles than older agents, but also because pharmaceutical companies are not motivated to fund such studies.

The most notable TCA study was a prospective RCT comparing imipramine with the hypnotic chloral hydrate among children and adolescents hospitalized because of severe burn injuries. Such patients are at very high risk for acute stress disorder and subsequent PTSD. In this study, burn victims randomized to the imipramine group had a significantly lower incidence of acute stress disorder than those treated with chloral hydrate (Robert et al. 1999).

Monoamine Oxidase Inhibitors

Monoamine oxidase inhibitors (MAOIs) block the intraneuronal metabolic breakdown of serotonin, norepinephrine, dopamine, and other monoamines, thereby making more neurotransmitter available for presynaptic release. An RCT using the MAOI phenelzine with Vietnam combat veterans was extremely successful in reducing reexperiencing and arousal PTSD symptoms (Kosten et al. 1991). Results have been mixed in open-label trials (see Friedman and Davidson 2007), and a small, 5-week crossover study with questionable methodology had negative results (Shestatzky et al. 1988). Finally, an open-label trial with moclobemide, a reversible monoamine oxidase A inhibitor (Neal et al. 1997), detected improvement in all three PTSD symptom clusters (i.e., reexperiencing, avoidance and numbing, and hyperarousal symptoms).

Other Second-Generation Antidepressants

Mirtazapine has serotonergic actions (blockade of postsynaptic 5-HT_2 and 5-HT_3 receptors), as well as action at presynaptic alpha-2 adrenergic receptors. Mirtazapine was significantly more effective than placebo in one RCT (Davidson et al. 2003). In an open-label 8-week trial in Korea (Bahk et al. 2002), mirtazapine effectively reduced PTSD symptom severity. Additionally, Lewis (2002) reported on the usefulness of mirtazapine for traumatic nightmares (or for post-waking memory of such nightmares) among 300 refugees who had previously failed to benefit from other medications.

Venlafaxine blocks presynaptic reuptake of norepinephrine and serotonin and has a much less potent effect on blocking dopamine reuptake. Two large multicenter trials of extended-release venlafaxine have shown superiority relative to placebo, in both 12-week (Davidson et al. 2006b) and 6-month RCTs (Davidson et al. 2006a). Furthermore, patients receiving venlafaxine exhibited significantly more resilience, or the ability to deal with daily stress, than did patients given placebo. Finally, as with SSRIs (Londborg et al. 2001), a substantial percentage of patients in the 6-month trial did not achieve remission until they had received several months of treatment.

Bupropion blocks presynaptic reuptake of norepinephrine and dopamine, but not of serotonin. Although anecdotal evidence and open-label trials suggest that bupropion may be effective in PTSD (Canive et al. 1998), a fairly recent RCT had negative results (Becker et al. 2007).

Antiadrenergic Agents

Despite favorable clinical reports on the efficacy of both propranolol and clonidine 25 years ago (Kolb et al. 1984), few studies have been done of antiadrenergic agents in treating PTSD. RCTs with this class of medications have focused mostly on the postsynaptic alpha 1 antagonist prazosin. This research has consistently indicated that prazosin reduces PTSD nightmares. Success against other PTSD symptoms has been inconsistent, possibly because the medication was prescribed for only once-daily administration rather than divided doses, due to prazosin's relatively short half-life (Raskind et al. 2003, 2007). A large-scale multisite trial is currently in progress.

Cahill and McGaugh (1996) showed that the beta-adrenergic antagonist propranolol reduced enhancement of emotional memories among human volunteers. In small clinical studies, propranolol has had beneficial effects on PTSD symptoms, including intrusive recollections and reactivity to traumatic stimuli (Famularo et al. 1988). Propranolol has also shown promise as a prophylactic agent for the prevention of developing PTSD in acutely traumatized individuals. Propranolol prevented subsequent (e.g., 1- and 3-month) posttraumatic physiological hyperreactivity but not PTSD when administered to acutely traumatized emergency room patients (Pitman et al. 2002; Taylor and

Cahill 2002; Vaiva et al. 2003). Finally, Brunet et al. (2008) conducted a provocative experiment in which subjects with PTSD described their traumatic experience during a script preparation session, after which they were randomized to 1 day of treatment with propranolol or placebo. One week later, after evocation of the traumatic event by script-driven imagery, the propranolol group exhibited significantly less physiological arousal. The investigators speculated that propranolol may have interfered with reconsolidation of the traumatic memory. This intriguing finding certainly merits further study.

Alpha-2-adrenergic agonists such as clonidine and guanfacine (which reduce the presynaptic release of norepinephrine) might also be expected to improve PTSD symptom severity. The sparse literature on the clinical efficacy of these agents in treating PTSD is generally favorable (Kinzie and Friedman 2004; Kolb et al. 1984). In an RCT with older veterans, however, guanfacine performed no better than placebo in reducing PTSD severity (Neylan et al. 2006).

Anticonvulsant/Mood Stabilizer Agents

Anticonvulsant/mood stabilizer agents have been sporadically tested in small single-site studies since the 1990s. Interest in this class of medications was prompted initially by their antikindling actions, because of interest in the sensitization/kindling hypothesis of PTSD. Detection of abnormalities in glutamatergic and GABAergic systems among patients with PTSD has also raised the level of interest in this class of medications. Finally, the development of several new anticonvulsants/mood stabilizers in recent years has motivated the pharmaceutical industry to support clinical trials using these agents with PTSD patients. Despite promising open-label studies with several anticonvulsants, two recent large-scale RCTs with tiagabine and valproate have had negative results (Davidson et al. 2007; L. L. Davis et al. 2008). Thus, current evidence does not favor the use of these agents in treating PTSD, despite significant theoretical interest.

D-Cycloserine

A second-line agent for the treatment of tuberculosis is D-cycloserine (DCS). DCS is also pharmacologically active as a partial agonist at the glutamatergic

N-methyl-D-aspartate (NMDA) receptor, which mediates learning and memory. An understanding of this research with DCS is aided by consideration of the Pavlovian fear conditioning model of PTSD.

According to the fear conditioning model, PTSD develops in reaction to a traumatic event (unconditioned stimulus), and PTSD symptoms are elicited by traumatic reminders (conditioned stimuli). Extrapolating from animal research, amelioration of conditioned fear must be accomplished through extinction. Extinction occurs when new responses to conditioned stimuli are learned and stimuli no longer elicit PTSD symptoms. This model is the theoretical rationale for exposure therapy, which is, in effect, a clinical paradigm for extinguishing conditioned fear.

Extinction involves new learning, primarily mediated by NMDA receptors. Because DCS acts at NMDA receptors and animal research has shown that DCS facilitates extinction of conditioned fear, it was hypothesized that DCS would enhance the efficacy of exposure therapy and reduce the number of therapeutic sessions needed to achieve clinical remission (M. Davis et al. 2006). In successful RCTs, DCS accelerated successful exposure therapy for acrophobia (fear of heights) and social phobia (Hofmann et al. 2006; Ressler et al. 2004). Research currently in progress will determine whether DCS will also accelerate PTSD treatment with exposure therapy.

Benzodiazepines

Benzodiazepines have not proved efficacious for PTSD. An RCT with alprazolam did not reduce core reexperiencing or avoidant/numbing symptoms, although it did lead to improvement in insomnia and generalized anxiety (Braun et al. 1990). Treatment of recently traumatized emergency room patients with clonazepam (Gelpin et al. 1996) or the hypnotic benzodiazepine temazepam (Mellman et al. 2002) did not prevent the later development of PTSD. Other open-label trials with benzodiazepines have also been unsuccessful (Friedman et al. 2000).

Although there is theoretical reason to expect that medications acting at $GABA_A$ receptors, such as benzodiazepines (or the aforementioned ineffective anticonvulsants/mood stabilizers tiagabine and valproate), would share efficacy in PTSD treatment, little research evidence is available to support this hypothesis. One possible explanation is that any beneficial pharmacological effects are more than offset by benzodiazepine-induced interference with cognitive mechanisms necessary for therapeutic processing of traumatic material.

Atypical Antipsychotic Medications

A small but growing literature shows that atypical antipsychotic agents have favorable results in treating PTSD. Most noteworthy about these findings are signs of efficacy in treatment-resistant patient groups (e.g., older chronic patients receiving treatment at U.S. Veterans Affairs Medical Centers).

In PTSD treatment, atypical antipsychotics have typically been used as adjunctive agents for patients who are refractory to SSRIs or other antidepressants. Reports have been published on three antipsychotic medications (risperidone, olanzapine, and quetiapine) as adjuncts to ongoing antidepressant pharmacotherapy. Results from four randomized trials (Bartzokis et al. 2005; Hamner et al. 2003; Monnelly et al. 2003; Reich et al. 2004) and several case reports using risperidone as adjunctive therapy show reduction in overall PTSD symptom severity and reductions in dissociative flashbacks and aggressive behavior. Similar findings were obtained in an RCT with olanzapine (Stein et al. 2002), indicating effectiveness as an adjunctive agent in reducing PTSD symptoms among chronic SSRI-refractory patients; however, another RCT with olanzapine as adjunctive treatment for PTSD had negative results (Butterfield et al. 2001). Positive results have also been obtained with quetiapine as an adjunctive agent in an open-label trial (Hamner et al. 2003), a retrospective medical record review (Sokolski et al. 2003), and several case reports.

Hypothalamic-Pituitary-Adrenocortical System

Corticotropin-Releasing Factor Antagonists

PTSD is associated with elevated levels of CRF. Given CRF's key role in mobilizing the human stress response, as well as its increased expression among PTSD patients, there is good reason to predict that CRF antagonists might have beneficial clinical effects on PTSD-related symptoms. Preclinical studies with the CRF receptor antagonist antalarmin have demonstrated reductions in cerebrospinal fluid CRF, reduced stress-induced fearful behavior, and suppression of both adrenergic and HPA responses to stress (Habib et al. 2000). To date, CRF antagonists have not been tested with PTSD patients.

Glucocorticoids

Whether cortisol levels are elevated or glucocorticoid receptors are supersensitive, excessive HPA activity may exacerbate PTSD symptoms and promote neurotoxicity through activation of excitatory amino acids and intraneuronal calcium influx. HPA dysregulation has frequently been observed in individuals with PTSD, although cortisol levels have sometimes been elevated and at other times reduced (Southwick et al. 2007). Therefore, it is useful to consider pharmacological strategies that might either prevent or ameliorate PTSD-related symptom exacerbation and neurotoxic effects hypothesized to result from excessive HPA activity. With regard to early intervention, potential treatments theoretically might include CRF antagonists aimed at reducing the intensity of the acute stress response. (It should be noted that currently no CRF antagonists have been tested with acutely traumatized patients or patients with PTSD.) If the problem is excessive cortisol levels, a medication that inhibits cortisol synthesis (e.g., ketoconazole) or that blocks glucocorticoid receptors (e.g., mifepristone) might be considered. If the problem is reduced cortisol and supersensitive glucocorticoid receptors, glucocorticoids could be administered to downregulate supersensitive glucocorticoid receptors. Indeed, acute hydrocortisone treatment for septic shock has been shown to effectively prevent the later development of PTSD (Schelling et al. 2001).

Applicability to Military and Veteran Populations

In studies of Vietnam veterans in VA hospital treatment settings, negative findings initially caused speculation that PTSD due to combat trauma is less responsive to pharmacotherapy than PTSD due to other causes (Friedman et al. 2007). This conclusion was repudiated in RCTs with paroxetine and fluoxetine. In studies with paroxetine (Marshall et al. 2001; Tucker et al. 2001), veterans who had been recruited from the general population (rather than from VA hospital treatment settings) exhibited as much benefit from SSRI treatment as did male and female nonveterans. Positive results also were found in an RCT with fluoxetine (Martényi et al. 2002b), which recruited mostly male veterans of then-recent United Nations and North Atlantic Treaty Organization (NATO) deployments. Indeed, exposure to combat trauma actually predicted a successful response to fluoxetine pharmacotherapy in that study.

These findings illustrate three things. First, people with PTSD due to combat trauma are as likely to respond to SSRI treatment as those with PTSD due to other traumatic events. Second, both men and women can benefit from SSRI treatment. Third, male Vietnam veterans in VA settings with chronic and severe PTSD may be overall less likely than other veterans to benefit from pharmacotherapy or from psychosocial treatments (Friedman 1997; Friedman et al. 2007; Schnurr et al. 2003). These findings are a strong argument for early detection and treatment of PTSD, because decades of chronicity appear to reduce the likelihood of a favorable outcome.

Gaps in Current Knowledge

Several important gaps in knowledge limit generalizability of current findings. First, there is insufficient information on nonwhite subjects both within the United States and from other nations. This deficiency is particularly true for refugees or internally displaced people, who are at very high risk for PTSD (Green et al. 2003).

A second serious gap in knowledge concerns children and adolescents. Childhood sexual, physical, or emotional abuse and exposure to accidents are major causes of PTSD. Mounting concern about increased suicides among children and adolescents treated with SSRIs for depression (U.S. Food and Drug Administration 2004), however, has generated caution and resistance to conducting clinical trials with medications for younger people with PTSD.

Data are also scant on the efficacy of medications for older individuals with PTSD. Concerns about safety, age-related pharmacokinetic capacity, drug-drug interactions, and comorbid medical conditions must always be factored into decisions for treating older individuals. Given that PTSD is a risk factor for medical illness (Schnurr and Green 2003) and primary care practitioners have just begun to identify PTSD among older patients, attention to PTSD among older individuals is beginning to emerge as an important clinical challenge about which very little evidence is available to guide current practice.

Combined Therapy

Two promising combined therapy approaches (both reviewed above) have received attention in clinical trials: augmentation of exposure therapy with DCS to accelerate the pace of treatment (by facilitating extinction of fear-conditioned, PTSD-related symptoms) and augmentation of SSRI partial responders with atypical antipsychotics. In clinical practice, patients often receive more than one treatment, although research showing the effectiveness of such approaches is limited. Most frequently, patients are treated with both psychotherapy and pharmacotherapy.

Gerardi et al. (in press) review several different strategies for combining pharmacotherapy and psychotherapy, and some challenges and advantages to each. When combining antidepressants with CBT, one needs to consider that the medications usually require 4 or more weeks to take effect. Therefore, it makes more sense to combine these approaches sequentially, beginning with administration of the antidepressant for at least 4 weeks before commencing the psychotherapy. CBT should be added only for those with a partial response to the medication, as in Rothbaum et al.'s (2006) sertraline and CBT trial. In that trial, 88 male and female outpatients with PTSD, initially treated with open-label sertraline (up to 200 mg), were subsequently randomly assigned to receive continuation with sertraline alone or to receive augmentation with prolonged exposure (10 twice-weekly sessions of 90–120 minutes). The major finding was that patients who had previously had only a partial response to sertraline exhibited significant improvement following prolonged exposure augmentation. Prolonged exposure had no added benefit when complete remission had previously been achieved with sertraline alone.

In a trial with almost a mirror design to Rothbaum et al.'s (2006) study, Simon et al. (2008) started participants with eight sessions of prolonged exposure over 4–6 weeks and then randomly assigned them to receive either controlled-release paroxetine plus five additional sessions of prolonged exposure or placebo plus five additional sessions of prolonged exposure. The largest reductions of PTSD symptoms occurred following prolonged exposure, with no significant differences between placebo and paroxetine in the augmentation phase. In other words, SSRI augmentation of prolonged exposure was not effective (Simon et al. 2008), whereas prolonged exposure augmentation of SSRI therapy was significantly beneficial (Rothbaum et al. 2006).

There are few data to guide us regarding other augmentation strategies. Extrapolating from the general effects of different medications for PTSD patients, it is common practice to augment SSRI or SNRI treatment with trazodone for patients with insomnia. Prazosin appears very effective for reducing traumatic nightmares and insomnia. Regarding other augmentation strategies, Friedman (2006, p. 60) has made the following suggestions, with the caveat that no direct empirical evidence is available to support these recommendations:

1. Antiadrenergic agents might be useful for excessively aroused, hyperreactive, or dissociating patients.
2. Anticonvulsants might benefit labile, impulsive, and/or aggressive patients.
3. Atypical antipsychotics might be effective for fearful, hypervigilant, paranoid, and psychotic patients.

Key Clinical Points

- The best current treatment for PTSD is cognitive-behavioral therapy (CBT).
- CBT is currently more effective than pharmacotherapy; however, further research to improve understanding of the key systems altered in PTSD will likely provide better and more effective medications than those currently available.
- The SSRIs paroxetine and sertraline have been FDA approved for the treatment of PTSD, but the entire SSRI class has at least some evidence of effectiveness in PTSD.
- Trazodone as monotherapy has limited efficacy but is often used in conjunction with SSRIs for treatment.
- MAOIs and some TCAs, including imipramine and amitriptyline, have shown efficacy in reducing PTSD symptoms, but the use of TCAs and MAOIs is limited because of their side effects.
- Mirtazapine and venlafaxine have both been shown to have efficacy in reducing PTSD symptoms, including specific utility for mirtazapine in treating traumatic nightmares.

- Bupropion has not been shown to be effective in the treatment of PTSD.
- The antiadrenergic agent prazosin appears to be effective in treating nightmares associated with PTSD and may have other uses in PTSD management.
- Current evidence does not favor the use of anticonvulsant/mood stabilizer agents or benzodiazepines in the treatment of PTSD.
- Atypical antipsychotics appear to have a role in the treatment of PTSD as adjunctive agents.
- Glucocorticoids, CRF antagonists, and D-cycloserine may all have applicability in the treatment of PTSD, but further research is needed.
- For prevention of the later development of PTSD, propranolol, hydrocortisone, and imipramine have shown promise in preliminary trials.
- Much more research is needed on pharmacotherapy for nonwhite populations, children and adolescents, and older individuals with PTSD.

References

Bahk WM, Pae CU, Tsoh J, et al: Effects of mirtazapine in patients with posttraumatic stress disorder in Korea: a pilot study. Hum Psychopharmacol 17:341–344, 2002

Bartzokis G, Lu PH, Turner J, et al: Adjunctive risperidone in the treatment of chronic combat-related posttraumatic stress disorder. Biol Psychiatry 57:474–479, 2005

Becker ME, Hertzberg MA, Moore SD, et al: A placebo-controlled trial of bupropion SR in the treatment of chronic posttraumatic stress disorder. J Clin Psychopharmacol 27:193–197, 2007

Brady K, Pearlstein T, Asnis GM, et al: Efficacy and safety of sertraline treatment of posttraumatic stress disorder: a randomized controlled trial. JAMA 283:1837–1844, 2000

Braun P, Greenberg D, Dasberg H, et al: Core symptoms of posttraumatic stress disorder unimproved by alprazolam treatment. J Clin Psychiatry 51:236–238, 1990

Brunet A, Orr SP, Tremblay J, et al: Effect of post-retrieval propranolol on psychophysiologic responding during subsequent script-driven traumatic imagery in posttraumatic stress disorder. J Psychiatr Res 42:503–506, 2008

Butterfield MI, Becker ME, Connor KM, et al: Olanzapine in the treatment of posttraumatic stress disorder: a pilot study. Int Clin Psychopharmacol 16:197–203, 2001

Cahill L, McGaugh JL: Modulation of memory storage. Curr Opin Neurobiol 6:237–242, 1996

Canive JM, Clark RD, Calais LA, et al: Bupropion treatment in veterans with posttraumatic stress disorder: an open study. J Clin Psychopharmacol 18:379–383, 1998

Davidson JR, Kudler H, Smith R, et al: Treatment of posttraumatic stress disorder with amitriptyline and placebo. Arch Gen Psychiatry 47:259–266, 1990

Davidson JR, Pearlstein T, Londborg P, et al: Efficacy of sertraline in preventing relapse of posttraumatic stress disorder: results of a 28-week double-blind, placebo-controlled study. Am J Psychiatry 158:1974–1981, 2001a

Davidson JR, Rothbaum BO, van der Kolk BA, et al: Multicenter, double-blind comparison of sertraline and placebo in the treatment of posttraumatic stress disorder. Arch Gen Psychiatry 58:485–492, 2001b

Davidson JR, Weisler RH, Butterfield MI, et al: Mirtazapine vs. placebo in posttraumatic stress disorder: a pilot trial. Biol Psychiatry 53:188–191, 2003

Davidson JR, Baldwin D, Stein DJ, et al: Treatment of posttraumatic stress disorder with venlafaxine extended release: a 6-month randomized controlled trial. Arch Gen Psychiatry 63:1158–1165, 2006a

Davidson JR, Rothbaum BO, Tucker P, et al: Venlafaxine extended release in posttraumatic stress disorder: a sertraline- and placebo-controlled study. J Clin Psychopharmacol 26:259–267, 2006b

Davidson JR, Brady K, Mellman TA, et al: The efficacy and tolerability of tiagabine in adult patients with posttraumatic stress disorder. J Clin Psychopharmacol 27:85–88, 2007

Davis LL, Davidson JRT, Ward LC, et al: Divalproex in the treatment of posttraumatic stress disorder: a randomized, double-blind, placebo-controlled trial in a veteran population. J Clin Psychopharmacol 28:84–88, 2008

Davis M, Ressler K, Rothbaum BO, et al: Effects of D-cycloserine on extinction: translation from preclinical to clinical work. Biol Psychiatry 60:369–375, 2006

Famularo R, Kinscherff R, Fenton T: Propranolol treatment for childhood posttraumatic stress disorder, acute type. Am J Dis Child 142:1244–1247, 1988

Foa EB, Keane TM, Friedman MJ, et al (eds): Effective Treatments for PTSD: Practice Guidelines From the International Society for Traumatic Stress Studies, 2nd Edition. New York, Guilford, 2009

Friedman MJ: Drug treatment for PTSD: answers and questions. Ann N Y Acad Sci 821:359–371, 1997

Friedman MJ (ed): Post-traumatic and Acute Stress Disorders: The Latest Assessment and Treatment Strategies, 4th Edition. Kansas City, KS, Compact Clinicals, 2006

Friedman MJ, Davidson JR: Pharmacotherapy for PTSD, in Handbook of PTSD: Science and Practice. Edited by Friedman MJ, Keane TM, Resick PA. New York, Guilford, 2007, pp 376–405

Friedman MJ, Davidson JR, Mellman TA, et al: Pharmacotherapy, in Effective Treatments for PTSD: Practice Guidelines From the International Society for Traumatic Stress Studies. Edited by Foa EB, Keane TM, Friedman MJ. New York, Guilford, 2000, pp 84–105

Friedman MJ, Marmar CR, Baker DG, et al: Randomized, double-blind comparison of sertraline and placebo for posttraumatic stress disorder in a Department of Veterans Affairs setting. J Clin Psychiatry 68:711–720, 2007

Friedman MJ, Davidson JR, Stein DJ: Psychopharmacotherapy for adults, in Effective Treatments for PTSD: Practice Guidelines From the International Society for Traumatic Stress Studies, 2nd Edition. Edited by Foa EB, Keane TM, Friedman MJ, et al. New York, Guilford, 2009, pp 245–268

Gelpin E, Bonne OB, Peri T, et al: Treatment of recent trauma survivors with benzodiazepines: a prospective study. J Clin Psychiatry 57:390–394, 1996

Gerardi M, Ressler K, Rothbaum BO: Combined treatment of anxiety disorders, in Textbook of Anxiety Disorders, 2nd Edition. Edited by Stein DJ, Hollander E, Rothbaum BO. Washington, DC, American Psychiatric Publishing, 2010, pp 147–156

Green BL, Friedman MJ, De Jong JTVM, et al: Trauma Interventions in War and Peace: Prevention, Practice, and Policy. New York, Kluwer Academic/Plenum, 2003

Habib KE, Weld KP, Rice KC, et al: Oral administration of a corticotropin-releasing hormone receptor antagonist significantly attenuates behavioral, neuroendocrine, and autonomic responses to stress in primates. Proc Natl Acad Sci U S A 97:6079–6084, 2000

Hamner MB, Faldowski RA, Ulmer HG, et al: Adjunctive risperidone treatment in post-traumatic stress disorder: a preliminary controlled trial of effects on comorbid psychotic symptoms. Int Clin Psychopharmacol 18:1–8, 2003

Hofmann SG, Meuret AE, Smits JA, et al: Augmentation of exposure therapy with D-cycloserine for social anxiety disorder. Arch Gen Psychiatry 63:298–304, 2006

Kinzie JD, Friedman MJ: Psychopharmacology for refugee and asylum seeker patients, in Broken Spirits: The Treatment of Asylum Seekers and Refugees With PTSD. Edited by Wilson JP, Drozdek B. New York, Brunner-Routledge Press, 2004, pp 579–600

Kolb LC, Burris BC, Griffiths S: Propranolol and clonidine in the treatment of the chronic post-traumatic stress disorders of war, in Posttraumatic Stress Disorder: Psychological and Biological Sequelae. Edited by van der Kolk BA. Washington, DC, American Psychiatric Press, 1984, pp 97–107

Kosten TR, Frank JB, Dan E, et al: Pharmacotherapy for posttraumatic stress disorder using phenelzine or imipramine. J Nerv Ment Dis 179:366–370, 1991

Lewis JD: Mirtazapine for PTSD nightmares (letter). Am J Psychiatry 159:1948–1949, 2002

Londborg PD, Hegel MT, Goldstein S, et al: Sertraline treatment of posttraumatic stress disorder: results of weeks of open-label continuation treatment. J Clin Psychiatry 62:325–331, 2001

Marshall RD, Beebe KL, Oldham M, et al: Efficacy and safety of paroxetine treatment for chronic PTSD: a fixed-dose, placebo-controlled study. Am J Psychiatry 158:1982–1988, 2001

Martényi F, Brown EB, Zhang H, et al: Fluoxetine versus placebo in posttraumatic stress disorder. J Clin Psychiatry 63:199–206, 2002a

Martényi F, Brown EB, Zhang H, et al: Fluoxetine v. placebo in prevention of relapse in post-traumatic stress disorder. Br J Psychiatry 181:315–320, 2002b

Mellman TA, Bustamante V, David D, et al: Hypnotic medication in the aftermath of trauma (letter). J Clin Psychiatry 63:1183–1184, 2002

Monnelly EP, Ciraulo DA, Knapp C, et al: Low-dose risperidone as adjunctive therapy for irritable aggression in posttraumatic stress disorder. J Clin Psychopharmacol 23:193–196, 2003

Neal LA, Shapland W, Fox C: An open trial of moclobemide in the treatment of post-traumatic stress disorder. Int Clin Psychopharmacol 12:231–237, 1997

Neumeister A, Henry S, Krystal JH: Neurocircuitry and neuroplasticity, in Handbook of PTSD: Science and Practice. Edited by Friedman MJ, Keane TM, Resick PA. New York, Guilford, 2007, pp 166–189

Neylan TC, Lenoci MA, Samuelson KW, et al: No improvement of posttraumatic stress disorder symptoms with guanfacine treatment. Am J Psychiatry 163:2186–2188, 2006

Pitman RK, Sanders KM, Zusman RM, et al: Pilot study of secondary prevention of posttraumatic stress disorder with propranolol. Biol Psychiatry 51:189–192, 2002

Rapaport MH, Endicott J, Clary CM: Posttraumatic stress disorder and quality of life: results across 64 weeks of sertraline treatment. J Clin Psychiatry 63:59–65, 2002

Raskind MA, Peskind ER, Kanter ED, et al: Reduction of nightmares and other PTSD symptoms in combat veterans by prazosin: a placebo-controlled study. Am J Psychiatry 160:371–373, 2003

Raskind MA, Peskind ER, Hoff DJ, et al: A parallel group placebo controlled study of prazosin for trauma nightmares and sleep disturbances in combat veterans with posttraumatic stress disorder. Biol Psychiatry 61:928–934, 2007

Reich DB, Winternitz S, Hennen J, et al: A preliminary study of risperidone in the treatment of posttraumatic stress disorder related to childhood abuse in women. J Clin Psychiatry 65:1601–1606, 2004

Reist C, Kauffmann CD, Haier RJ, et al: A controlled trial of desipramine in 18 men with posttraumatic stress disorder. Am J Psychiatry 146:513–516, 1989

Ressler KJ, Rothbaum BO, Tannenbaum L, et al: Cognitive enhancers as adjuncts to psychotherapy: use of D-cycloserine in phobic individuals to facilitate extinction of fear. Arch Gen Psychiatry 61:1136–1144, 2004

Robert RS, Blakeney PE, Villarreal C, et al: Imipramine treatment in pediatric burn patients with symptoms of acute stress disorder: a pilot study. J Am Acad Child Adolesc Psychiatry 38:873–882, 1999

Rosen CS, Chow HC, Finney JF, et al: VA practice patterns and practice guidelines for treating posttraumatic stress disorder. J Trauma Stress 17:213–222, 2004

Rothbaum BO: Critical parameters for D-cycloserine enhancement of cognitive-behavioral therapy for obsessive-compulsive disorder. Am J Psychiatry 165:293–296, 2008

Rothbaum BO, Cahill SP, Foa EB, et al: Augmentation of sertraline with prolonged exposure in the treatment of posttraumatic stress disorder. J Trauma Stress 19:625–638, 2006

Saygin MZ, Sungur MZ, Sabol EU, et al: Nefazodone versus sertraline in treatment of posttraumatic stress disorder. Bulletin of Clinical Psychopharmacology 12:1–5, 2002

Schelling G, Briegel J, Roozendaal B, et al: The effect of stress doses of hydrocortisone during septic shock on posttraumatic stress disorder in survivors. Biol Psychiatry 50:978–985, 2001

Schnurr PP, Green BL (eds): Trauma and Health: Physical Health Consequences of Exposure to Extreme Stress. Washington, DC, American Psychological Association, 2003

Schnurr PP, Friedman MJ, Foy DW, et al: Randomized trial of trauma-focused group therapy for posttraumatic stress disorder. Arch Gen Psychiatry 60:481–489, 2003

Shestatzky M, Greenberg D, Lerer B: A controlled trial of phenelzine in posttraumatic stress disorder. Psychiatry Res 24:149–155, 1988

Simon NM, Connor KM, Lang AJ, et al: Paroxetine CR augmentation for posttraumatic stress disorder refractory to prolonged exposure therapy. J Clin Psychiatry 69:400–405, 2008

Sokolski KN, Denson TF, Lee RT, et al: Quetiapine for treatment of refractory symptoms of combat-related post-traumatic stress disorder. Mil Med 168:486–489, 2003

Southwick SM, Davis LL, Aikins DE, et al: Neurobiological alterations associated with PTSD, in Handbook of PTSD: Science and Practice. Edited by Friedman MJ, Keane TM, Resick PA. New York, Guilford, 2007, pp 190–206

Stein MB, Kline NA, Matloff JL: Adjunctive olanzapine for SSRI-resistant combat-related PTSD: a double-blind, placebo-controlled study. Am J Psychiatry 159:1777–1779, 2002

Taylor F, Cahill L: Propranolol for reemergent posttraumatic stress disorder following an event of retraumatization: a case study. J Trauma Stress 15:433–437, 2002

Tucker P, Zaninelli R, Yehuda R, et al: Paroxetine in the treatment of chronic posttraumatic stress disorder: results of a placebo-controlled, flexible-dosage trial. J Clin Psychiatry 62:860–868, 2001

U.S. Food and Drug Administration: FDA launches a multi-pronged strategy to strengthen safeguards for children treated with antidepressant medications. FDA news release, U.S. Food and Drug Administration, October 15, 2004

Vaiva G, Ducrocq F, Jezequel K, et al: Immediate treatment with propranolol decreases posttraumatic stress disorder two months after trauma. Biol Psychiatry 54:947–949, 2003

van der Kolk BA, Dreyfuss D, Michaels MJ, et al: Fluoxetine in posttraumatic stress disorder. J Clin Psychiatry 55:517–522, 1994

7

Psychosocial Treatments

Katherine M. Iverson, Ph.D.

Kristin M. Lester, Ph.D.

Patricia A. Resick, Ph.D.

In this chapter, we provide a broad overview of the literature on psychosocial treatment research for posttraumatic stress disorder (PTSD) among adults. The vast majority of treatment outcome research has focused on adaptations of cognitive-behavioral therapy (CBT), which consistently has been shown to be efficacious in the reduction of PTSD symptoms and has been tested in more randomized controlled trials (RCTs) than other treatment procedures (Benish et al. 2008; Cahill et al. 2008). Thus, CBT interventions are the primary focus of this chapter. After providing a general overview of CBT theo-

Dr. Iverson's contribution to the writing of this manuscript was supported by a training grant from the National Institute of Mental Health (T32 MH019836) awarded to Terence M. Keane.

retical approaches, we briefly delineate specific CBT interventions and review their empirical support. In view of the abundance of CBT interventions, we review only published RCTs that uphold the highest methodological standards and target PTSD symptoms among adults. We conclude this chapter by raising awareness of future directions in several important areas pertaining to psychosocial treatments for PTSD. For a quick reference to the abbreviations used throughout this chapter to refer to psychosocial approaches for PTSD and relevant research methodology, please refer to Table 7–1.

Theoretical Foundations of Cognitive-Behavioral Treatments for PTSD

There are multiple CBT theoretical models that attempt to explain the development and maintenance of PTSD. These models represent the views of a diverse group of clinical scientists who concern themselves with different survivor populations and trauma symptoms while placing an emphasis on empiricism and processes of new learning. Although the purpose of this chapter is not to provide a unifying definition of CBT for PTSD, the theoretical models of PTSD have many similarities. These models have resulted in theoretically driven CBTs for PTSD. We describe each of the major models in the following subsections.

Learning Theories

One of the first CBT theories applied to the understanding and treatment of PTSD was Mowrer's (1960) two-factor learning theory (Keane et al. 1985; Kilpatrick et al. 1982, 1985). According to this theory, the first factor consists of a fear response (conditioned fear and other aversive emotions) that is learned through association via classical (respondent) conditioning mechanisms. The second factor consists of learned behaviors that function as avoidance or escape from cues stimulating aversive emotions via operant (instrumental) conditioning. In relating this model to PTSD, Mowrer posited that neutral cues associated with the traumatic event acquire the capacity to trigger conditioned emotional (fearful) responses even in the absence of aversive stimuli. This mechanism is meant to promote future safety and survival. However, avoidance of the conditioned stimuli is negatively reinforced, thereby preventing

Table 7–1. Abbreviations used to refer to PTSD treatment approaches and research methodologies

Abbreviation	Definition
CBCT	Cognitive-behavioral conjoint therapy
CBT	Cognitive-behavioral therapy
COMB	Combination of cognitive-behavioral intervention strategies
CPT	Cognitive processing therapy
CPT-C	Cognitive processing therapy–cognitive therapy portion only
CT	Cognitive therapy
CTT-BW	Cognitive trauma therapy for battered women
EMDR	Eye movement desensitization and reprocessing
EX	exposure therapy (or exposure-based treatment)
ITT	Intent-to-treat (analysis of clinical trial results that includes all data from participants in the groups to which they were randomized even if they never received the treatment or dropped out prematurely)
M-CET	Multiple channel exposure therapy
PCT	Present-centered therapy
Prolonged EX	Prolonged exposure therapy
PTSD	Posttraumatic stress disorder
RCT	Randomized controlled trial
RLX	Relaxation training
SC	Supportive counseling
SIT	Stress inoculation training
SPAARS	Schematic, propositional, analogue, and associative representational systems model of PTSD
STAIR	Skills training in affective and interpersonal regulation
WL	Wait-list control group

extinction of the link between the trauma cues and anxiety and thus maintaining PTSD symptoms. Strengths of Mowrer's theory (1960) include the fact that it is relatively uncomplicated and parsimonious. Additionally, learning theory accounts for much of the development and maintenance of fear and avoidance symptoms in PTSD; however, it does not fully explain other PTSD symptoms, specifically intrusive symptoms or the development of other strong emotions. Nor does this model account for individual factors, such as childhood experiences, that predate the trauma and may impact the likelihood of developing PTSD.

Keane and Barlow (2002) developed a comprehensive learning model of the etiology of PTSD. This model builds on Mowrer's (1960) two-factor learning theory by accounting for individual differences in terms of childhood experiences that may also impact stress responses. According to this model, individuals carry various psychological and biological vulnerabilities into the traumatic exposure. At the time of the traumatic event, individuals experience a "true alarm," in which their physiology is highly active and they experience strong basic emotions, such as fear, anxiety, and anger, in addition to thoughts about what is happening to them or someone else. These true alarms subsequently lead to "learned alarms," in which individuals experience ("reexperience") similar physiological, emotional, and cognitive responses to situations that symbolize or resemble an aspect of the traumatic event. The learned alarms then lead to a general anxious apprehension (i.e., hyperarousal symptoms) about reexperiencing symptoms, which results in avoidance of thoughts, feelings, or memories of the event. Over time, such avoidance of learned alarms may lead to a general shutdown of emotional responsiveness, typically referred to as numbing symptoms. These avoidance strategies, in turn, maintain the PTSD symptoms (Resick et al. 2007). Many CBT evidence-based exposure interventions for PTSD can be understood from this model.

Information and Emotional Processing Theories

Numerous CBT clinical scientists have highlighted the important role of cognitive factors and schemas in the development and maintenance of PTSD symptoms (Brewin et al. 1996; Chemtob et al. 1988; Foa et al. 1989; Resick and Schnicke 1993; Resick et al. 2007). Drawing on Lang's (1977) information processing theory of anxiety development, Foa et al. (1989) suggested that PTSD emerges secondary to the mechanisms by which trauma-related information is encoded and recalled (Foa and Kozak 1986; Foa et al. 1989). Fear structures contain information about the feared stimulus, including information about verbal, physiological, and overt behavioral responses, as well as interpretive information about the meaning of stimulus and response elements of the fear structure (Foa et al. 1989). This theory posits that during trauma, information processing is interrupted and, as a result, traumatic memories are disorganized and fragmented. Over time, trauma survivors encounter situations that activate their trauma memory structures. When the fear network is subsequently activated by trauma cues, the information in the network enters consciousness, resulting in reexperiencing symptoms (i.e., intrusive thoughts, flashbacks, and emotional distress). For most trauma survivors, natural recovery occurs because the survivor learns that these situations during which the fear structures are activated are safe and the feared consequences (e.g., repeat trauma) do not occur. These experiences lead to habituation to the intrusive symptoms and allow for corrective information to be incorporated into the fear structures (i.e., emotional processing).

According to Foa and Kozak (1986), an inability to emotionally process the traumatic memory leads to the development of chronic PTSD. This inability to process the trauma results from inadequate activation of the fear structure and/or a failure to incorporate corrective information into the fear network when activated. Understandably, individuals who have experienced a trauma may attempt to avoid activation of these processes; however, such attempts at avoiding activation result in the avoidance symptoms of PTSD, which in turn maintains PTSD. One important limitation of emotional processing theory is its emphasis on fear as the primary emotion underlying the development and maintenance of PTSD; however, other emotions, such as anger, guilt, and shame, are also relevant to the development and maintenance of PTSD (Brewin et al. 2000; Rizvi et al. 2008).

Cognitive Theories

The cognitive theories are also concerned with information and emotional processing; however, cognitive theories focus primarily on the impact of trauma on a person's beliefs about the self, other people, and the world (Ehlers and Clark 2000; McCann and Pearlman 1990; Resick and Schnicke 1992, 1993; Resick et al. 2007). Ehlers and Clark (2000) proposed a cognitive model of PTSD, emphasizing cognitions pertaining to perceptions of current and future threat. According to this model, PTSD becomes chronic when individuals appraise the event or its sequelae in a manner that suggests they are in danger. In turn, the traumatized individuals tend to overgeneralize from the event and overestimate the probability of a similar event occurring in the future.

In theories based on Jean Piaget's concepts, Hollon and Garber (1988) and Resick and colleagues (Resick and Schnicke 1992; Resick et al. 2008b) posited that there are two ways to respond to event information. Individuals may assimilate the information, by which they maintain their previous schemas either because the event matches those schemas or by distorting the event in order to match those previous beliefs (Resick et al. 2008b). Conversely, individuals may accommodate the information, which occurs when an event is schema discrepant and individuals must alter their preexisting beliefs about themselves and the world in order to incorporate and accept this new information. Accommodation represents balanced thinking and acceptance of the traumatic event. Resick and Schnicke (1992, 1993) proposed that overaccommodation results when individuals modify the information excessively, resulting in maladaptive overgeneralizations about themselves or the world. Both assimilation and overaccommodation can result in manufactured (secondary) emotions, such as guilt and shame. Therefore, social-cognitive models focus not only on natural (primary) emotions (e.g., fear, sadness), but also on secondary emotional responses, such as shame, that may result from cognitive distortions. Despite the emphasis on thoughts and emotions stemming from the traumatic event, Cahill and Foa (2007) suggested that cognitive theories do not place enough emphasis on the role of avoidance and the importance of confronting traumatic memories.

Dual-Representation Theory

Dual-representation theory attempts to integrate the information processing and social-cognitive theories (Brewin et al. 1996). It also emphasizes the importance of primary emotions (e.g., fear), which are conditioned during the trauma, and secondary emotions (e.g., shame, anger), which result from the "meaning" elements stemming from cognitive processes following the traumatic event. Additionally, the dual-representation theory suggests that memories of traumatic events are stored in two ways. Some memories are "verbally accessed," which refers to autobiographical information the individual attended to before, during, and after the trauma that received sufficient conscious attention to be stored in long-term memory. These memories are more readily retrieved from memory. Other memories are "situationally accessed"; these include nonconscious sensory information about the traumatic event that cannot be deliberately accessed or easily modified. Thus, successful emotional processing ("integration") necessitates activation of both the verbally and situationally accessed memories. During activation of these memories, resolution of schema conflicts can occur through a conscious search for meaning, which also leads to reductions in strong negative affect. It remains to be seen whether dual-representation theory provides a better account of PTSD than other available models.

In the SPAARS model of PTSD, Dalgleish (2004) proposed four levels of mental representation systems: the Schematic, Propositional, Analogue, and Associative Representational Systems. The model expands on the dual-representation theory and incorporates many of the previous theories of PTSD. The SPAARS model accounts for the processing of trauma-related information during the time of a traumatic event and explains how this information and the individual's reactions to it are processed in various mental representational systems following the event, thereby contributing to the development of PTSD. At the time of the traumatic event, the individual appraises information at the schematic level in a threat-related manner due to the intense fear associated with the event. At the same time, the person's thoughts and sensory information, such as sounds and images, are stored at the propositional and analogue levels. Propositional-level information is memory that is verbally accessible, whereas analogue information may not be verbally accessible but rather presents in the form of reexperiencing symptoms in response to trauma cues. Associative representations are similar to the fear structures hypothesized in emotional processing theory and represent the connections between other types of mental representations. Trauma-related information is incongruent with previous beliefs about one's self, the world, and others. As such, this information is poorly integrated into representations during encoding. The trauma memory exists across different levels of mental representation but is not fully incorporated with other mental representations. Because the memory of the traumatic event represents an ongoing threat to goals, the person is left with high vulnerability to fear activation, cognitive biases toward attending to threat appraisals, intrusive symptoms, and cognitive distortions. Such strong memory, emotional intrusions, and cognitive biases result in efforts to cope through avoidance. Despite the comprehensive nature of the SPAARS model of PTSD, research is needed to determine its precision in accounting for the development and maintenance of PTSD.

Summary

These cognitive-behavioral theoretical models of the etiology and maintenance of PTSD have yielded productive and theoretically driven approaches to the psychosocial treatment of PTSD. Similarly, these theories have driven the research into the clinical efficacy of CBT for PTSD. Before reviewing the research on treatment outcome for PTSD, we describe some of the widely studied treatment protocols below.

CBT Treatments and Techniques for PTSD

Five predominant forms of CBT treatments for PTSD have been well defined and systematically studied: coping skills–focused treatments; exposure-based treatments; eye movement desensitization and reprocessing (EMDR); cognitive therapy; and combinations, which typically consist of some portion of a combination of CBT approaches, such as exposure-based treatment, cognitive therapy, and coping skills. These treatment approaches directly address the sequelae following exposure to a traumatic event and are the primary empirically supported CBT treatments used with trauma survivors. We briefly describe each of these treatment types.

Coping Skills–Focused Interventions

Stress Inoculation Training

Stress inoculation training (SIT) was originally developed by Meichenbaum (1974) as a general anxiety management treatment and subsequently modified to treat rape survivors (Kilpatrick et al. 1982). SIT is a flexible approach that can be tailored to problems faced by each individual patient and can be delivered in an individual or group format. The theory underlying SIT emphasizes anxiety responses that become conditioned during the traumatic exposure and then generalize to other situations. SIT is essentially training in fear management techniques, including relaxation and cognitive coping strategies. The treatment protocol consists of three phases: education, anxiety management skills building, and application and generalization of skills. Anxiety management skills include muscle relaxation, breathing retraining, role-playing, covert modeling, self-dialogue, graduated in vivo exposure, and thought stopping. As part of SIT, the patient is taught to visualize a fearful stimulus and to imagine confronting it successfully. Patients learn to manage anxiety by using these new skills, thereby reducing avoidance and allowing opportunities for the habituation of anxiety responses.

Relaxation Training

Relaxation training (RLX) has been used to treat PTSD as part of a comprehensive program, such as SIT. It has also been used as a primary mode of intervention as a comparison treatment modality in a handful of studies (discussed in the treatment outcome research section below). Similar to SIT, RLX is intended to help patients learn to reduce their anxiety, particularly anxiety and distress elicited by trauma-related stimuli.

Exposure Therapy

Exposure therapy (EX) is another form of CBT. The various types of EX, including flooding, imaginal, in vivo, and directed exposure therapy, have distinguishing features; however, in this chapter, for the purpose of maintaining consistency, we use the term *exposure therapy* broadly. Generally, in EX, the patient engages in exposure to anxiety-provoking stimuli without engaging in relaxation or other anxiety-reducing strategies. There are many derivations of the delivery of EX.

Most EX interventions are modeled on the prolonged EX protocol of Foa and co-workers (Foa et al. 1991, 2007; Rothbaum and Foa 1992), which is conducted in 9 to 12 individual weekly or biweekly 90-minute sessions. Prolonged EX consists of four components: education/rationale, breathing retraining, behavioral EX, and imaginal EX. The first two sessions cover assessment, treatment planning, and explanation of the rationale for exposure, as well as breathing retraining. Additionally, a hierarchy of uncomfortable stimuli (i.e., feared and avoided) is generated. Patients are then asked to confront fear cues for at least 45 minutes a day, starting with a moderately anxiety-provoking stimulus. Beginning with the third session, the patient reviews homework assignments; participates in imaginal exposure for 45–60 minutes (while reliving the trauma scene imaginally, the patient is asked to describe it aloud in the present tense); and finally processes the exposure with nondirective statements (e.g., education about trauma reactions, normalizing reactions, reiterating the rationale for exposure). The patient determines the level of detail for the first two sessions, but thereafter the therapist encourages further details, such as thoughts, physiological responses, and feared consequences. Imaginal exposure therapy sessions are recorded, and patients are assigned homework to listen to the tape and allow their emotional arousal to increase while listening to their account. At the end of each session, the therapist and patient ensure significant reduction of session-induced anxiety prior to the patient's departure (Foa et al. 2007).

Eye Movement Desensitization and Reprocessing

EMDR has received increasing attention from both clinicians and researchers. It involves a number of techniques, including imaginal EX (Shapiro 1995). The patient is instructed to recall trauma-related memories and associated features (i.e., negative thoughts) while attending to external oscillatory stimulation. This stimulation is typically in the form of lateral eye movements induced by the therapist's moving his or her finger across the patient's visual field. Specifically, the patient is instructed to select 1) a disturbing image associated with the traumatic memory, 2) a negative thought associated with the memory, and 3) bodily sensations associated with the memory. The patient is asked to keep these features in awareness during the eye movement procedures. This process is continued until the distress associated with the memory decreases and new adaptive cognitions are installed regarding the experience. This new material becomes the focus on each new set of eye movements, and new adaptive behaviors, coping strategies, and alternative cognitions arise.

Cognitive Therapy

Cognitive therapy (CT), originally developed by Beck (1976) for the treatment of depression, seeks to modify maladaptive or dysfunctional interpretations that result in negative emotional states. In cognitive therapies, patients and therapists collaboratively identify and challenge maladaptive thoughts with the goal of replacing them with more balanced, healthy cognitions. CT has been adapted for the treatment of anxiety disorders, including PTSD (Ehlers and Clark 2000; Ehlers et al. 2003; Marks et al. 1998; Tarrier et al. 1999).

Cognitive processing therapy (CPT) is one type of cognitive therapy that has been tested in several RCTs. CPT is a 12-session manualized CT developed by Resick and colleagues (Resick and Schnicke 1993; Resick et al. 2008b) for the treatment of PTSD. The overall goals of CPT are to help patients identify what assumptions and interpretations about the event have interfered with recovery from PTSD and systematically process their trauma. Using the original protocol, patients are given two major writing assignments to help them identify and challenge "stuck points" (distorted or unrealistic beliefs regarding the event itself) and to facilitate processing of the traumatic event and its impact. In the first major assignment, the impact statement, the patient writes why the trauma happened and its impact on five major themes (safety, trust, power/control, esteem, and intimacy) found to be significantly disrupted for patients with PTSD (McCann and Pearlman 1990; Owens et al. 2001). The second major writing assignment, the trauma account, is a description of the traumatic event, including thoughts and feelings at the time of the event and as much sensory detail as possible. Early on, there is a greater focus on using Socratic dialogue to examine assimilated stuck points, often reflecting aspects of undoing and blame. As treatment progresses, the focus turns to overaccommodated stuck points and overgeneralized negative beliefs that reflect current and futuristic thinking about self and others. During the course of treatment, stuck points are targeted through in- and out-of-session practice worksheets designed to help patients challenge distorted beliefs and generate alternative statements for the purpose of reducing associated negative emotional states. A recent adaptation of the CPT protocol by Resick et al. (2008a) has eliminated the written account portion of treatment (which resembles EX approaches) and, therefore, CPT can be considered a type of cognitive therapy.

Combination Treatments and Additive Treatments

Combination treatments have been developed as an intended aggregation of therapies or may reflect additive studies in which a new component is added to an existing treatment to determine if the extra component adds value to an existing therapy. For example, Cloitre et al. (2002, 2006) proposed that victims of child abuse, in addition to their PTSD, have problems related to affect regulation and interpersonal effectiveness that compromise their ability to fully benefit from trauma-focused interventions. Thus, these authors developed a protocol, called skills training in affective and interpersonal regulation (STAIR), that included treatment for these problems prior to implementing a modification of EX (Foa et al. 2007). In the first phase of the intervention, therapists assist the patients in learning emotion management and interpersonal skills for 8 weeks; the second phase of treatment involves imaginal EX. The imaginal EX phase also includes post-exposure emotional management and CT.

Treatment Outcome Research in PTSD

Extensive clinical research efforts over the past two decades have resulted in a number of evidence-based treatments for adults with PTSD. Within the last decade, treatment outcome studies for PTSD have incorporated more rigorous methodology to ensure the validity of inferences drawn from the findings. Foa and Meadows (1997) outlined seven features of well-controlled trials: 1) clearly defined treatment targets (symptoms); 2) reliable and valid measures; 3) use of blind/independent evaluators; 4) reliable and valid assessor training; 5) manualized, replicable, specific treatment programs; 6) unbiased (randomized) assignment to treatment; and 7) treatment adherence. Randomized group assignment, blind assessments, and credible comparison groups reduce the risk of bias in treatment outcome research (Harvey et al. 2003). Foa et al. (2008) outlined two additions to these original gold standards of treatment outcome research for PTSD. The first addition is the inclusion of intent-to-treat (ITT) analyses. ITT analyses include everyone who was randomized into the trial and do not rely on last observation carried forward (Institute of Medicine 2008). The second addition is the comparability of therapist background, experience, allegiance, and training and supervision for all treatments in comparative outcome trials, with the goal of increasing the credibility of comparison groups and improving the strength of significant effects for treatment approaches. Excellent discussions of treatment outcome methodology for PTSD are also provided by Resick et al. (2007) and Schnurr (2007).

Finally, research designs should include enough statistical power to detect clinically meaningful treatment effects. Sufficient statistical power can be accomplished either with large enough sample sizes to obtain medium to small effect sizes when comparing two active treatments or by obtaining enough data points to ensure sufficient power using longitudinal analysis methods, such as mixed effects regression analysis or hierarchical linear modeling. Unfortunately, thus far the only studies in the PTSD field that have accomplished this goal are those of Resick et al. (2002, 2008a) and Schnurr et al. (2003, 2007). The rest of the studies reviewed here were only powered for large effect size differences. Studies finding no differences between two active treatments are subject to the alternative explanation of an insufficient sample size to detect a meaningful difference.

Each treatment outcome study evaluated in this chapter is examined in light of these methodological standards. Due to the large number of treatment outcome studies for PTSD, we review only those studies that were RCTs with 30 or more participants and that met five or more standards of treatment outcome research in PTSD as defined by Foa and colleagues (Foa and Meadows 1997; Foa et al. 2008). Because RCTs for PTSD have focused on treating PTSD associated with a wide range of traumatic exposure types, each section below is organized by type of trauma. Although not exhaustive, Table 7–2 provides a general overview of the primary CBT interventions for PTSD, the trauma populations studied, and a summary of evidence for each approach.

Interpersonal Victimization

Physical and Sexual Assault and Abuse

A number of the most methodologically sound studies have examined PTSD secondary to interpersonal assault victimization occurring in childhood and/or adulthood. Several of these studies have compared EX to SIT, CT, or some combination of various CBTs for survivors of interpersonal victimization. In one of the first methodologically rigorous RCTs for PTSD, Foa et al. (1991) compared EX to a modified SIT, supportive counseling (SC), and a wait-list (WL) control group for 55 female rape survivors. All patients were seen individually, and 45 participants completed treatment. To prevent overlapping techniques in their comparison, Foa et al. eliminated the in vivo EX component (confronting feared cues) from SIT. Completer analyses revealed significant improvements from pretreatment to posttreatment for all three active treatments. SIT was found to be the most effective treatment modality at posttreatment in reducing PTSD symptoms, anxiety, and depression. The small sample size in the completer sample may have limited the power to find an effect for one treatment over the others. At a 3.5-month follow-up, however,

Table 7–2. Overview of cognitive-behavioral therapies for PTSD[a]

	Coping skills–focused therapy	Exposure-based interventions	EMDR	Cognitive interventions	Combination/additive approaches
Overall goals of the class of interventions	Reduction of PTSD symptoms, particularly anxiety and distress elicited by trauma-related stimuli Typically involves training in fear management techniques, to include relaxation, SIT, and cognitive coping strategies	Reduction of PTSD symptoms through imaginal and/or behavioral exposure to anxiety-provoking trauma-related stimuli without engaging in relaxation or other anxiety-reducing strategies	Reduction of PTSD symptoms through imaginal exposure to trauma-related memories and associated features (i.e., negative thoughts) Imaginal exposure conducted while patient is attending to external oscillatory stimulation, typically in the form of lateral eye movement induced by the therapist moving his or her finger across the patient's visual field	Reduction of PTSD symptoms by modifying trauma-based maladaptive or dysfunctional interpretations resulting in negative emotional states	Intended aggregation of therapies such as EX and SIT. Also reflects additive studies in which a new component is added to an existing treatment to determine if the extra component adds value.

Table 7–2. Overview of cognitive-behavioral therapies for PTSD[a] *(continued)*

	Coping skills–focused therapy	Exposure-based interventions	EMDR	Cognitive interventions	Combination/additive approaches
Trauma populations studied	Interpersonal victimization, mixed trauma samples	Interpersonal victimization, military-related trauma, natural disasters, mixed trauma samples	Interpersonal victimization, mixed trauma samples	Interpersonal victimization, military-related trauma, motor vehicle accidents, refugees, mixed trauma samples	Interpersonal victimization, motor vehicle accidents, mixed trauma samples
RCTs supporting this approach	Foa et al. 1991, 1999	Basoglu et al. 2005; Foa et al. 1991, 1999, 2005; Neuner et al. 2004; Schnurr et al. 2007; Tarrier et al. 1999; Taylor et al. 2003	Power et al. 2002; Rothbaum et al. 2005; Vaughan et al. 1994	Bryant et al. 2008; Duffy et al. 2007; Ehlers et al. 2003; Kubany et al. 2003, 2004; Monson et al. 2006; Resick et al. 2002, 2008a; Tarrier and Sommerfield 2004; Tarrier et al. 1999	Blanchard et al. 2003; Bryant et al. 2003; Cloitre et al. 2002, 2004; Hinton et al. 2005; Maercker et al. 2006

Table 7–2. Overview of cognitive-behavioral therapies for PTSD[a] *(continued)*

	Coping skills–focused therapy	Exposure-based interventions	EMDR	Cognitive interventions	Combination/additive approaches
Unique findings		EX has been evaluated in 25 RCTs for PTSD. It has support for its use across a wide range of traumatized populations. Prolonged EX is effective in reducing symptoms of complex PTSD (Resick et al. 2003).	EMDR and EX have been found effective at reducing PTSD symptoms; however, participants with multiple comorbidities did not fare as well with EMDR (Rothbaum et al. 2005).	In treatment of rape victims, CPT compared with prolonged EX has been shown to be particularly effective at reducing guilt (Resick et al. 2002) as well as health symptoms (Galovski et al. 2009). In a dismantling study of CPT for treatment of rape victims, the full CPT protocol did not differ from either of the two components (written account vs. CT alone), suggesting that CT without direct reexperiencing of the traumatic memory can be effective (Resick et al. 2008a).	Mixed results have been reported regarding the benefit of augmenting EX with CT among mixed trauma samples (Bryant et al. 2008; Foa et al. 2005; Marks et al. 1998).

Table 7–2. Overview of cognitive-behavioral therapies for PTSD[a] *(continued)*

Note. CPT=cognitive processing therapy; CT=cognitive therapy; EMDR=eye movement desensitization and reprocessing; EX=exposure-based therapy; prolonged EX=prolonged exposure therapy; RCT=randomized controlled trial; SIT=stress inoculation training.

[a]Studies reviewed were methodologically sound and mostly found large pretreatment to posttreatment changes in PTSD, clearly demonstrating that CBT is an effective treatment for PTSD for a wide range of traumas. Generally, in comparative treatment studies, no large differences were found when two active PTSD treatments were compared to one another (i.e., EX vs. EMDR or CPT).

there was a trend toward EX showing greater efficacy than the other modalities. It is notable that this study also found no significant differences across therapists in treatment outcome.

Foa et al. (1999) then conducted an additive study in which they compared EX, modified SIT, and a combination of EX and SIT in treating 96 female sexual and nonsexual assault survivors with PTSD. Seventy-nine participants completed treatment. Results indicated that the combination did not improve the results over EX or SIT alone. However, the combination may have performed at less than optimal levels due to treatment design, given that participants only received half as much EX or SIT as participants in the groups receiving only EX or SIT. Similar to the study by Foa et al. (1991), this study is likely underpowered due to the small sample size, which was probably insufficient to find small and medium effect sizes (Resick et al. 2007).

In another small additive study, Bryant et al. (2003) compared imaginal EX, imaginal EX+CT, and SC in treating 58 males and females with chronic PTSD following a physical assault (n=31) or motor vehicle accident (MVA) (n=27). Forty-five participants completed treatment. Results from the completer analyses indicated that both of the EX modalities led to more improvement than SC; however, this finding did not hold in the ITT analyses, which found no differences among the three treatment groups. Completer analyses did indicate, however, that EX+CT appeared to have the added benefit of reducing intrusion symptoms and depression. Treatment gains were maintained at a 6-month follow-up.

Kubany et al. (2003) developed a treatment for PTSD, cognitive trauma therapy for battered women (CTT-BW), and have tested its efficacy in two RCTs. CTT-BW is used to treat formerly battered women with extensive CT as well as EX. In the first study, Kubany et al. (2003) assigned 37 female survivors of domestic violence with PTSD to a CTT-BW group or a WL control group. ITT analyses indicated a reduction of PTSD symptoms in the CTT-BW group relative to the WL group. CTT-BW also resulted in decreased depression, trauma-related guilt, and shame, as well as increased self-esteem. Participants in the WL group were subsequently given the active treatment, leading to replication of the findings. Results were maintained at a 3-month follow-up.

In a subsequent larger trial, Kubany et al. (2004) assigned 125 female survivors of domestic violence with PTSD to a CTT-BW group or a WL control group. Replicating their previous study results (Kubany et al. 2003), ITT analyses indicated that compared with the WL group, the CTT-BW group experienced a reduction in PTSD, depression, trauma-related guilt, and shame, and improved self-esteem. Participants in the WL group were subsequently given CTT-BW, leading to another replication of the findings. Results were maintained at both 3-month and 6-month follow-ups.

Foa et al. (2005) compared EX, EX+CT, and WL conditions in 179 female sexual or physical assault survivors treated in either a community rape crisis center or an academic treatment center. ITT analyses with last observation carried forward indicated that both the EX and EX+CT conditions were superior to the WL in reducing PTSD and depression. However, in contrast to other studies demonstrating an additive effect for EX+CT (e.g., Bryant et al. 2003), Foa et al. (2005) found no significant differences in outcomes between EX and EX+CT, indicating that they performed equally well. An important innovation in the Foa et al. study was the use of a flexible dosing rule, in which participants who achieved at least a 70% reduction of self-reported PTSD severity by session 8 were scheduled to terminate at session 9. The remaining participants were offered additional sessions (up to five more sessions). Among participants who received additional sessions (58% of the original sample), participants tended to experience additional improvements between session 8 and their final session.

In another well-controlled RCT, 74 female rape survivors with PTSD were randomly assigned to EMDR, EX, or a WL group (Rothbaum et al. 2005). ITT analyses indicated that both treatments were very effective at reducing PTSD symptoms. There were no differences between EMDR and EX in PTSD outcome at posttreatment or at 6-month follow-up. Participants with multiple comorbidities, however, did not fare as well with EMDR as the EX participants with similar comorbidities, suggesting that EX may have targeted more underlying psychopathology.

In a large, well-controlled study, Resick et al. (2002) randomly assigned 171 female rape survivors to cognitive processing therapy (CPT), EX, or a WL control group. ITT analyses with mixed effects regression indicated that both CPT and EX were very effective in reducing PTSD symptoms relative to the WL. Participants in the WL group were subsequently randomly assigned to one of the two active treatments, allowing for a replication of the initial findings. A small effect size (i.e., strength of treatment effect) difference favored

CPT over EX. Additionally, CPT was superior in reducing aspects of guilt among rape survivors. Of note, secondary analyses indicated significant decreases in depressive symptoms, anger, and dissociation with both CPT and EX modalities (Resick et al. 2003), and CPT was found to be superior with regard to perceived health (Galovski et al. 2009). Such findings suggest the utility of CPT and EX in addressing complex comorbid problems common among interpersonal trauma survivors.

More recently, Resick et al. (2008a) conducted another well-controlled RCT, in which 150 female sexual and/or physical assault survivors were randomly assigned to either full CPT, a CT-only version of CPT (CPT-C), or a written account in a dismantling study of CPT. Dismantling studies are designed to evaluate the primary active components of treatment relative to the full package of treatment, with the goal of determining the necessary and sufficient aspects of a particular therapy. In this dismantling study, ITT analyses indicated that all three versions of treatment resulted in significant reductions in PTSD symptoms. All three interventions also resulted in reduced depression, anxiety, anger, trauma-related cognitions, guilt, and shame. Results were maintained at a 6-month follow-up. It is important to note that the CPT-C intervention performed significantly better than the written account intervention in reducing PTSD. The full CPT protocol did not differ from either of the two components, suggesting that the CT condition alone was effective and the written account component may not be necessary for reducing PTSD. The findings from this study are consistent with those of the earlier studies of Marks et al. (1998) and Tarrier et al. (1999) and a more recent Ehlers et al. (2003) study, reviewed below, which found CT without an emphasis on EX to be effective in reducing PTSD.

To summarize, each of the studies reviewed above was methodologically sound and found large pretreatment to posttreatment changes in PTSD. The data clearly demonstrate that CBT is an effective treatment for PTSD subsequent to interpersonal violence, including physical and sexual assault or abuse. Generally, in comparative treatment studies, no large differences were found when two active PTSD treatments were compared with one another (i.e., EX vs. EMDR or CPT). For one study, the addition of CT to EX led to greater improvements in outcomes (Bryant et al. 2003); however, Foa et al. (1999) did not find the addition of CT to enhance treatment outcomes for EX.

Child Sexual and Physical Abuse

Several RCTs have demonstrated the efficacy of CBT approaches designed specifically for childhood sexual and/or physical abuse survivors. Chard (2005) developed and tested an adaptation of CPT (Resick and Schnicke 1993; Resick et al. 2008b) and compared it with a WL control. This adaptation of CPT includes a combination of group and individual treatment, with the processing of written accounts occurring in individual treatment and cognitive interventions conducted in a group context. This adaptation of CPT also adds group modules that focus on developmental issues, communication skills, and social support seeking. Of 71 female survivors of childhood sexual abuse with PTSD who began the study, 55 participants completed the study. Completer analyses indicated that compared with the WL group, participants treated with the 17-week CPT intervention experienced clinically significant improvements in PTSD, often resulting in full remission. Additionally, treatment gains were maintained at the 1-year follow-up.

Cloitre et al. (2002) assigned 58 adult female survivors of childhood physical and/or sexual abuse to either a two-phase treatment composed of 8 weekly individual therapy sessions using STAIR, followed by eight twice-weekly sessions of imaginal EX, or a WL control. Forty-six participants completed treatment. Completer analyses indicated that compared with WL controls, participants completing the STAIR and EX treatment experienced significantly greater reductions on measures of PTSD severity. Additionally, the intervention resulted in decreased anger expression, dissociation, alexithymia (i.e., the inability to accurately label and express emotions), depression, and anxiety, as well as an increased ability to regulate negative affect. Additional analyses indicated that the STAIR portion of treatment was most useful in reducing anger, depression, and anxiety, and in improving negative mood regulation. Importantly, this portion of the treatment did not lead to significant reductions in PTSD symptoms. The EX portion, however, was effective in reducing PTSD symptoms, dissociation, and alexithymia. The authors also found that participants continued to improve at 3- and 9-month follow-ups. In a secondary analysis of this study, Cloitre et al. (2004) found that early formation of a therapeutic alliance led to greater affect regulation in Phase 1 (STAIR), which resulted in better treatment outcome following EX.

In another well-controlled trial, McDonagh et al. (2005) randomly assigned 74 female survivors of childhood sexual abuse with PTSD to one of three conditions: a combination (COMB) intervention of EX and CT, a present-centered therapy (PCT), or a WL control. PCT specifically excluded CBT interventions while focusing on here-and-now problem solving. Fifty-seven participants completed treatment. Completer analyses indicated that both active treatments were superior to WL in reducing PTSD, anxiety, and trauma-related cognitions; however, there may have been too little power to detect differences between the COMB and PCT conditions due to the high rate (41.4%) of treatment noncompletion in the COMB condition relative to PCT and WL. The ITT analyses indicated that PCT was superior to the WL in terms of reducing trauma-related cognitions. Treatment gains were maintained at 3- and 6-month follow-ups. Significantly fewer participants in the COMB modality continued to meet criteria for PTSD at the follow-up assessments, indicating that although both treatments were effective in reducing PTSD, the COMB treatment appeared to be superior in sustaining recovery. Compared with noncompletion rates of similar PTSD studies, the high dropout rate in this study suggests that women were less able or willing to complete the particular CBT protocol used in this study (e.g., Chard 2005; Foa et al. 1991, 1999; Marks et al. 1998; Resick et al. 2002, 2008a).

Other RCTs in childhood sexual abuse samples have upheld various standards of treatment outcome research. In a study involving 48 adult female child sexual abuse survivors with PTSD, Zlotnick et al. (1997) compared an affect management group intervention based on dialectical behavior therapy skills (Linehan 1993) with a WL control. Weaknesses of the study design include 1) the lack of clinician ratings of PTSD severity administered by a blind evaluator at posttreatment and 2) no report of treatment adherence. The content of the group sessions focused on education and practice of various emotion regulation skills, including emotion identification and labeling, anger management, self-soothing, and distress tolerance. Thirty-three participants completed treatment. Completer analyses indicated that compared with the WL condition, the group treatment resulted in superior reductions in self-reported PTSD severity and dissociation.

Bradley and Follingstad (2003) compared a group COMB treatment and a WL control for 49 incarcerated women with histories of exposure to childhood sexual and/or physical abuse. The COMB sessions consisted of education and teaching of affect regulation skills, followed by sessions focused on structured writing assignments. The writing assignments were designed not to function as exposure to traumatic events, but instead to help the women examine associations between past experiences (including trauma) and current feelings. Completer analyses revealed greater improvement in six out of seven trauma symptoms for the 31 participants who completed the study than for the WL control group.

Motor Vehicle Accidents

A few well-controlled studies have examined the treatment of PTSD resulting from MVAs. Blanchard et al. (2003) compared a COMB intervention (combination of EX and some CT), to SC and a WL control with 98 men and women with PTSD or subsyndromal PTSD following an MVA within the past 6–24 months. Sixty-eight participants completed treatment. Completer and ITT analyses indicated that the COMB treatment was superior to either the SC or the WL control on measures of PTSD, depression, and anxiety. These results were maintained at a 3-month follow-up. A very similar study conducted by Maercker et al. (2006) compared the COMB treatment used by Blanchard et al. (2003), with additional emphasis on CT, with a WL control for 48 male and female MVA survivors. Forty-two participants completed treatment. The completer analyses indicated that the COMB treatment was superior to WL on reductions in PTSD, depression, anxiety, and trauma-related cognitions. These gains were maintained at a 3-month follow-up.

In another study of MVA survivors, Ehlers et al. (2003) compared CT, a self-help booklet (consisting of CBT principles and psychoeducation), and repeated assessments with 97 men and women after a 3-week period of self-monitoring. Eighty participants completed treatment. Completer analyses indicated that a small percentage of patients (12%) improved with self-monitoring alone. Those with persistent PTSD symptoms were randomly assigned to one of the three groups approximately 3 months after an MVA. CT was far superior to both the self-help booklet and the repeated assessment conditions, which both showed improvement but were not significantly different from each other in terms of outcome. Additionally, the CT group did not have any dropouts. This study used a structured interview of PTSD administered by blind, independent assessors; however, because the authors did not report on treatment fidelity, it is unknown if CT was delivered as it was meant to be delivered. Overall, findings from these studies indicate that CT participants experienced greater benefit than those in self-help and WL groups.

Mixed Trauma Samples

Several well-controlled studies have been conducted with mixed trauma samples. Tarrier et al. (1999) compared imaginal EX with CT in a study of 72 men and women with chronic PTSD. Sixty-two participants completed treatment. Both treatments resulted in reductions in PTSD and depressive symptoms; however, the investigators did not find a difference between the two treatment conditions at posttreatment or follow-up. In the longest PTSD treatment follow-up study to date, Tarrier and Sommerfield (2004) completed a 5-year follow-up and were able to reassess 52% of their original sample. Interestingly, they found that none of the patients who received CT were diagnosed with PTSD at this 5-year follow-up, compared with nearly 30% of those receiving EX. Additionally, participants in the EX group reported significantly more PTSD and depressive symptoms than those treated with CT. These follow-up findings provide strong support for the long-lasting benefits of changing one's thought patterns through CT.

Bryant et al. (2008) investigated the extent to which CT augments treatment response when provided in conjunction with EX. In this study, 118 men and women with PTSD from various civilian traumas were assigned to one of four treatment groups: 1) imaginal EX, 2) in vivo EX, 3) imaginal EX+in vivo EX, or 4) imaginal EX+in vivo EX+CT. The study did not include a CT-only group. ITT analyses indicated that combining exposure therapy with cognitive therapy (imaginal EX+in vivo EX+CT) resulted in the greatest treatment effects for PTSD and depressive symptoms. ITT analyses also indicated that fewer participants continued to meet criteria for PTSD in this treatment (31%) than in the imaginal EX (75%), in vivo EX (69%), and imaginal EX+in vivo EX (63%) groups at a 6-month follow-up assessment. Findings from this study further support the notion that cognitive change is an important mechanism underlying recovery from PTSD.

The study by Bryant et al. (2008) provides some evidence of the benefits of additive treatments for PTSD; however, these findings contrast with those of other studies in which CT did not provide additive gains relative to those provided by EX in the treatment of PTSD (e.g., Foa et al. 2005; Marks et al. 1998; Paunovic and Öst 2001). For example, Marks et al. (1998) compared EX, CT, EX combined with CT, and RLX for 87 men and women who had PTSD from a range of civilian traumas. Among the 77 participants who completed treatment, completer analyses indicated no significant differences between CT, EX, and COMB treatments; however, all three treatment modalities were more effective than RLX. The treatment gains were maintained through a 6-month follow-up. These findings suggest that PTSD symptoms can be improved through emotional and/or cognitive-focused intervention. More research is needed to clarify what types of patients benefit from various combinations of EX and CT.

Rothbaum et al. (2006) conducted an innovative two-phase study in which they provided 10 weeks of open-label sertraline treatment to 88 men and women with chronic PTSD from a range of civilian traumas. Following the initial 10 weeks, the researchers randomly assigned participants to either continue taking sertraline ($n = 31$) or continue sertraline and receive 10 EX sessions administered twice weekly ($n = 34$) for 5 additional weeks. Because the authors did not evaluate treatment fidelity for EX, the integrity of the EX intervention delivered in this study remains unknown. Sertraline was associated with significant improvement in PTSD, depression, and anxiety symptoms; during the first 10 weeks of treatment. ITT analyses indicated that participants treated in the sertraline-only group maintained their gains. Participants who also received EX continued to improve in terms of PTSD symptoms; however, the differences were not statistically significant relative to the medication-only group. A post hoc analysis conducted by dividing participants into two groups based on their initial response to sertraline (excellent responders vs. partial responders) found that the augmentation effect of EX occurred for those participants who were considered partial responders.

In a study of 84 males and females with PTSD from a range of traumas, Hollifield et al. (2007) randomly assigned participants to one of three conditions: a group COMB treatment that incorporated education, behavioral activation, CT, image rehearsal therapy, and systematic desensitization; acupuncture; or a WL control. Because the researchers did not report on assessor training or treatment fidelity, the validity of assessment measures and fidelity to treatment remain uncertain. ITT analyses indicated that compared with the WL control, both the COMB and acupuncture modalities resulted in significant reduction of self-reported PTSD severity, depression, anxiety, and functional impairment. The two active treatments, however, did not differ in terms of their effectiveness. Treatment gains were maintained for both groups at a 3-month follow-up.

A few well-controlled trials have compared EMDR with EX and other treatments in mixed trauma samples. Taylor et al. (2003) compared in vivo EX, RLX, and EMDR in 60 men and women with chronic PTSD. Among the 45 participants who completed treatment, EX was statistically superior to EMDR in reducing PTSD, and EMDR was not statistically different from RLX. Vaughan et al. (1994) compared EMDR to image habituation training (a form of EX) and applied muscle relaxation (a form of RLX) in 36 men and women with PTSD or subsyndromal PTSD (78% met full criteria for PTSD) from a range of civilian traumatic events. The study did include ITT analyses; however, aside from the small sample, a significant weakness of this study was that the researchers did not report on treatment adherence. All treatments led to modest improvements, but EMDR had the largest effect size.

Power et al. (2002) assigned 105 men and women with a range of civilian trauma exposures to one of three groups: EMDR, a combination of EX and CT, or a WL control. Seventy-two participants completed treatment. Completer analyses indicated that both active treatment groups were superior to the WL control group. Although the two active treatments showed no significant differences, Power et al. (2002) reported effect size advantages for EMDR in terms of reducing the frequency and intensity of PTSD symptoms.

In general, within mixed trauma samples, active treatments did not differ in efficacy and were superior to WL controls. This lack of findings between treatment conditions may again be a reflection of limited power from relatively small sample sizes and minimal assessment administrations. There appear to be mixed results regarding the benefit of augmenting EX with CT in mixed trauma samples.

Natural Disasters

Two well-controlled trials involving natural disaster samples met criteria for review. The first study is reviewed here, and the second study (Basoglu et al. 2007) is reviewed later in "Technology-Assisted Interventions for PTSD." Basoglu et al. (2005) compared a single session of self-directed in vivo EX to a WL control in 59 male and female earthquake survivors with chronic PTSD. ITT analyses indicated that single-session EX produced significantly greater reductions in PTSD, depression, and anxiety than the WL condition. Treatment gains were maintained at a 1- to 2-year follow-up, indicating a long-lasting effect for a very brief and focused intervention.

Military-Related Trauma Samples

Results from three well-controlled RCTs have demonstrated the efficacy of CBT for veterans with PTSD. Monson et al. (2006) assigned 60 male and female veterans with chronic military-related PTSD to receive CPT or to a WL control group. ITT analyses indicated that CPT was superior to WL in reducing PTSD and anxiety; 40% of the CPT participants no longer met criteria for a PTSD diagnosis at the end of treatment. Notably, the researchers also found that PTSD-related disability status was not related to treatment outcome.

In one of the largest well-controlled RCTs reported to date, Schnurr et al. (2003) conducted a multisite study within the Veterans Affairs hospitals, comparing group COMB treatment with a present-centered problem-solving group treatment in 360 male Vietnam War veterans. ITT analyses indicated that approximately 38% of each group exhibited clinically significant improvements after treatment and 44% showed improvement at 1 year after beginning treatment, but there were no differences between the two treatment groups on any of the measures. In considering the modest findings and lack of differences between the active and control conditions, the investigators questioned 1) whether the number of exposures in the group setting was adequate, 2) whether more experienced CBT therapists might have made a difference, and 3) whether veterans with multiple comorbid conditions might be a more difficult population to treat. Additionally, the length of time since the traumatic exposure may have had an impact on treatment.

In another large, well-controlled RCT, Schnurr et al. (2007) conducted a second multisite study within Veterans Affairs hospitals, comparing EX to PCT in 284 female veterans with chronic PTSD. Unlike the first multisite study (Schnurr et al. 2003), which used an untested CBT group treatment, this study implemented individual treatment with prolonged EX (Foa et al. 1991, 1999, 2005), which has been established as efficacious. ITT analyses indicated that relative to PCT, the EX group experienced superior symptom reduction on measures of PTSD, depression, and anxiety at posttreatment and 3-month follow-up, but not at a 6-month follow-up. Although the EX group maintained gains at the 6-month follow-up, the PCT group continued to improve following termination of therapy, leading to results similar to those of the EX group at a 6-month follow-up. Similar to the findings of Monson et al. (2006), 41% of PCT participants no longer met criteria for PTSD as a result of treatment. Schnurr et al. (2007) also found that PTSD-related disability status was not related to treatment outcome or to having been the victim of military sexual trauma.

Taken together, these trials of CBT for PTSD provide some of the most encouraging results to date in the treatment of veterans with chronic military-related PTSD. However, more research is warranted to enhance treatment efficacy.

Refugees, Terrorism, and Civil Conflict

Hinton et al. (2005) compared a COMB CBT with a crossover design for 40 male and female Cambodian refugees meeting criteria for current PTSD and panic attacks. Of note, each of the participants had been taking a selective serotonin reuptake inhibitor and receiving supportive therapy for 1 year but continued to meet criteria for PTSD. Thus, participants in this study were considered to have treatment-resistant PTSD. Participants were randomly assigned to receive treatment immediately or delayed treatment (WL followed by the COMB treatment). The COMB treatment included education, diaphragmatic breathing, EX, CT, and SIT. ITT analyses indicated that the COMB intervention was superior to the WL in reducing PTSD, anxiety sensitivity, depression, and anxiety. Additionally, COMB participants experienced a decrease in the severity of their panic attacks. Results were replicated with the delayed-treatment group as well. Treatment gains were maintained at a 5-month follow-up.

Duffy et al. (2007) conducted an RCT in Northern Ireland comparing CT to a WL control condition in a study of 58 men and women with PTSD from exposure to terrorism and civil conflict. ITT analyses indicated that CT significantly improved self-reported PTSD, depression, and social adjustment relative to the WL control condition. Gains were maintained up to a 12-month follow-up. Neuner et al. (2008) replicated and extended these findings by comparing narrative EX with flexible trauma counseling or an assessment-only control condition for 277 Sudanese refugees with chronic PTSD living in a Ugandan refugee settlement. Both treatments were administered by lay counselors. ITT analyses indicated that both active treatments were effective in reducing PTSD symptoms relative to the assessment-only control condition. No significant differences in effectiveness were found between groups, with only 30% of the narrative EX group and 35% of the flexible trauma counseling group still meeting criteria for PTSD. Both treatments also resulted in improved self-reported physical health symptoms. However, the narrative EX condition resulted in significantly fewer dropouts (4%) than the flexible trauma counseling condition (21%).

The three studies described in this section upheld high methodological standards. However, an important caveat is that treatment adherence was not sufficiently addressed.

Special Applications of CBT

As demonstrated in the review above, various forms of CBT are effective in the treatment of PTSD and comorbid problems. Researchers have begun to develop and test special applications of CBT to address more complex comorbidities and posttrauma symptoms. Researchers have also tested treatment applications in new, innovative settings. The majority of these studies upheld high methodological standards, with the limitations noted in each review.

Nightmares

Krakow et al. (2001) compared image rehearsal therapy with a WL control among 168 female sexual assault survivors with PTSD or subsyndromal PTSD. This study has two methodological limitations: the authors did not report on assessor training or treatment fidelity. ITT analyses indicated that image rehearsal therapy resulted in significant reductions in nightmares, sleep disruptions, and PTSD symptom frequency and severity. PTSD symptoms decreased by at least one level of clinical severity for 65% of the treatment group, whereas symptoms worsened or stayed the same for 69% of the control group. Results were maintained at a 3- to 6-month follow-up. Notably, the treatment group improved from the moderately severe to the moderate range of PTSD during treatment. These findings indicate that PTSD symptoms were still in the distressed range at posttreatment and follow up.

Davis and Wright (2007) tested a COMB treatment, consisting of a modified image rescripting therapy with RLX, EX (writing and talking about the nightmares), and education about common trauma-related themes typically explored in CPT. The COMB treatment was administered individually or in small groups for three weekly sessions. Forty-three men and women with PTSD or subsyndromal PTSD from a range of traumas were randomly assigned to the COMB treatment or to a WL control. Similar to Krakow et al.'s

(2001) findings, ITT analyses indicated that COMB treatment was associated with greater reductions in nightmares, sleep disruption, and PTSD severity than the WL condition. Treatment gains were maintained at 3- and 6-month follow-ups. The study did not report on certain aspects of the assessment protocol, including evaluator training and the use of blind assessments. Treatment adherence was also not reported. Therefore, more methodologically rigorous trials are needed for the treatment of PTSD-related nightmares.

Comorbid Panic Attacks

Falsetti et al. (2001) integrated components of panic control therapy (Barlow and Craske 1994), interoceptive (i.e., confronting feared bodily symptoms associated with anxiety, such as shortness of breath) and in vivo EX exercises, and CPT to develop multiple channel exposure therapy (M-CET). M-CET was delivered in group format for the treatment of PTSD with comorbid panic attacks in 22 females with a range of civilian traumas. Eighteen women completed the treatment. Completer analyses indicated that relative to a WL control, the intervention was effective in reducing PTSD and panic symptoms. Treatment adherence was monitored but not reported in this study. Falsetti et al. (2008) conducted a subsequent study in which they compared M-CET and a delayed-treatment WL control for 53 females with PTSD and comorbid panic attacks from a range of civilian traumas. ITT analyses indicated that the intervention was effective in reducing PTSD and panic attacks, as well as fear associated with panic attacks and panic-related distress. These findings were replicated in the delayed-treatment group. Completer analyses showed that results were maintained at 3- and 6-month follow-ups.

Serious Mental Illness

In a very well-controlled trial, Mueser et al. (2007) developed and tested a COMB CBT program for the treatment of PTSD. Participants were 108 males and females with PTSD and a comorbid serious mental illness, including schizophrenia, schizoaffective disorder, severe depression, and bipolar disorder. The COMB treatment focused primarily on education, coping skills, and CT. This intervention was compared to treatment as usual consisting of medication management, case management, vocational rehabilitation, and SC. ITT analyses indicated that the COMB treatment resulted in superior improvements on measures of PTSD, depression, anxiety, and trauma-related cognitions. Results were maintained at 3- and 6-month follow-ups. The effects of the COMB intervention on PTSD were found to be strongest for participants with the most severe PTSD symptoms. Additionally, the COMB treatment was successful in changing trauma-related cognitions, which in turn led to improvements in PTSD in the COMB group.

Technology-Assisted Interventions for PTSD

Computerized interventions provide an alternative form of treatment for individuals who may have difficulty accessing treatment (Green and Iverson 2009). Lange et al. (2003) developed a treatment program called Interapy, which uses the Internet to provide pretreatment and posttreatment assessments in conjunction with written assignments and exercises that provide education, EX, and CT. Participants complete written assignments and receive feedback from a therapist who has read the assignments. Lange et al. (2003) randomly assigned 184 men and women with PTSD or subsyndromal PTSD following a range of civilian traumas to either Interapy or a WL control group. Of these participants, 101 completed the study. ITT analyses indicated that relative to WL, Interapy significantly reduced PTSD symptoms, depression, anxiety, somatization, and sleep disturbances. Treatment gains were maintained at a 6-week follow-up.

Basoglu et al. (2007) compared an earthquake simulator intervention (EX) to a WL control for 31 male and female earthquake survivors with chronic PTSD. The earthquake simulator intervention includes education about EX as well as EX sessions in the simulator, consisting of a small house based on a movable platform that mimics earthquake tremors. The intensity of the tremors could be controlled by participants. ITT analyses indicated that relative to the WL control, the treatment resulted in significant reductions in PTSD, fear, depression, and anxiety and improvements in global functioning. Improvement rates were 40% at 4 weeks posttreatment, 72% at week 12, and 80% at week 24, and these gains were maintained at a 1- to 2-year follow-up. Postsession reduction in fear of earthquakes and increased sense of control over fear at follow-up were prospectively related to improvement in PTSD.

Litz et al. (2007) conducted a well-controlled trial of a COMB Internet therapy for PTSD. This treatment was compared with supportive counseling in Department of Defense service members with PTSD related to the attack on the Pentagon or military personnel with combat-related PTSD from serving in Iraq and/or Afghanistan. Study therapists administered the pretreatment assessment of PTSD severity, whereas an independent evaluator blind to the participant's study group administered the posttreatment assessment. Following one face-to-face meeting between a participant and a study therapist, the remainder of the intervention was administered via the Internet. The CBT comprised a combination of anxiety management, cognitive restructuring, in vivo exposure, and exposure to the trauma memory via writing. Although no significant differences were found between groups in the ITT analysis, the COMB Internet therapy resulted in greater improvement among completers at the 6-month follow-up.

Virtual reality interventions are another form of technology that is receiving increased empirical and clinical attention (Rothbaum 2009). Virtual reality interventions are a form of in vivo EX that integrates real-time computer graphics, body-tracking devices, and visual, audio, and other sensory input devices to simulate a virtual environment into which the participant is immersed. Rothbaum et al. (2001) developed and evaluated a virtual reality EX intervention in an open trial for 16 male Vietnam veterans with combat-related PTSD. Due to the dearth of large-scale research on virtual reality interventions for PTSD, this study warrants a brief review despite the lack of a comparison group and the small sample size. Veterans participated in 8–16 sessions (90 minutes each) of virtual reality in which they were exposed to two virtual environments: a helicopter flying over a virtual Vietnam and a clearing surrounded by jungle. Ten participants completed treatment. There was a trend for a significant reduction in PTSD from pretreatment to posttreatment; however, a significant reduction in PTSD occurred from pretreatment to 3-month follow-up, and significant reductions in PTSD and self-reported depression occurred from pretreatment to 6-month follow-up. Additional research is currently under way to further evaluate virtual reality interventions in the treatment of PTSD.

Conjoint Therapy

Intimate relationships may have an important role in the development, maintenance, and exacerbation of PTSD, leading researchers and clinicians to encourage the inclusion of intimate partners in treatment (Riggs 2008). Unfortunately, there is a lack of controlled research on such interventions, so no firm conclusions can yet be made. Glynn et al. (1999) provided the most methodologically rigorous study of a family-based skills intervention. The researchers randomly assigned 42 male Vietnam War veterans with chronic combat-related PTSD, as well as a family member each (90% domestic partners), to one of three conditions: COMB treatment (ET+CT), COMB followed by behavioral family therapy, or a WL control. Thirty-six participants completed treatment. At the end of the COMB phase, completer analyses indicated that both active interventions were superior to the WL condition in reducing positive PTSD symptoms (e.g., reexperiencing and hyperarousal), but the interventions did not reduce negative PTSD symptoms (e.g., avoidance and numbing). Treatment gains were maintained at a 6-month follow-up. The addition of the behavioral family therapy did not further improve PTSD symptoms but did lead to significant improvements in self-reported problem solving in the relationship.

Monson et al. (2004) developed and evaluated cognitive-behavioral conjoint therapy (CBCT) for PTSD. Despite the lack of a comparison group and the small sample size, this pilot study warrants a brief mention due to the dearth of research on couple-focused interventions for PTSD. Seven couples in which the husband was diagnosed with combat-related PTSD from service in Vietnam completed the treatment. Veterans demonstrated significant improvements from pretreatment to posttreatment in assessor- and partner-rated PTSD symptoms, as well as in veterans' self-reported depression and anxiety. The veterans' partners also reported increased relationship satisfaction. Interestingly, veterans' self-reported PTSD and relationship satisfaction did not change significantly during treatment. Further research is currently under way on the efficacy of CBCT for couples (and other dyads, such as with friends or family members) in which one person has PTSD.

Summary of Evidence for CBT

The treatment outcome research clearly suggests that psychosocial interventions, particularly CBT approaches, are effective in ameliorating PTSD in adults. In summary, EX and CT have received the most empirical attention, and much of this science has conformed to the highest standards of clinical research. Thus, the evidence supporting EX and CT for PTSD is very strong. CBTs are generally equivalent to each other, with some possible exceptions in the maintenance of treatment gains and treatment of comorbidities. When designing future clinical trials, researchers should include larger, more diverse samples; more data collection points to increase power to detect differences between active treatments; and longer follow-up assessments to better understand the robustness of treatment gains. Although CBT for PTSD treatment outcome research has clearly demonstrated efficacy over the past two decades, many unanswered questions remain and need further study.

Future Directions for Treatment Outcome Research

What Treatment Components Are Necessary and Sufficient?

Despite the clear evidence of effective psychosocial PTSD treatments, it remains to be seen what components of the various CBT approaches are necessary and sufficient for effective treatment of PTSD. Direct comparisons and meta-analyses (Benish et al. 2008) have generally shown many CBT treatments to be comparable in terms of their effectiveness. As a result, researchers have begun to focus attention on what components of available therapies are necessary for PTSD recovery. For instance, some researchers have investigated whether exposure to traumatic memories via writing and reading a trauma narrative (or some other variant) is necessary for recovery from PTSD, whereas others have examined if CT is sufficient alone. Dismantling studies and component analyses may help determine the necessary and sufficient treatment components for the effective treatment of PTSD. Such research would allow therapists to deliver more efficient treatment by eliminating unnecessary aspects of therapy. For instance, the recent results from a dismantling study by Resick et al. (2008a) suggest that the written account may not improve results over cognitive therapy. These findings suggest CT may be a preferable treatment choice for at least some individuals with PTSD; however, much more research is necessary to identify who would most benefit from CT, from EX, or from a combination of both treatment modalities.

Similarly, to refine theoretical assumptions of PTSD treatment, research designs should include examinations of mechanisms of change in treatment. For example, to test cognitive models, researchers should measure cognitions before treatment, at various time points throughout treatment, and following treatment. Such work would have implications for furthering the understanding of the etiology and maintenance of PTSD and for developing more efficient PTSD treatment. Likewise, treatment research on different modes of therapy with functional magnetic resonance imaging might elucidate whether there is more than one mechanism of change and might lead to more efficient interventions. Finally, there is a dearth of research on medications that might facilitate new learning in PTSD treatment. As noted earlier, preliminary evidence indicates that prolonged EX is helpful for individuals who do not fully respond to sertraline (Rothbaum et al. 2006). Research is needed to determine when to combine psychotherapy with medications, and how to best sequence medications and psychotherapy for the treatment of PTSD.

What Demographic Variables Affect PTSD Treatment?

Research examining the associations among demographic variables and PTSD treatment is scarce. In particular, there is much to be learned about the influence of gender, ethnicity, culture, and developmental issues in the treatment of PTSD.

More research is needed to examine gender differences in PTSD treatment outcome. Although several treatment outcome studies have included both men and women, small sample sizes have hindered statistical power to detect gender differences in treatment response (Kimerling et al. 2007). Although some evidence suggests that women may experience superior treatment response compared with men (Cason et al. 2002), it is unclear whether these responses are a reflection of women being generally more responsive to treatment or whether factors such as baseline symptoms and trauma type (both of which are related to gender) account for the data in Cason et al.'s study.

Likewise, although much of the extant literature indicates disparities in mental health care treatment negatively impacting engagement and retention for ethnic minorities, the existing literature is inconclusive as to whether individuals from diverse ethnic backgrounds respond differently to treatments (Miranda et al. 2005). Future studies should be designed specifically for the study of ethnic differences. These studies should determine what differences exist, if any, and examine factors contributing to those differences. For example, the role of coping style, cultural stigma, and client-therapist match should be furthered explored. Some evidence, for instance, suggests that the ethnicity of the therapist does not impact treatment outcome (e.g., Kubany et al. 2004). To elucidate this issue, researchers should take into account the role of client acculturation and other factors that might impact therapy engagement and treatment outcome.

Additionally, cultural issues in PTSD treatment are in need of further scientific inquiry (Osterman and de Jong 2007). For example, it is unknown whether current CBTs will meet the needs of individuals with PTSD across the globe. The majority of treatment studies to date have been conducted in Western countries, and therefore more research is needed to examine the generalizability of treatments to other cultures. Moreover, there is much to be learned about whether certain cultures, such as military culture, differentially impact treatment outcome.

Similarly, little is known about the relationship between age and PTSD treatment response, particularly among older adults. Some evidence suggests that patients who are younger may be more open to changing beliefs and established patterns of thinking than older clients (Donnellan and Lucas 2008), and therefore may benefit more from treatment. Interestingly, three studies of female patients have shown that younger patients are more likely than older patients to drop out of PTSD treatment (Cloitre et al. 2004; Foa et al. 2005; Rizvi et al. 2009). Rizvi et al. (2009) found that younger age in CPT and older age in prolonged EX were related to the best outcomes, whereas older age in CPT and younger age in prolonged EX were related to relatively worse outcomes (although all age groups demonstrated significant symptom reduction over time). Differences in the focus of the two different CBTs might account for this finding. More research is needed to replicate and expand these findings to inform treatment matching.

How Do Comorbidities Affect Treatment of PTSD?

The co-occurrence of psychiatric disorders in PTSD treatment is currently an important focus of treatment outcome research because PTSD is associated with numerous and complex comorbidities (Keane et al. 2007; Najavits et al. 2008). Relatively little is known, however, about the effect of comorbidity on the efficacy of treatment for PTSD, about the effect of treatment for PTSD on comorbid conditions, and about how comorbidities may inform treatment matching (for an excellent review, see Najavits et al. 2008). The majority of CBT approaches reviewed in this chapter have been shown to reduce depression and anxiety, in addition to improving PTSD; however, less is known about the effect of treatment on other comorbidities. For example, CPT has been successfully combined with panic control treatment for the treatment of PTSD with comorbid panic attacks (Falsetti et al. 2001), yet it is unclear whether standard CBT approaches would reduce panic as well. The literature on treating PTSD and other comorbid anxiety disorders appears to be inconclusive. For example, the limited data on PTSD treatment for patients with comorbid generalized anxiety disorder (GAD) are mixed, with one study demonstrating poorer outcomes (Tarrier et al. 1999) and another study finding that reductions in PTSD reduced incidences of GAD (Blanchard et al. 2003). There have also been some promising results in the treatment of comorbid PTSD and serious mental illness. Mueser et al. (2007) found that an intervention that integrated several common components of CBT was successful in reducing PTSD and distress among individuals with serious mental illness.

Substance use disorders also commonly co-occur with PTSD (Najavits et al. 2008); however, because most RCTs for PTSD exclude participants with substance dependence, relatively little is known about how substance use impacts treatment outcome. In *Seeking Safety: A Treatment Manual for PTSD and Substance Abuse*, Najavits (2002) describes a CBT for co-occurring substance use disorders and PTSD that has received growing support as an effective treatment (Najavits et al. 2008). Additional research is needed to determine whether development or implementation of such integrated treatments is necessary (or optimal) to address PTSD comorbidities.

Although a heterogeneous mix of Axis II disorders appear to co-occur with PTSD (Keane et al. 2007), less is known about how Axis II traits impact treatment outcome (Najavits et al. 2008; Resick et al. 2007). Several secondary analyses of RCTs suggest that individuals with borderline personality disorder traits are able to participate fully in treatment (i.e., their dropout rates are not significantly different from those of participants without borderline traits) and experience significant reductions in PTSD with CBT (Clarke et al. 2008; Feeny et al. 2002; Hembree et al. 2004). Additionally, Clark et al. (2008) found that CBT was associated with improvements in borderline symptoms. These studies, however, excluded individuals with suicidality, self-harm behaviors, and substance dependence; therefore, it remains unknown whether existing CBTs would be as efficacious when applied to patients with more severe disorders. Likewise, more research is needed to understand the effect of PTSD treatment on other personality disorders, such as antisocial and obsessive-compulsive personality disorders.

What About Research in Real-World Settings?

Now that the clinical efficacy of psychosocial treatments for PTSD has been established, more effectiveness research is needed to examine the utility of such interventions in real-world settings. Even when the inclusion and exclusion criteria are set to be as inclusive as possible and to represent typical clinical populations, treatment research is typically conducted under highly controlled settings with expert therapists who are closely monitored and supervised. A serious concern is transporting evidence-based treatments into practice settings in which no quality assurance process is in place to ensure the integrity of the treatment delivery. We do not know how well clinicians can be trained to implement these therapy protocols in busy practice settings or whether or how well the treatments will be implemented and adopted as part of routine clinical care. Research on alternative delivery systems, such as the Internet or telemental health services (Moreland et al. 2004), is in its infancy but appears very promising. More attention is currently being paid to these dissemination issues in the literature, but a great deal of research is needed to assess whether the efficacious treatments for PTSD have the same effectiveness in practice settings and to determine the best ways to teach therapists to adopt the protocols without losing the fidelity. For example, the Department of Veterans Affairs is currently disseminating evidence-based PTSD treatments via the CPT and Prolonged Exposure Training Initiative Programs. Program evaluation efforts for these programs are under way.

Conclusion

Tremendous movement has been made over the last two decades toward developing and evaluating theoretically derived psychosocial interventions for PTSD and its extensive comorbidities. We have attempted to demonstrate the significant advances that have been made, particularly among CBT therapists, in developing treatments and testing them in a methodologically sound manner. We hope that this chapter provides practical information on the available empirically supported and theoretically driven interventions for clinicians interested in treating patients with PTSD. Because traumatic events will never be fully eliminated from the human experience, and PTSD is on the rise among veterans returning from Iraq and Afghanistan, it is essential that clinicians have access to treatments that work. This chapter highlights the fact that clinicians can choose from theoretically sound and effective clinical interventions to successfully ameliorate PTSD and numerous other trauma symptoms subsequent to all types of traumatic events.

Key Clinical Points

- Five predominant forms of CBT treatments have been well defined and systematically studied: coping skills–focused treatments, exposure-based treatments, cognitive therapy, eye movement desensitization and reprocessing, and combination therapies.
- Coping skills–focused treatments include relaxation training and stress inoculation training; respectively, these treatments focus on anxiety management and the reconditioning of anxiety responses.
- Exposure and prolonged exposure therapy are methods of reexperiencing the trauma in a controlled environment as a means of reducing an individual's response to the trauma and incorporating corrective information into existing fear structures.
- EMDR uses external oscillatory stimulation (typically lateral eye movements following a device or the provider's finger) while the individual recounts the traumatic experience, in order to decrease the distress associated with the trauma.
- Cognitive therapy seeks to modify maladaptive or dysfunctional interpretations of events that result in negative emotional states; the CPT subtype of cognitive therapy, in particular, has been shown to be effective in treating PTSD.
- Current evidence most strongly supports cognitive therapy and exposure therapy for PTSD.
- Different aspects of various current interventions are being studied to understand which portions of each are most effective and how such interventions could be recombined to most effectively treat PTSD.
- Alternative modes of treatment delivery, including computer-assisted and telemental health models , appear to have benefit in PTSD symptom reduction.

References

Barlow DH, Craske MG: Mastery of Your Anxiety and Panic II: Treatment Manual. Albany, NY, Graywind, 1994

Basoglu M, Salcioglu E, Livanou M, et al: Single-session behavioral treatment of earthquake-related posttraumatic stress disorder: a randomized waiting list controlled trial. J Trauma Stress 18:1–11, 2005

Basoglu M, Salcioglu E, Livanou M: A randomized controlled study of single-session behavioral treatment of earthquake-related post-traumatic stress disorder using an earthquake simulator. Psychol Med 37:203–213, 2007

Beck AT: Cognitive Therapy and the Emotional Disorders. New York, International Universities Press, 1976

Benish SG, Imel ZE, Wampold BE: The relative efficacy of bona fide psychotherapies for treating post-traumatic stress disorder: a meta-analysis of direct comparisons. Clin Psychol Rev 28:746–758, 2008

Blanchard EB, Hickling EJ, Devineni T, et al: A controlled evaluation of cognitive behavioral therapy for posttraumatic stress in motor vehicle accident survivors. Behav Res Ther 41:79–96, 2003

Bradley RG, Follingstad DR: Group therapy for incarcerated women who experienced interpersonal violence: a pilot study. J Trauma Stress 16:337–340, 2003

Brewin CR, Dalgleish T, Joseph S: A dual representational theory of posttraumatic stress disorder. Psychol Rev 103:670–686, 1996

Brewin CR, Andrews B, Rose S: Fear, helplessness, and horror in posttraumatic stress disorder: investigating DSM-IV criterion A2 in victims of violent crime. J Trauma Stress 13:499–509, 2000

Bryant RA, Moulds ML, Guthrie RM, et al: Imaginal exposure alone and imaginal exposure with cognitive restructuring in treatment of posttraumatic stress disorder. J Consult Clin Psychol 71:706–712, 2003

Bryant RA, Moulds ML, Guthrie RM, et al: A randomized controlled trial of exposure therapy and cognitive restructuring for posttraumatic stress disorder. J Consult Clin Psychol 76:695–703, 2008

Cahill SP, Foa EB: Psychological theories of PTSD, in Handbook of PTSD: Science and Practice. Edited by Friedman MJ, Keane TM, Resick PA. New York, Guilford, 2007, pp 55–77

Cahill SP, Rothbaum BO, Resick PA, et al: Cognitive-behavioral therapy for adults, in Effective Treatments for PTSD: Practice Guidelines From the International Society for Traumatic Stress Studies, 2nd Edition. Edited by Foa EB, Keane TM, Friedman MJ, et al. New York, Guilford, 2008, pp 139–222

Cason D, Grubaugh A, Resick P: Gender and PTSD treatment: efficacy and effectiveness, in Gender and PTSD. Edited by Kimerling R, Oiumette P, Wolfe J. New York, Guilford, 2002, pp 305–334

Chard KM: An evaluation of cognitive processing therapy for the treatment of posttraumatic stress disorder related to childhood sexual abuse. J Consult Clin Psychol 73:965–971, 2005

Chemtob C, Roitblatt HL, Hamada RS, et al: A cognitive action theory of posttraumatic stress disorder. J Anxiety Disord 2:253–275, 1988

Clarke SB, Rizvi SL, Resick PA: Borderline personality characteristics and treatment outcome in cognitive-behavioral treatments for PTSD in female rape victims. Behav Ther 39:72–78, 2008

Cloitre M, Koenen KC, Cohen LR, et al: Skills training in affective and interpersonal regulation followed by exposure: a phase-based treatment for PTSD related to childhood abuse. J Consult Clin Psychol 70:1067–1074, 2002

Cloitre M, Stovall-McClough KC, Miranda R, et al: Therapeutic alliance, negative mood regulation, and treatment outcome in child abuse-related posttraumatic stress disorder. J Consult Clin Psychol 72:411–416, 2004

Cloitre M, Cohen LR, Koenen KC: Treating Survivors of Childhood Sexual Abuse: Psychotherapy for an Interrupted Life. New York, Guilford, 2006

Dalgleish T: Cognitive approaches to posttraumatic stress disorder: the evolution of multirepresentational theorizing. Psychol Bull 130:228–260, 2004

Davis JL, Wright DC: Randomized clinical trial for treatment of chronic nightmares in trauma exposed adults. J Trauma Stress 20:123–133, 2007

Donnellan MB, Lucas RE: Age differences in the Big Five across the life span: evidence from two national samples. Psychol Aging 23:558–566, 2008

Duffy M, Gillespie K, Clark DM: Post-traumatic stress disorder in the context of terrorism and other civil conflict in Northern Ireland: randomised controlled trial. BMJ 334:1147–1150, 2007

Ehlers A, Clark DM: A cognitive model of posttraumatic stress disorder. Behav Res Ther 38:319–345, 2000

Ehlers A, Clark DM, Hackmann A, et al: A randomized controlled trial of cognitive therapy, a self-help booklet, and repeated assessment as early interventions for posttraumatic stress disorder. Arch Gen Psychiatry 60:1024–1032, 2003

Falsetti SA, Resnick HS, Davis J, et al: Treatment of posttraumatic stress disorder with comorbid panic attacks: combining cognitive processing therapy with panic control treatment techniques. Group Dyn 5:252–260, 2001

Falsetti SA, Resnick HS, Davis J: Multiple channel exposure therapy for women with PTSD and comorbid panic attacks. Cogn Behav Ther 37:117–130, 2008

Feeny NC, Zoellner LA, Foa EB: Treatment outcome for chronic PTSD among female assault victims with borderline personality characteristics: a preliminary examination. J Pers Disord 16:30–40, 2002

Foa EB, Kozak MJ: Emotional processing of fear: exposure to corrective information. Psychol Bull 99:20–35, 1986

Foa EB, Meadows EA: Psychosocial treatments for post-traumatic stress disorder: a critical review, in Annual Review of Psychology, Vol 48. Edited by Spence J, Darley JM, Foss DJ. Palo Alto, CA, Annual Reviews, 1997, pp 449–480

Foa EB, Steketee G, Rothbaum BO: Behavioral/cognitive conceptualizations of post-traumatic stress disorder. Behav Ther 20:155–176, 1989

Foa EB, Rothbaum BO, Riggs D, et al: Treatment of post-traumatic stress disorder in rape victims: a comparison between cognitive-behavioral procedures and counseling. J Consult Clin Psychol 59:715–723, 1991

Foa EB, Dancu CV, Hembree EA, et al: A comparison of exposure therapy, stress inoculation training, and their combination for reducing posttraumatic stress disorder in female assault victims. J Consult Clin Psychol 67:194–200, 1999

Foa EB, Hembree EA, Cahill SE, et al: Randomized trial of prolonged exposure for posttraumatic stress disorder with and without cognitive restructuring: outcome at academic and community clinics. J Consult Clin Psychol 73:953–964, 2005

Foa EB, Hembree EA, Rothbaum BO: Prolonged Exposure Therapy for PTSD: Emotional Processing of Traumatic Experiences. New York, Oxford University Press, 2007

Foa EB, Keane TM, Friedman MJ, et al: Introduction: cognitive-behavioral therapy for adults, in Effective Treatments for PTSD: Practice Guidelines From the International Society for Traumatic Stress Studies, 2nd Edition. Edited by Foa EB, Keane TM, Friedman MJ, et al. New York, Guilford, 2008, pp 1–20

Galovski TE, Monson C, Bruce SE, et al: Does cognitive-behavioral treatment for PTSD improve perceived health and sleep impairment? J Trauma Stress 22:197–204, 2009

Glynn SM, Eth S, Randolph ET, et al: A test of behavioral family therapy to augment exposure for combat-related PTSD. J Consult Clin Psychol 67:243–251, 1999

Green K, Iverson KM: Computerized cognitive-behavioral therapy in a stepped care model of treatment. Prof Psychol Res Pr 40:96–103, 2009

Harvey AG, Bryant RA, Tarrier N: Cognitive behavior therapy for posttraumatic stress disorder. Clin Psychol Rev 23:501–522, 2003

Hembree EA, Cahill SE, Foa EB: Impact of personality disorders on treatment outcome for assault survivors with chronic posttraumatic stress disorder. J Pers Disord 18:117–127, 2004

Hinton DE, Chhean D, Pich V, et al: A randomized controlled trial of cognitive-behavior therapy for Cambodian refugees with treatment-resistant PTSD and panic attack: a cross-over design. J Trauma Stress 18:617–629, 2005

Hollifield M, Sinclair-Lian N, Warner TD, et al: Acupuncture for posttraumatic stress disorder: a randomized controlled pilot trial. J Nerv Ment Dis 195:504–513, 2007

Hollon SD, Garber J: Cognitive therapy, in Social Cognition and Clinical Psychology: A Synthesis. Edited by Abramson LY. New York, Guilford, 1988, pp 204–253

Institute of Medicine: Treatment of Posttraumatic Stress Disorder: An Assessment of the Evidence. Washington, DC, National Academies Press, 2008

Keane TM, Barlow DH: Posttraumatic stress disorder, in Anxiety and Its Disorders: The Nature and Treatment of Anxiety and Panic. Edited by Barlow DH. New York, Guilford, 2002, pp 418–452

Keane TM, Zimering RT, Caddell JM: A behavioral formulation of posttraumatic stress disorder in Vietnam veterans. Behavior Therapist 8:9–12, 1985

Keane TM, Brief DJ, Pratt EM, et al: Assessment of PTSD and its comorbidities in adults, in Handbook of PTSD: Science and Practice. Edited by Friedman MJ, Keane TM, Resick PA. New York, Guilford, 2007, pp 279–305

Kilpatrick DG, Veronen LJ, Resick PA: Psychological sequelae to rape: assessment and treatment strategies, in Behavioral Medicine: Assessment and Treatment Strategies. Edited by Dolcys DM, Meredith RL, Ciminero AR. New York, Plenum, 1982, pp 473–497

Kilpatrick DG, Veronen LJ, Best CL: Factors predicting psychological distress among rape victims, in Trauma and Its Wake. Edited by Figley CR. New York, Brunner/Mazel, 1985, pp 114–141

Kimerling R, Ouimette P, Weitlauf JC: Gender issues in PTSD, in Handbook of PTSD: Science and Practice. Edited by Friedman MJ, Keane TM, Resick PA. New York, Guilford, 2007, pp 207–228

Krakow B, Hollifield M, Johnston L, et al: Imagery rehearsal therapy for chronic nightmares in sexual assault survivors with posttraumatic stress disorder: a randomized controlled trial. JAMA 286:537–545, 2001

Kubany ES, Hill EE, Owens JA: Cognitive trauma therapy for battered women with PTSD: preliminary findings. J Trauma Stress 16:81–91, 2003

Kubany ES, Hill EE, Owens JA, et al: Cognitive trauma therapy for battered women with PTSD (CTT-BW). J Consult Clin Psychol 72:3–18, 2004

Lang PJ: Imagery in therapy: an information processing analysis of fear. Behav Ther 8:862–886, 1977

Lange A, Rietdijk D, Hudcovicova M, et al: Interapy: a controlled randomized trial of the standardized treatment of posttraumatic stress through the Internet. J Consult Clin Psychol 71:901–909, 2003

Linehan MM: Cognitive-Behavioral Treatment of Borderline Personality Disorder. New York, Guilford, 1993

Litz BT, Engel CC, Bryant RA, et al: A randomized, controlled proof-of-concept trial of an Internet-based, therapist-assisted self-management treatment for posttraumatic stress disorder. Am J Psychiatry 164:1676–1683, 2007

Maercker A, Zöllner T, Menning H, et al: Dresden PTSD treatment study: randomized controlled trial of motor vehicle accident survivors. BMC Psychiatry 6:1–8, 2006

Marks I, Lovell K, Noshirvani H, et al: Treatment of posttraumatic stress disorder by exposure and/or cognitive restructuring: a controlled study. Arch Gen Psychiatry 55:317–325, 1998

McCann IL, Pearlman LA: Psychological Trauma and the Adult Survivor: Theory, Therapy and Transformation. New York, Brunner/Mazel, 1990

McDonagh A, Friedman M, McHugo G, et al: Randomized trial of cognitive-behavioral therapy for chronic posttraumatic stress disorder in adult female survivors of childhood sexual abuse. J Consult Clin Psychol 73:515–524, 2005

Meichenbaum D: Self-instructional methods, in Helping People Change. Edited by Kanfer FH, Goldstein AP. New York, Pergamon Press, 1974, pp 357–391

Miranda J, Bernal G, Lau A, et al: State of the science on psychosocial interventions for ethnic minorities. Annu Rev Clin Psychol 1:113–142, 2005

Monson CM, Schnurr PP, Stevens SP, et al: Cognitive-behavioral couple's treatment for posttraumatic stress disorder: initial findings. J Trauma Stress 17:341–344, 2004

Monson CM, Schnurr PP, Resick PA, et al: Cognitive processing therapy for veterans with military-related posttraumatic stress disorder. J Consult Clin Psychol 74:898–907, 2006

Moreland LA, Pierce K, Wong MY: Telemedicine and coping skills groups for Pacific Island veterans with post-traumatic stress disorder: a pilot study. J Telemed Telecare 10:286–289, 2004

Mowrer OA: Learning Theory and Behavior. New York, Wiley, 1960

Mueser KT, Bolton E, Carty PC, et al: The Trauma Recovery Group: a cognitive-behavioral program for post-traumatic stress disorder in persons with severe mental illness. Community Ment Health J 43:281–304, 2007

Najavits LM: Seeking Safety: A Treatment Manual for PTSD and Substance Abuse. New York, Guilford, 2002

Najavits LM, Ryngala D, Back SE, et al: Treatment for PTSD and comorbid disorders: a review of the literature, in Effective Treatments for PTSD: Practice Guidelines From the International Society for Traumatic Stress Studies, 2nd Edition. Edited by Foa EB, Keane TM, Friedman MJ, et al. New York, Guilford, 2008, pp 508–535

Neuner F, Schauer M, Klaschik C, et al: A comparison of narrative exposure therapy, supportive counseling, and psychoeducation for treating posttraumatic stress disorder in an African refugee settlement. J Consult Clin Psychol 72:579–587, 2004

Neuner F, Enyutt PL, Ertl V, et al: Treatment of posttraumatic stress disorder by trained lay counselors in an African refugee settlement: a randomized controlled trial. J Consult Clin Psychol 76:686–694, 2008

Osterman JE, de Jong JT: Cultural issues and trauma, in Handbook of PTSD: Science and Practice. Edited by Friedman MJ, Keane TM, Resick PA. New York, Guilford, 2007, pp 425–446

Owens GP, Pike JL, Chard KM: Treatment effects of cognitive processing therapy on cognitive distortions of female child sexual abuse survivors. Behav Ther 32:413–424, 2001

Paunovic N, Öst LG: Cognitive-behavior therapy versus exposure therapy in the treatment of PTSD in refugees. Behav Res Ther 39:1183–1197, 2001

Power K, McGoldrick T, Brown K, et al: A controlled comparison of eye movement desensitization and reprocessing versus exposure plus cognitive restructuring versus waiting list in the treatment of posttraumatic stress disorder. Clin Psychol Psychother 9:299–318, 2002

Resick PA, Schnicke MK: Cognitive processing therapy for sexual assault victims. J Consult Clin Psychol 60:748–756, 1992

Resick PA, Schnicke MK: Cognitive Processing Therapy for Rape Victims: A Treatment Manual. Thousand Oaks, CA, Sage, 1993

Resick PA, Nishith P, Weaver TL, et al: A comparison of cognitive-processing therapy with prolonged exposure and a waiting condition for the treatment of chronic posttraumatic stress disorder in female rape victims. J Consult Clin Psychol 70:867–879, 2002

Resick PA, Nishith P, Griffin MG: How well does cognitive-behavioral therapy treat symptoms of complex PTSD? An examination of child sexual abuse survivors within a clinical trial. CNS Spectr 8:340–355, 2003

Resick PA, Monson CM, Gutner C: Psychosocial treatment for PTSD, in Handbook of PTSD: Science and Practice. Edited by Friedman MJ, Keane TM, Resick PA. New York, Guilford, 2007, pp 330–358

Resick PA, Galovski TE, O'Brien Uhlmansiek M, et al: A randomized clinical trial to dismantle components of cognitive processing therapy for posttraumatic stress disorder in female victims of interpersonal violence. J Consult Clin Psychol 76:243–258, 2008a

Resick PA, Monson CM, Chard KM: Cognitive Processing Therapy: Veteran/Military Version. Washington, DC, Department of Veterans Affairs, 2008b

Riggs DS: Marital and family therapy, in Effective Treatments for PTSD: Practice Guidelines From the International Society for Traumatic Stress Studies, 2nd Edition. Edited by Foa EB, Keane TM, Friedman MJ, et al. New York, Guilford, 2008, pp 354–355

Rizvi S, Kaysen D, Gutner C, et al: Beyond fear: the role of peritraumatic responses in posttraumatic stress and depressive symptoms among female crime victims. J Interpers Violence 23:853–868, 2008

Rizvi SL, Vogt DS, Resick PA: Cognitive and affective predictors of treatment outcome in cognitive processing therapy and prolonged exposure for posttraumatic stress disorder. Behav Res Ther 47:737–743, 2009

Rothbaum BO: Using virtual reality to help our patients in the real world. Depress Anxiety 26:209–211, 2009

Rothbaum BO, Foa EB: Exposure therapy for rape victims with post-traumatic stress disorder. Behavior Therapist 15:219–222, 1992

Rothbaum BO, Hodges L, Ready D, et al: Virtual reality exposure therapy for Vietnam veterans with posttraumatic stress disorder. J Clin Psychiatry 62:617–622, 2001

Rothbaum BO, Astin MC, Marsteller F: Prolonged exposure versus eye movement desensitization and reprocessing (EMDR) for PTSD rape victims. J Trauma Stress 18:607–617, 2005

Rothbaum BO, Cahill SP, Foa EB, et al: Augmentation of sertraline with prolonged exposure in the treatment of posttraumatic stress disorder. J Trauma Stress 19:625–638, 2006

Schnurr PP: The rocks and hard places in psychotherapy outcome research. J Trauma Stress 20:779–792, 2007

Schnurr PP, Friedman MJ, Foy DW, et al: Randomized trial of trauma-focused group therapy for posttraumatic stress disorder: results from a Department of Veterans Affairs cooperative study. Arch Gen Psychiatry 60:481–489, 2003

Schnurr PP, Friedman MJ, Engel CC, et al: Cognitive behavioral therapy for posttraumatic stress disorder in women: a randomized controlled trial. JAMA 297:820–830, 2007

Shapiro F: Eye Movement Desensitization and Reprocessing: Basic Principles, Protocols, and Procedures. New York, Guilford, 1995

Tarrier N, Sommerfield C: Treatment of chronic PTSD by cognitive therapy and exposure: 5-year follow-up. Behav Ther 35:231–246, 2004

Tarrier N, Pilgrim H, Sommerfield C, et al: A randomized trial of cognitive therapy and imaginal exposure in the treatment of chronic posttraumatic stress disorder. J Consult Clin Psychol 67:13–18, 1999

Taylor S, Thordarson DS, Maxfield L, et al: Comparative efficacy, speed, and adverse effects of three PTSD treatments: exposure therapy, EMDR, and relaxation training. J Consult Clin Psychol 71:330–338, 2003

Vaughan K, Armstrong MS, Gold R, et al: A trial of eye movement desensitization compared to image habituation training and applied muscle relaxation in post-traumatic stress disorder. J Behav Ther Exp Psychiatry 25:283–291, 1994

Zlotnick C, Shea TM, Rosen K, et al: An affect management group for women with posttraumatic stress disorder and histories of childhood sexual abuse. J Trauma Stress 10:425–436, 1997

8

Violence and Aggression

Thomas A. Grieger, M.D., D.F.A.P.A.
David M. Benedek, M.D., D.F.A.P.A.
Robert J. Ursano, M.D., D.F.A.P.A.

During and after the war in Vietnam, clinicians observed that a substantial portion of soldiers experienced protracted problems with readjustment into civilian society. The constellation of symptoms reported by many of these veterans became the basis for diagnostic criteria for posttraumatic stress disorder (PTSD). Other difficulties were also observed, however. Among these were intermittent acts of aggression or violence, impaired interpersonal relationships, impaired affect modulation, self-destructive and impulsive behaviors, feeling threatened, and changes in personality characteristics. The American Psychiatric Association's practice guidelines note that some individuals with PTSD have an increased expectation of danger, resulting in an "anticipatory bias" toward their environment and an increased readiness for "flight, fight, or freeze" responses (Ursano et al. 2004). This increased readiness for aggression may reduce tolerance of mild or moderate slights, resulting in acts disproportionate to the degree of provocation. Models of the association between PTSD and aggression include heightened levels of arousal (Taft et al. 2007) and the loss of behavioral inhibition in response to punishment (Casada and Roache 2005). Although avoidance and numbing are not associated with commonly thought-of acts of aggression (e.g., fights, threats, the use of weapons), numbing may be associated with aggression toward the patient's children (Lauterbach et al. 2007; Taft et al. 2007).

Early studies of aggression and violence in patients with PTSD were conducted among combat veterans from the Vietnam era. Among participants in the National Vietnam Veterans Readjustment Study (NVVRS; Kulka et al. 1990), male veterans with PTSD reported an average of 13.3 acts of violence in the preceding year, whereas those without PTSD reported 3.5 acts of violence. The veterans with PTSD were also 1.5 times more likely to have been arrested or jailed and 3 times more likely to have been convicted of a felony crime. In another analysis of the NVVRS data, premilitary behaviors and experiences and postservice PTSD were both associated with postmilitary antisocial behavior (Fontana and Rosenheck 2005).

Violent behaviors of individuals who develop PTSD in response to sexual assaults, physical assaults, motor vehicle crashes, acts of terrorism, or exposure to natural and man-made disasters have not been as well studied. In contrast to individuals with noncombat PTSD, war veterans may have experienced periods of heightened vigilance and arousal lasting weeks to months and may have experienced extreme and repeated interpersonal violence during their traumatic exposure. This violence may include small arms battle with enemy forces, killing of enemy forces, wounding or killing of noncombatants, and repeated unexpected attacks with mortars, grenades, and other explosive devices. Some veterans may have also witnessed or participated in repeated nonwarfare acts of abusive violence, such as the killing of prisoners or civilians (Laufer et al. 1984). Some civilian law enforcement officers and other emergency responders may experience similar exposures but generally to a lesser degree and almost always for a shorter duration.

Psychiatric conditions commonly comorbid with PTSD include major depression, substance abuse disorders, and other anxiety disorders (American Psychiatric Association 2000). Elevated rates of PTSD and depression have been found among veterans from the current conflicts in Afghanistan and

Iraq, indicating that a new cohort of veterans is potentially at risk for elevated levels of aggression and violence, social impairments, and chronic physical problems, which may include traumatic brain injury (Grieger et al. 2006; Hoge et al. 2004, 2007, 2008; Lapierre et al. 2007). Among a small sample of such veterans, anger, hostility, and aggression were elevated in those who met full PTSD criteria, as well as in those who met subthreshold study criteria (Jakupcak et al. 2007). The four elements of aggression evaluated were destruction of property, threatened use of violence (with and without a weapon), and physical assault.

A meta-analysis of 39 studies, including those of nonveteran populations (e.g., battered women, refugees, those with physical illnesses), found a strong association between PTSD and anger and aggression (Orth and Wieland 2006). Military war experience, compared with other traumas, increased the effect size of the association. An increase in passage of time since the traumatic event also increased the effect size, suggesting that those with chronic PTSD are at greater risk of aggression and violent acts.

Compared with other populations, veterans with PTSD often demonstrate higher levels of anger, difficulty regulating anger, increased levels of criminality, increased levels of violence, and greater potential for serious acts of violence. Domains of anger problems include inaccurate perception and processing of environmental cues, heightened physiological and emotional activation, and behavioral inclinations to act in antagonistic or confrontative ways. Patients with regulatory deficits in all three domains display anger and aggression that has been labeled as a "ball of rage" (Chemtob et al. 1997).

In the 4 months prior to hospitalization, veterans hospitalized with severe PTSD were 7 times more likely than other psychiatric inpatients to have engaged in one or more acts of violence, 6 times more likely to have destroyed property, 6 times more likely to have threatened others without a weapon, 4 times more likely to have engaged in physical fights, and 3 times more likely to have made threats with a weapon (McFall et al. 1999). Severity of PTSD symptoms was also associated with increased risk of making threats of violence without a weapon, engaging in physical fights, and making threats with a weapon. Among veteran psychiatric inpatients with any diagnosis, veterans with combat exposure were more likely to engage in assaults or assault-related behavior during hospital admission than were veterans without such experiences (Yesavage 1983). Among elderly veterans in a chronic care setting, prior trauma and symptoms of PTSD were associated with increased anger, irritability, and observed aggressive behaviors (Carlson et al. 2008).

Among Vietnam War veterans with PTSD, premilitary problems, exposure to war-zone atrocities, and postwar problems were common. One-third of veterans reported childhood physical abuse, and approximately one-half endorsed one or more significant adolescent behavioral problems. Eighty-six percent endorsed witnessing abusive war-zone violence, and 91% both witnessed and participated in abusive violence (hurting, killing, or mutilating of Vietnamese people). Postmilitary problems in those with PTSD included violence toward one's spouse, 58%; violence toward others, 71%; drug problems, 62%; and alcohol problems, 73%. Interestingly, in this study, no association was found between premilitary factors and postmilitary violence or criminal behavior. Participation in killing during war was associated with postmilitary violence toward others and toward spouses (Hiley-Young et al. 1995).

Childhood traumas, level of combat exposure, presence and severity of PTSD symptoms, number of combat roles, exposure to atrocities, and preservice antisocial behaviors have all been examined in relation to later antisocial behavior and violence. The studies often used different measures, controlled for different potentially contributing variables, and sometimes had conflicting findings. When examined together, preservice antisocial behavior and the level of combat exposure were associated with postservice antisocial behavior, which included incidents of violence, other nonviolent illegal behaviors, occupational problems, and nonviolent interpersonal problems (Resnick et al. 1989). In another study, the number of combat roles, subjective stress in combat, the number of specific stress exposures, and total PTSD symptom severity were found to be associated with postservice assault and weapons charges (Wilson and Zigelbaum 1983).

Studies of PTSD and violence suggest multiple possible explanations for this association. Remaining questions include the extent to which troubled childhoods, exposure to violence itself, and comorbid substance use or other psychiatric conditions mediate the association. Perhaps due to the complex number of pathways to violence, models to predict future acts of violence among veterans with PTSD have not been successfully developed. Among one group of hospitalized veterans with PTSD, demographic variables, exposure to atrocities, severity of PTSD symptoms, severity of drug and alcohol problems, past violent behaviors, past suicidal behaviors, and prior treatment information were used in an attempt to develop such a model (Hartl et al. 2005). Only prior violence history was useful in predicting postdischarge violence; PTSD and depression severity both performed poorly in predicting high- and low-risk group membership.

General Risk Factors for Violence or Aggression

One of the few studies examining the association between PTSD and violence in individuals with PTSD as a consequence of mostly nonwartime experiences was conducted in a population of 1,140 incarcerated male felons (Collins and Bailey 1990). Prison arrest records indicated that 14% were currently incarcerated for acts of expressive violence (homicide, rape, or aggravated assault). Only 2.3% of the sample met study criteria for presence of PTSD. Of those, 31% reported combat trauma. Although most inmates did not meet criteria for the disorder, 795 (70%) endorsed at least one of nine symptoms of PTSD. When controlling for demographic variables, antisocial characteristics, and substance abuse, the researchers found that those who met criteria for the diagnosis of PTSD were 4.58 times more likely to be currently incarcerated for homicide, rape, or assault, and 6.75 times more likely to have been arrested for violence within the past year. Among those who did not meet full criteria for PTSD, the presence of each additional symptom of PTSD increased risk of current incarceration for a violent crime (odds ratio = 1.22) and of arrest for violence in the past year (odds ratio = 1.26). Of those arrested for a violent crime who endorsed at least 1 symptom of PTSD ($n = 80$), most reported that the PTSD symptoms began 1 or more years prior to the arrest, suggesting that the presence of symptoms may have contributed to the commission of the crime.

Risk of Family Violence

PTSD appears to contribute to direct aggression toward intimate partners, impaired relationships with children, and possible violence against children. On the Standard Family Violence Index (throwing something at someone, pushing, grabbing, shoving, slapping, kicking, biting, hitting, beating up, threatening with a gun or knife, or using a gun or knife on someone), veterans with PTSD endorsed an average of 22 such acts in the past year (Beckham et al. 1997). In contrast, combat veterans without PTSD endorsed an average of 0.2 such acts in the past year. Socioeconomic status, patterns of aggressive responding, and PTSD severity were associated with increased violence. Another study found that the presence of PTSD may actually mediate the effect of combat exposure on later intimate partner violence (Orcutt et al. 2003). Among multiple studies of Vietnam veterans, past-year partner violence rates ranged from 13% to 58%, with higher rates generally seen among inpatients with substance dependence, PTSD, or other psychiatric disorders (A. D. Marshall et al. 2005). PTSD severity was also correlated with partner abuse severity. Partner physical abuse has also been associated with alcohol consumption (frequency and amounts) and severity of hyperarousal symptoms (Savarese et al. 2001). Higher rates of depression and drug abuse, often comorbid with PTSD, were seen in veterans who have engaged in partner violence (Taft et al. 2005).

In a study of veterans with either PTSD or depression, but not both conditions, there were similar rates of partner violence (roughly 80%) and severe partner violence (roughly 40%) during the previous year (Sherman et al. 2006). Compared with control couples, in which the veteran did not currently meet criteria for a serious psychiatric illness, those couples in which the veteran had either depression or PTSD were twice as likely to endorse any act of partner violence and 4 times as likely to endorse an act of severe partner violence. The study did not include veterans with comorbid depression and PTSD, so the authors did not assess the relationship of comorbid illness to partner violence.

Among Vietnam veterans, the severity of PTSD symptoms was associated with negative satisfaction with parenting (perceived efficacy, enjoyment, quality of the relationship, satisfaction, and problems presented by the children) (Samper et al. 2004). After controlling for combat exposure, depression, and substance abuse, Ruscio et al. (2002) found that of the PTSD symptom clusters, emotional numbing was most positively associated with child misbehavior and disagreement with children, and most negatively associated with sharing experiences, contact, and overall quality of the parent-child relationship. Numbing was also most strongly associated with poorer parent relationships with children and with parent-on-child aggression (predominantly psychological, such as refusing to communicate or saying something spiteful) (Lauterbach et al. 2007). Although not tied to the presence of PTSD symptoms, increased rates of substantiated child maltreatment have occurred within military families in the period following the initiation of conflicts and frequent deployments to Iraq and Afghanistan (Rentz et al. 2007). This trend suggests that further study is needed to better understand whether PTSD or other deployment-related psychiatric conditions, including depression and substance abuse, are contributing to child maltreatment.

Risk Related to Firearm Ownership and Firearms Behaviors

Possession of firearms or the presence of firearms within a household may increase the risk of potential serious violence toward others or may elevate the risk of successful suicide. Compared with veterans who have substance use problems, veterans with PTSD reported owning over 4 times as many total firearms (3.2 vs. 0.72), over 5 times as many handguns (1.6 vs. 0.28), and 5 times as many rifles or shotguns (4.3 vs. 0.86). Interestingly, there was no difference in overall gun ownership between the two groups prior to military service (1.69 vs. 1.68) (Freeman and Roca 2001). Of the veterans with PTSD, 22% endorsed aiming a gun at a family member; 21% endorsed firing a gun in their house; 39% endorsed firing a gun to protect home, self, or family; and 54% endorsed holding a loaded gun with suicide in mind. In a separate study, 33% of the PTSD group endorsed carrying a gun on their person at least some of the time, and 33% endorsed killing or mutilating an animal "in a fit of rage" (not while hunting) (Freeman et al. 2003). Both studies were conducted among clinical samples of veterans with chronic combat-related PTSD. The combination of firearm-related aggressive acts and the presence of numerous firearms in homes of veterans with PTSD suggests a strong potential for lethal violence against others or successful suicide.

Risk of Suicide

Patients with PTSD are also at increased risk of suicide attempts or completions. Comorbidity of PTSD and other psychiatric conditions is common, and many patients with PTSD are diagnosed with three or more additional psychiatric conditions (Brady et al. 2000a). The most commonly comorbid conditions are depressive disorders, substance use disorders, and other anxiety disorders, all of which are associated with an increased risk of suicide. In one study, patients with comorbid depression and PTSD were at increased risk of suicide attempts compared with patients with only depression (Oquendo et al. 2003). In a second study, the presence of Cluster B personality disorders (paranoid, narcissistic, borderline, or antisocial personality) in addition to PTSD and depression further increased the risk of suicide attempts (Oquendo et al. 2005). In both of these studies, the majority of subjects were nonveteran women. Among veterans with schizophrenia or schizoaffective disorders, those with comorbid PTSD had higher rates of both suicidal ideation and suicidal behaviors (Strauss et al. 2006). In a large community sample (*N*=36,984), after adjusting for other mental disorders and physical disorders, PTSD was associated with increased suicide attempts (Sareen et al. 2007).

Subthreshold PTSD can also develop following exposure to traumatic events. Individuals not meeting full diagnostic criteria for the disorder experience comparable levels of impairment and suicidality when compared with patients who meet full criteria for the disorder (Zlotnick et al. 2002). In one large national screening study, roughly one in four subjects reported at least one PTSD symptom of at least 1 month in duration (R.D. Marshall et al. 2001b). Functional impairment, number of comorbid disorders, presence of a depressive disorder, and current suicidal ideation increased linearly and statistically with each additional PTSD symptom. Individuals with subthreshold PTSD were at greater risk of suicidal ideation even after controlling for the presence of a depressive disorder. These studies highlight the importance of screening all patients for a history of trauma and violence and for the presence of PTSD symptoms that may increase the risk of suicide or suicide attempts.

Assessment and Management of PTSD and Violence

Various guidelines have been published for the assessment and clinical management of PTSD (National Center for Posttraumatic Stress Disorder 2004; Ursano et al. 2004; Veterans Health Administration, Department of Defense 2004). Generally, the guidelines suggest that management be prioritized based on the degree to which each symptom or behavior is causing distress or loss of function or may have an impact on future safety. A high percentage of patients with PTSD experience comorbid conditions such as depression or substance abuse. Such comorbid conditions must also be evaluated and may need to be addressed first, because they may be the source of increased risk of morbidity or future risk. Friedman (2006) specifically addressed approaches to assessment and treatment of military veterans of the recent wars in Afghanistan and Iraq.

Knowing the nature of the events leading to the development of PTSD is of key importance in assessing potential future dangerousness. Exposures to combat and direct interpersonal violence, such as physical assault, appear much more likely to lead to PTSD-associated violence than traumas such as motor vehicle crashes or natural disasters. Risk factors to assess in combat veterans or others who have experienced extreme acts of interpersonal violence are outlined in Table 8–1. Patients should be asked to elaborate on the details, frequency, and duration of each endorsed experience to help the clinician fully understand and assess for potential and future violence.

As in all psychiatric evaluations, clinicians should question patients with PTSD about current suicidal ideation and past suicidal behaviors. High rates of comorbid depression, substance use disorders, or other psychiatric conditions and the tendency toward firearm ownership all increase the risk of suicide, as well as the risk of harm to others. Each of these areas should be carefully assessed in both acute and chronic inpatient and outpatient care settings. Because spouses and children are often the most available targets of violence, patients should be asked about patterns of interaction and conflict resolution within these relationships. If their responses are guarded or inconsistent, the clinician may need to contact family members for corroborating information. If spousal abuse is active and severe, court protective orders or

Table 8–1. Historical violence risk factor assessment in the evaluation of patients with PTSD

1. Have you been the victim of violent sexual or physical assault?
2. How many times have you been assaulted, and in what settings?
3. Did the assault(s) involve use of a weapon?
4. Have you been in combat?
5. Have you killed or wounded another in combat?
6. Did you participate in or observe killing, mutilation, or torture of civilians?
7. Are there specific settings or events that cause you to become irritable or "on guard"?
8. What are your patterns of substance use?
9. What access do you have to dangerous weapons?

other protective actions may be needed until other solutions can be developed. Nonviolent relationship difficulties should also be evaluated and addressed proactively because they may lead to escalating and potentially violent interactions. Numbing and social withdrawal should be assessed carefully, because this cluster of symptoms seems strongly associated with interpersonal difficulties within families, including emotionally and potentially physically abusive behaviors.

If patients endorse chronic angry or hostile attitudes or are the victims of violent interpersonal assault, they should be asked about their own history of violent acts. Information about the frequency and severity of these acts and the time duration since the most recent episode should be obtained. Potential screening questions and follow-on elaboration questions are provided in Table 8–2. For each past act of violence, patients should be questioned about the specific events leading up to the incident, specific provocation by the target of their violence, and possible involvement of alcohol or drugs. Patients should also be asked how their situation, condition, attitudes, and recent behaviors differ from those present at the time of the prior act. If current conditions closely parallel those present at the time of past acts of violence, specific behavioral "trigger avoidance" or "emotional defusing" plans should be developed and rehearsed in the clinician's office. Shortened intervals between treatment sessions, warnings to individuals specifically at risk, and possibly hospitalization or other protective interventions should also be considered. In all instances, the treatment record should reflect the components of the risk assessment and management decision process.

Clinicians should always be vigilant for their own safety. In emergency department settings, agitated or intoxicated patients with PTSD may need to be relocated to quieter and less stimulating settings. Personal belongings and clothing should be checked for firearms or other weapons both in the emergency department and upon admission, if required. All personnel should be trained in emergency response and restraint techniques. Hospitalized patients with PTSD should be carefully assessed for a history of prior violence; prior to discharge, a thorough assessment of potential future violence should be performed. Follow-up visits should be scheduled to occur shortly after discharge, preferably with a provider known to the patient. Family members should be educated on signs of pending violent behavior and methods of obtaining an emergent reevaluation or engaging in other safety plans (e.g., leaving the

Table 8–2. Acts of aggression inventory

Event inventory

1. In the past year, have you been involved in a physical or verbal altercation with a stranger?
2. In the past year, have you been involved in a physical or verbal altercation with an acquaintance?
3. In the past year, have you been involved in a physical or verbal altercation with a spouse or relative?
4. In the past year, have you hit, kicked, or otherwise harmed or killed an animal in anger?
5. In the past year, have you damaged property as a consequence of being angry?
6. In the past year, have you contemplated or attempted suicide?
7. Have you been involved in a physical altercation within the past 6 months?
8. In the past year, have you threatened, struck, or been emotionally aggressive toward your spouse/significant other or any of your children?
9. Do you own a firearm?
    a. Where do you keep it?
    b. Do you keep it loaded?
    c. Do you carry a firearm or other weapon on your person or keep one "at arm's length"?
    d. Have you ever pointed a firearm or brandished another weapon at another individual as a warning or threat?

For each positive event response:

- a. Were you under the influence of alcohol or drugs at the time?
- b. Did you have in your possession a firearm, knife, or other weapon?
- c. Did you use or consider using the weapon?
- d. When was the last time such an incident occurred?
- e. What were the specific circumstances that led up to the event?
- f. What was the outcome of the event?
- g. How did it end?
- h. Did you feel your behavior was appropriate under the circumstances?
- i. Would you likely respond the same way in a similar situation?
- j. How commonly would you encounter similar situations?

home or calling police) if they perceive a threat of violence. Involvement of family members in treatment can offer both increased support and early identification of potential problem behaviors.

Schoenfeld et al. (2004) and Friedman (2006) provide overviews of pharmacological treatments for PTSD. Most studies of treatment for PTSD have been in nonveteran populations and have not specifically examined the efficacy on symptoms of aggression or irritability. Selective serotonin reuptake inhibitors (SSRIs) have been shown to be effective, well tolerated, and safe in treatment of non-combat-related PTSD. Sertraline was effective during the acute and continuation stages of treatment, with improvements seen in intrusive symptoms, avoidance symptoms, and arousal symptoms (Brady et al. 2000b; Davidson et al. 2001b; Londborg et al. 2001). Continued treatment was also effective in preventing relapse of PTSD (Davidson et al. 2001a), and study participants reported improvements in quality of life and functional measures, whereas discontinuation was associated with a worsening of symptoms and a decline in quality of life (Rapaport et al. 2002). Similar response rates and improvements in symptoms and function were seen in controlled studies of paroxetine versus placebo in the treatment of PTSD (R. D. Marshall et al. 2001a). Fluoxetine has also been shown to reduce the symptoms of PTSD; however, the response was not as robust as in studies with other SSRIs (Martenyi et al. 2002). Because an increase in symptoms is associated with increased rates of violent acts, the use of SSRIs in the management of PTSD symptoms may result in lower rates of violence among patients with PTSD.

The antihypertensive prazosin may also be helpful in reducing nightmares, improving sleep quality, reducing psychological responses to trauma cues, and improving global clinical status (Daly et al. 2005; Raskind et al. 2007; Taylor et al. 2006). Reduced response to trauma cues suggests that prazosin may also be of benefit in reducing irritability and aggressive behavior.

Other antidepressants, mood stabilizers, and atypical antipsychotic medications may also be helpful for augmentation treatment of refractory symptoms of PTSD—including anger and irritability, which are often tied to potential acts of violence (Friedman 2006; Schoenfeld et al. 2004). Although studies have shown the efficacy of these medications in managing aggression, these studies have primarily evaluated aggression related to disorders other than PTSD (e.g., pervasive developmental disorders, traumatic brain injury, dementia) (Aupperle 2006; Bellino et al. 2006; Findling 2008; Kim and

Bijlani 2006; McDougle et al. 2008; Pappadopulos et al. 2006). In view of the potentially serious side effects of these medications and the safer profile of the SSRI medications, atypical antipsychotic medications should generally not be considered for initial treatment or single-agent therapy unless a severe or unusual symptom profile is present. Short-term treatment may be of benefit for severe agitation, sleep disturbance, aggression, or pervasive paranoia.

Among available psychotherapeutic choices, cognitive-behavioral therapies have been shown to be most effective in treating patients with PTSD (Ursano et al. 2004). Within this class of treatments, both prolonged exposure therapy (guided imagery of the events and in vivo experiences) and cognitive therapy or cognitive processing therapy (correction of distorted perceptions or appraisal of events) have been shown to have benefit in trauma survivors (Foa 2006; Foa and Meadows 1998; Foa et al. 2005; Monson et al. 2006). Virtual reality is also currently being examined as a component of the exposure (Gerardi et al. 2008; Ready et al. 2008). In addition, many patients prefer psychosocial treatments over pharmacological treatments (Zoellner et al. 2003). Cognitive therapies are highly adaptable to specific patient problems. If anger, hostility, and aggression are prominent, these functional difficulties can be addressed and reduced effectively by using behavioral rehearsal, cognitive processing, and/or prolonged exposure to the cues that elicit these emotions or behaviors.

Marital and/or family therapy may also be needed if these relationships have deteriorated or if aggression toward a spouse or child has been demonstrated. Reestablishment of communication, definition of family roles, and education of family members would all be beneficial in decreasing interpersonal aggression and hostility, thereby reducing the risk of further deterioration of existing social supports and aggression within and outside the family.

Key components of evaluation, treatment planning, and management of aggression and violence associated with PTSD are summarized in Table 8–3.

Conclusion

Although older studies of associations between PTSD, violence, and aggression typically focused on combat veterans from the Vietnam War, newer studies have included nonveteran populations and veterans from more recent conflicts. In contrast to patients with PTSD evolving from single-event

Table 8–3. Summary of assessment and management of aggression or violence associated with PTSD

Assessment

1. Obtain a detailed psychiatric history, including substance use history.
2. Perform a comprehensive mental status examination, including an assessment of suicidal and homicidal ideation or behaviors, psychosis, or significant cognitive behaviors.
3. Identify comorbid conditions, such as active substance abuse, depression, or other anxiety disorders.
4. Determine historical risk factors (see Table 8–1).
5. Assess past violent or aggressive acts (see Table 8–2).
6. Obtain information from family members.

Management and treatment

1. Establish rapport and trust.
2. Establish the hierarchy of problems to be addressed.
3. Establish a risk reduction plan.
    a. Reduce/eliminate substance use/abuse.
    b. Reduce firearm access/use.
    c. Develop patient and family reaction plans in the event of imminent acts of violence or aggression.
    d. Ensure safety in hospital or clinic environments.
4. Consider pharmacological treatments.
    a. Consider initial treatment with a selective serotonin reuptake inhibitor.
    b. Depending on the symptom profile, consider the use of prazosin, an atypical antipsychotic, or other medication(s).
5. Consider psychotherapeutic treatments.
    a. Based on the hierarchy of problems, select from among behavioral, cognitive, or exposure therapies (recognizing that each includes components of the others).
    b. Adjust the focus of treatment as problems subside or others emerge.
    c. Consider couples, family, and interpersonal therapies.
    d. If substance use problems are present, consider the use of 12-step or similar community-based assistance programs.

trauma, those who develop PTSD as a consequence of repeated threats to life, threats from multiple sources, and observation of repeated acts of violence toward others over extended periods of time are more likely to display altered levels of vigilance, psychological numbing, and possibly aggressive or violent behaviors in future settings. Although reasonable evidence supports recommended treatments for PTSD in general, most of the validation of such treatments was not performed in combat veteran populations—that is, those most likely to experience aggression and display violence as a consequence of their experiences and illness. Furthermore, no controlled studies have specifically examined the effects of treatments on reducing aggression or violence in patients with PTSD. Areas that require further research include therapeutic interventions specifically targeting combat-related PTSD and PTSD-related violent behavior and aggression. Present knowledge and clinical experience suggest that assessment and management of aggression and violence in patients with PTSD include the use of pharmacological and psychotherapeutic treatments with demonstrated efficacy in other (e.g., noncombat) patients with PTSD. Effective management also requires treatment of other comorbid conditions, often the involvement of family members, and development of a hierarchy of problems and interventions.

Key Clinical Points

- Violence and aggression are common problems for people with PTSD.
- Individuals with PTSD, particularly those with PTSD from combat, are more likely than the general population to become violent, to be arrested, and to be convicted of a felony.
- Factors such as preservice antisocial behavior, combat exposure, the number of combat roles, subjective stress from combat, and PTSD symptom severity correlate to increased violent behavior.
- Combat veterans with PTSD own more firearms and are more likely to aim a gun at a family member, fire a gun in their house, and hold a loaded gun while contemplating suicide compared to combat veterans without PTSD.
- Individuals with PTSD are at a higher risk for self-harm, including a higher risk for suicide.

- Most guidelines for treating PTSD suggest management prioritized on which symptom or behavior is causing distress, loss of function, or diminished safety.
- Clinicians may need to address comorbid conditions prior to focusing on treatment of PTSD.
- Patients should be asked about patterns of interactions with family and friends and about conflict resolution within these relationships, with particular attention to any violent interactions.
- Previous violence is a strong predictor of future violence, so a thorough history of previous violence should be obtained from each patient, with attention to frequency, severity, and time since most recent episode.
- Providers should always ensure their own safety when interacting with potentially violent patients.
- Medication and therapies for patients with a history of violence should be instituted early in order to help manage future aggression.
- Management of violence and aggression should include the treatment of any comorbid conditions, involve family and friends in treatment plans as possible, and prioritize problems and interventions to ensure safety.

References

American Psychiatric Association: Diagnostic and Statistical Manual of Mental Disorders, 4th Edition, Text Revision. Washington, DC, American Psychiatric Association, 2000

Aupperle P: Management of aggression, agitation, and psychosis in dementia: focus on atypical antipsychotics. Am J Alzheimers Dis Other Demen 21:101–108, 2006

Beckham JC, Feldman ME, Kirby AC, et al: Interpersonal violence and its correlates in Vietnam veterans with chronic posttraumatic stress disorder. J Clin Psychol 53:859–869, 1997

Bellino S, Paradiso E, Bogetto F: Efficacy and tolerability of quetiapine in the treatment of borderline personality disorder: a pilot study. J Clin Psychiatry 67:1042–1046, 2006

Brady K, Killeen TK, Brewerton T, et al: Comorbidity of psychiatric disorders and posttraumatic stress disorder. J Clin Psychiatry 61 (suppl 7):22–32, 2000a

Brady K, Pearlstein T, Asnis GM, et al: Efficacy and safety of sertraline treatment of posttraumatic stress disorder: a randomized controlled trial. JAMA 283:1837–1844, 2000b

Carlson EB, Lauderdale S, Hawkins J, et al: Posttraumatic stress and aggression among veterans in long-term care. J Geriatr Psychiatry Neurol 21:61–71, 2008

Casada JH, Roache JD: Behavioral inhibition and activation in posttraumatic stress disorder. J Nerv Ment Dis 193:102–109, 2005

Chemtob CM, Novaco RW, Hamada RS, et al: Anger regulation deficits in combat-related posttraumatic stress disorder. J Trauma Stress 10:17–36, 1997

Collins JJ, Bailey SL: Traumatic stress disorder and violent behavior. J Trauma Stress 3:203–220, 1990

Daly CM, Doyle ME, Radkind M, et al: Clinical case series: the use of prazosin for combat-related recurrent nightmares among Operation Iraqi Freedom combat veterans. Mil Med 170:513–515, 2005

Davidson J, Pearlstein T, Londborg P, et al: Efficacy of sertraline in preventing relapse of posttraumatic stress disorder: results of a 28-week double-blind, placebo-controlled study. Am J Psychiatry 158:1974–1981, 2001a

Davidson JR, Rothbaum BO, van der Kolk BA, et al: Multicenter, double-blind comparison of sertraline and placebo in the treatment of posttraumatic stress disorder. Arch Gen Psychiatry 58:485–492, 2001b

Findling RL: Atypical antipsychotic treatment of disruptive behavior disorders in children and adolescents. J Clin Psychiatry 69 (suppl 4):9–14, 2008

Foa EB: Psychosocial therapy for posttraumatic stress disorder. J Clin Psychiatry 67 (suppl 2):40–45, 2006

Foa EB, Meadows EA: Psychosocial treatments for posttraumatic stress disorder, in Psychological Trauma. Edited by Yehuda R (Review of Psychiatry Series, Vol 17; Oldham JM and Riba MB, series eds). Washington, DC, American Psychiatric Press, 1998, pp 179–204

Foa EB, Hembree EA, Cahill SP, et al: Randomized trial of prolonged exposure for posttraumatic stress disorder with and without cognitive restructuring: outcome at academic and community clinics. J Consult Clin Psychol 73:953–964, 2005

Fontana A, Rosenheck R: The role of war-zone trauma and PTSD in the etiology of antisocial behavior. J Nerv Ment Dis 193:203–209, 2005

Freeman TW, Roca V: Gun use, attitudes toward violence, and aggression among combat veterans with chronic posttraumatic stress disorder. J Nerv Ment Dis 189:317–320, 2001

Freeman TW, Roca V, Kimbrell T: A survey of gun collection and use among three groups of veteran patients admitted to Veterans Affairs hospital treatment programs. South Med J 96:240–243, 2003

Friedman MJ: Posttraumatic stress disorder among military returnees from Afghanistan and Iraq. Am J Psychiatry 163:586–593, 2006

Gerardi M, Rothbaum BO, Ressler K, et al: Virtual reality exposure therapy using a virtual Iraq: case report. J Trauma Stress 21:209–213, 2008

Grieger TA, Cozza SJ, Ursano RJ, et al: Posttraumatic stress disorder and depression in battle-injured soldiers. Am J Psychiatry 163:1777–1783; quiz 1860, 2006

Hartl TL, Rosen C, Drescher KD, et al: Predicting high-risk behaviors in veterans with posttraumatic stress disorder. J Nerv Ment Dis 193:464–472, 2005

Hiley-Young B, Blake DD, Abueg FR, et al: Warzone violence in Vietnam: an examination of premilitary, military, and postmilitary factors in PTSD in-patients. J Trauma Stress 8:125–141, 1995

Hoge CW, Castro CA, Messer SC, et al: Combat duty in Iraq and Afghanistan, mental health problems, and barriers to care. N Engl J Med 351:13–22, 2004

Hoge CW, Terhakopian A, Castro CA, et al: Association of posttraumatic stress disorder with somatic symptoms, health care visits, and absenteeism among Iraq war veterans. Am J Psychiatry 164:150–153, 2007

Hoge CW, McGurk D, Thomas J, et al: Mild traumatic brain injury in U.S. soldiers returning from Iraq. N Engl J Med 358:453–463, 2008

Jakupcak M, Conybeare D, Phelps L, et al: Anger, hostility, and aggression among Iraq and Afghanistan War veterans reporting PTSD and subthreshold PTSD. J Trauma Stress 20:945–954, 2007

Kim E, Bijlani M: A pilot study of quetiapine treatment of aggression due to traumatic brain injury. J Neuropsychiatry Clin Neurosci 18:547–549, 2006

Kulka RA, Schlenger WE, Fairbank JA, et al: Trauma and the Vietnam War Generation: Report of Findings From the National Vietnam Veterans Readjustment Study. New York, Brunner/Mazel, 1990, pp 139–188

Lapierre CB, Schwegler AF, Labauve BJ: Posttraumatic stress and depression symptoms in soldiers returning from combat operations in Iraq and Afghanistan. J Trauma Stress 20:933–943, 2007

Laufer RS, Gallops MS, Frey-Wouters E: War stress and trauma: the Vietnam veteran experience. J Health Soc Behav 25:65–85, 1984

Lauterbach D, Bak C, Reiland S, et al: Quality of parental relationships among persons with a lifetime history of posttraumatic stress disorder. J Trauma Stress 20:161–172, 2007

Londborg PD, Hegel MT, Goldstein S, et al: Sertraline treatment of posttraumatic stress disorder: results of 24 weeks of open-label continuation treatment. J Clin Psychiatry 62:325–331, 2001

Marshall AD, Panuzio J, Taft CT: Intimate partner violence among military veterans and active duty servicemen. Clin Psychol Rev 25:862–876, 2005

Marshall RD, Beebe KL, Oldham M, et al: Efficacy and safety of paroxetine treatment for chronic PTSD: a fixed-dose, placebo-controlled study. Am J Psychiatry 158:1982–1988, 2001a

Marshall RD, Olfson M, Hellman F, et al: Comorbidity, impairment, and suicidality in subthreshold PTSD. Am J Psychiatry 158:1467–1473, 2001b

Martenyi F, Brown EB, Zhang H, et al: Fluoxetine versus placebo in posttraumatic stress disorder. J Clin Psychiatry 63:199–206, 2002

McDougle CJ, Stigler KA, Erickson CA, et al: Atypical antipsychotics in children and adolescents with autistic and other pervasive developmental disorders. J Clin Psychiatry 69 (suppl 4):15–20, 2008

McFall M, Fontana A, Raskind M, et al: Analysis of violent behavior in Vietnam combat veteran psychiatric inpatients with posttraumatic stress disorder. J Trauma Stress 12:501–517, 1999

Monson CM, Schnurr PP, Resick PA, et al: Cognitive processing therapy for veterans with military-related posttraumatic stress disorder. J Consult Clin Psychol 74:898–907, 2006

National Center for Posttraumatic Stress Disorder: Iraq War Clinician's Guide, 2nd Edition. Washington, DC, U.S. Department of Veterans Affairs, 2004

Oquendo MA, Friend JM, Halberstam B, et al: Association of comorbid posttraumatic stress disorder and major depression with greater risk for suicidal behavior. Am J Psychiatry 160:580–582, 2003

Oquendo M, Brent DA, Birmaher B, et al: Posttraumatic stress disorder comorbid with major depression: factors mediating the association with suicidal behavior. Am J Psychiatry 162:560–566, 2005

Orcutt HK, King LA, King DW: Male-perpetrated violence among Vietnam veteran couples: relationships with veterans' early life characteristics, trauma history, and PTSD symptomatology. J Trauma Stress 16:381–390, 2003

Orth U, Wieland E: Anger, hostility, and posttraumatic stress disorder in trauma-exposed adults: a meta analysis. J Consult Clin Psychol 74:698–706, 2006

Pappadopulos E, Woolston S, Chait A, et al: Pharmacotherapy of aggression in children and adolescents: efficacy and effect size. J Can Acad Child Adolesc Psychiatry 15:27–39, 2006

Rapaport MH, Endicott J, Clary CM: Posttraumatic stress disorder and quality of life: results across 64 weeks of sertraline treatment. J Clin Psychiatry 63:59–65, 2002

Raskind MA, Peskind ER, Hoff DJ, et al: A parallel group placebo controlled study of prazosin for trauma nightmares and sleep disturbance in combat veterans with posttraumatic stress disorder. Biol Psychiatry 61:928–934, 2007

Ready DJ, Thomas KR, Worley V, et al: A field test of group based exposure therapy with 102 veterans with war-related posttraumatic stress disorder. J Trauma Stress 21:150–157, 2008

Rentz ED, Marshall SW, Loomis D, et al: Effect of deployment on the occurrence of child maltreatment in military and nonmilitary families. Am J Epidemiol 165:1199–1206, 2007

Resnick HS, Foy DW, Donahoe CP, et al: Antisocial behavior and post-traumatic stress disorder in Vietnam veterans. J Clin Psychol 45:860–866, 1989

Ruscio AM, Weathers FW, King LA, et al: Male war-zone veterans' perceived relationships with their children: the importance of emotional numbing. J Trauma Stress 15:351–357, 2002

Samper RE, Taft CT, King DW, et al: Posttraumatic stress disorder symptoms and parenting satisfaction among a national sample of male Vietnam veterans. J Trauma Stress 17:311–315, 2004

Sareen J, Cox BJ, Stein MB, et al: Physical and mental comorbidity, disability, and suicidal behavior associated with posttraumatic stress disorder in a large community sample. Psychosom Med 69:242–248, 2007

Savarese VW, Suvak MK, King LA, et al: Relationships among alcohol use, hyperarousal, and marital abuse and violence in Vietnam veterans. J Trauma Stress 14:717–732, 2001

Schoenfeld FB, Marmar CR, Neylan TC, et al: Current concepts in pharmacotherapy for posttraumatic stress disorder. Psychiatr Serv 55:519–531, 2004

Sherman MD, Sautter F, Jackson MH, et al: Domestic violence in veterans with posttraumatic stress disorder who seek couples therapy. J Marital Fam Ther 32:479–490, 2006

Strauss JL, Calhoun PS, Marx CE, et al: Comorbid posttraumatic stress disorder is associated with suicidality in male veterans with schizophrenia or schizoaffective disorder. Schizophr Res 84:165–169, 2006

Taft CT, Pless AP, Stalans LJ, et al: Risk factors for partner violence among a national sample of combat veterans. J Consult Clin Psychol 73:151–159, 2005

Taft CT, Vogt DS, Marshall AD, et al: Aggression among combat veterans: relationships with combat exposure and symptoms of posttraumatic stress disorder, dysphoria, and anxiety. J Trauma Stress 20:135–145, 2007

Taylor FB, Lowe K, Thompson C, et al: Daytime prazosin reduces psychological distress to trauma specific cues in civilian trauma posttraumatic stress disorder. Biol Psychiatry 59:577–581, 2006

Ursano RJ, Bell C, Eth S, et al: Practice guideline for the treatment of patients with acute stress disorder and posttraumatic stress disorder. Am J Psychiatry 161 (suppl 11):3–31, 2004

Veterans Health Administration, Department of Defense: VA/DoD Clinical Practice Guideline for the Management of Post-Traumatic Stress, Version 1.0. Washington, DC, Veterans Health Administration, Department of Defense, 2004

Wilson JP, Zigelbaum SD: The Vietnam veteran on trial: the relation of post-traumatic stress disorder to criminal behavior. Behav Sci Law 1:69–83, 1983

Yesavage JA: Differential effects of Vietnam combat experiences vs. criminality on dangerous behavior by Vietnam veterans with schizophrenia. J Nerv Ment Dis 171:382–384, 1983

Zlotnick C, Franklin CL, Zimmerman M: Does "subthreshold" posttraumatic stress disorder have any clinical relevance? Compr Psychiatry 43:413–419, 2002

Zoellner LA, Feeny NC, Cochran B, et al: Treatment choice for PTSD. Behav Res Ther 41:879–886, 2003

9

Emerging and Alternative Therapies

Michael J. Roy, M.D., M.P.H.

Albert Rizzo, Ph.D.

Joann Difede, Ph.D.

Barbara O. Rothbaum, Ph.D., A.B.P.P.

Successful treatment of posttraumatic stress disorder (PTSD) should improve quality of life in multiple domains, such that patients experience improved functional status, decreased symptom severity, and reduced vulnerability to subsequent stress. The most proven pharmacological therapies are selective serotonin reuptake inhibitors (SSRIs), such as sertraline, which are safe and well tolerated, but reported response rates are only in the 40%–60% range and relapses are common (Brady et al. 2000; J.R. Davidson et al. 2001; Zohar et al. 2002). First-line nonpharmacological therapies, such as cognitive-behavioral therapy (CBT) with imaginal exposure therapy, have demonstrable benefit

(Ballenger et al. 2000; Foa et al. 1999; Rothbaum et al. 2000b), and a meta-analysis found a greater effect size and higher compliance rates for nonpharmacological therapies than for pharmacotherapy (Van Etten and Taylor 1998). However, even these well-validated approaches still leave many patients with persistent symptoms, because of either a reluctance to participate or an inability to effectively engage in the therapeutic process. Moreover, because many patients have an aversion to "traditional" psychotherapy as well as to pharmacotherapy, some may find alternative approaches more appealing.

Expert treatment guidelines and consensus statements in 1999 and 2000 recommended CBT and exposure therapy as first-line therapy for PTSD (Ballenger et al. 2000; Foa et al. 1999), and to date no evidence indicates that another therapy is more effective (Foa et al. 2003). In fact, a recent Institute of Medicine report concluded that CBT with exposure therapy is the only therapy with sufficient evidence to recommend it for PTSD (Berg et al. 2008). Imaginal exposure has been the most widely employed exposure approach. In this approach, the therapist asks the patient to repeatedly recall and narrate his or her traumatic experience in progressively greater detail, both to facilitate the therapeutic processing of related emotions and to decondition the learning cycle of the disorder via a habituation-extinction process. Prolonged exposure (Foa and Kozak 1986; Jaycox et al. 2002), one of the best-evidenced forms of exposure therapy, characteristically includes psychoeducation, controlled breathing techniques, and in vivo exposure as homework, in addition to prolonged imaginal exposure to traumatic memories during 9–12 therapy sessions of 90 minutes each. However, avoidance of reminders of the trauma is a defining feature of PTSD, so it is not surprising that many patients are unwilling or unable to effectively visualize and recount traumatic events. Some of the most promising emerging therapies, therefore, seek to broaden the appeal of exposure therapy to effectively engage more patients. The emerging therapies reviewed in this chapter do not yet have a sufficient evidence basis to fully endorse widespread use in clinical care. Most, however, have some preliminary supportive data, and ongoing trials aim to better define their clinical utility.

Virtual Reality Exposure Therapy

The most promising alternative to imaginal exposure is virtual reality exposure therapy (VRET), in which patients are immersed in simulated trauma-relevant environments that enable precise control of stimuli. Virtual reality proponents emphasize that technology facilitates the delivery of specific, consistent, and controllable stimuli that do not rely exclusively on the patient's imagination, and the success of several clinical applications has been documented (Glantz et al. 2003; Rizzo and Kim 2005; Rizzo et al. 2004; Rose et al. 2005). Virtual reality may be broadly defined as "a way for humans to visualize, manipulate, and interact with computers and extremely complex data" (Aukstakalnis and Blatner 1992, p. 2). Such advanced human-computer interaction is facilitated by the integration of computers, real-time graphics, visual displays, body tracking sensors, and specialized interface devices that serve to immerse a participant in a simulated world that changes in a natural way with head and body motion.

Virtual reality environments typically display computer graphics in a motion-tracked head-mounted display, which can be augmented by vibration platforms, localizable three-dimensional sounds, physical props such as rifles, and scent delivery technology, to facilitate a multisensory immersive experience for participants. This approach engenders a strong sense of presence, or of "being there," for those immersed in the virtual environment, and can enable greater clinical assessment and intervention than can traditional methods (Rizzo et al. 1998, 2004). Similar to an aircraft simulator that tests and trains pilots under various controlled conditions, virtual reality provides context-relevant simulated environments that can assess and treat cognitive and emotional conditions. The clinician can use virtual reality to precisely and systematically deliver complex, dynamic, and ecologically relevant stimuli, reinforced by behavioral tracking, performance recording, and physiological monitoring, to foster sophisticated interaction.

Diverse virtual environments have been used to treat a variety of phobias, including claustrophobia (Botella et al. 1998, 2000), fear of flying (Botella et al. 2004; Rothbaum et al. 1996, 2000b, 2002, 2006; Smith et al. 1999; Wiederhold and Wiederhold 2002), acrophobia (Emmelkamp et al. 2001; Rothbaum et al. 1995), arachnophobia (Carlin et al. 1997; Garcia-Palacios et al. 2002), and fear of driving after an automobile accident (Walshe et al. 2003); social anxiety disorder (Anderson et al. 2003; Klinger et al. 2005); and other anxiety disorders (Krijn et al. 2004; Powers and Emmelkamp 2008; Rothbaum and Hodges 1999). Virtual reality has also proven useful for treating addictive behaviors (Bordnick et al. 2005), for acute pain reduction (Gold et al.

2005), and for the assessment and rehabilitation of cognitive and motor impairments following stroke, brain injury, and other neurological disorders (Morrow et al. 2006; Rizzo et al. 2004; Rose et al. 2005; Stewart et al. 2007).

Virtual Vietnam

The first application of VRET to PTSD occurred in 1997 when Georgia Tech and Emory University researchers used a Virtual Vietnam environment with Vietnam veterans (Rothbaum et al. 2001). Even though this study occurred more than 20 years after the end of the Vietnam War, the disorder continued to significantly impair the psychological well-being, functional status, and quality of life of many veterans, despite valiant efforts to develop and apply traditional PTSD treatment methods. The virtual environment delivered via the head-mounted display featured rice fields, riverbanks, and perspectives from the inside and outside of a Huey helicopter, supplemented by visual and auditory stimuli, such as machine gun fire, rockets, explosions, and shouting. An initial case study of a 50-year-old male Vietnam veteran with PTSD (Rothbaum and Hodges 1999) documented posttreatment improvement on all measures of PTSD, and maintenance of these gains 6 months later: a 34% decrease in clinician-rated and a corresponding 45% decrease in self-reported symptoms of PTSD. In a subsequent open clinical trial, in which 16 male Vietnam veterans with PTSD participated in an average of 13 exposure therapy sessions over 5–7 weeks, Rothbaum et al. (2001) reported a significant reduction in PTSD and related symptoms. The degree of immersion was evidenced by patients who reported seeing things, such as enemy soldiers and burning vehicles, that were not in the virtual environment but were in fact part of their own memories.

Virtual World Trade Center

Difede and Hoffman (2002) treated a World Trade Center (WTC) survivor of the 9/11/2001 attack with VRET, effecting a complete remission. In a subsequent clinical trial, WTC survivors who completed VRET treatments demonstrated statistically and clinically significant decreases on the "gold standard" Clinician-Administered PTSD Scale (CAPS) relative to pretreatment and to the wait-list control group, with a between-groups posttreatment effect size of 1.54 (Difede et al. 2006, 2007). Seven of 10 completers in the virtual reality group achieved remission of PTSD, whereas none of the wait-list controls did;

treatment gains were maintained at 6 month follow-up. Also noteworthy was that five of the 10 virtual reality patients had previously participated in imaginal exposure treatment with no clinical benefit. This finding suggests that virtual reality may be a useful treatment option for PTSD related to combat or terrorist attacks. A predetermined sequence of events and stimuli was employed for all participants. The virtual environment included actual 9/11 audio recordings made by a national news network, as well as virtual humans (avatars), which, for example, could be seen falling from the burning World Trade Center towers.

Other Applications of Virtual Reality Following War or Terrorism

VRET may prove to be a better option for some populations than others. VRET might be ill suited for victims of rape or childhood sexual trauma, because graphic depiction of such assaults might be prohibitively uncomfortable for patient and therapist alike. On the other hand, VRET might have distinct advantages over imaginal exposure therapy for many active-duty military service members and combat veterans.

Studies addressing treatment failures with imaginal exposure have shown that a failure to engage emotionally is the best predictor of a poor treatment outcome (Cardena and Spiegel 1993; Foa et al. 1995; Jaycox et al. 1998; Koopman et al. 1994), and the machismo that succeeds on the battlefield may pose a significant obstacle to therapy requiring repeated acknowledgment of fears and emotions associated with traumatic memories. Although VRET does not obviate the need for such disclosures, a vivid, attractive medium may facilitate recall and expression. VRET offers a way to circumvent natural avoidance by directly delivering multisensory contextual cues that evoke the trauma without demanding that the patient actively engage in effortful memory retrieval. Within a virtual reality environment, the hidden world of the patient's imagination is not exclusively relied upon, which may be particularly relevant with PTSD, because avoidance of cues and reminders of the trauma is a cardinal symptom of the disorder.

In addition, VRET offers an appealing, nontraditional treatment approach that may be perceived with less stigma by "digital-generation" service members and veterans who are often reluctant to participate in traditional talk therapies. This sophisticated and highly realistic virtual environment may be especially appealing to service members who have shown distrust and reluctance toward traditional mental health services despite knowing they need help. Service members, particularly those returning with their units rather than alone, attach significantly greater stigma to psychological issues than to medical problems, which suggests that subjective norms influence stigma perceptions (Britt 2000). The challenges inherent in emotionally engaging with fear structures, as required in prolonged exposure, and the stigma associated with traditional talk therapies pose significant barriers to optimizing access to care that might be more effectively addressed through VRET. Although servicewide efforts have modestly reduced some of the more commonly cited obstacles to seeking mental health care, they nevertheless remain highly prevalent (Hoge et al. 2004; Warner et al. 2008). Even if the efficacy of VRET is no greater than for imaginal exposure, if the novelty or appeal is sufficient to attract greater numbers of service members and veterans to engage in treatment, VRET could significantly reduce the morbidity of PTSD. Also, VRET might achieve a higher rate of response and more rapid response, by facilitating recall of traumatic events and related feelings and reactions, thus enabling a therapist to more quickly identify and ameliorate disabling symptoms, especially for patients who are more avoidant or alexithymic.

Studies of several virtual environments to treat PTSD in survivors of war and terrorist attacks are under way. In one case series, Wood et al. (2008) described "partial remission" of PTSD symptoms in four of six Iraq war service members using virtual reality combined with meditation and attentional refocusing. However, the report did not include statistical analyses, and the mean pretreatment PTSD Checklist–Military Version (PCL-M) score was 47.3, lower than the conservative cutoff score of 50 that best identifies PTSD (Weathers et al. 1993). Portuguese researchers, addressing an estimated 25,000 survivors with PTSD from the 1961–1974 Portuguese Colonial War in Africa, modified a common PC-based combat game to develop a virtual reality exposure scenario (Gamito et al. 2007). An initial case report identified a participant who withdrew after experiencing a distressing flashback following the seventh session. Although this type of reaction is rarely reported in the exposure literature, and may be just a chance occurrence, it highlights the need for well-trained clinicians who can pace therapy appropriately and carefully monitor patient response. Meanwhile, Israeli researchers are beginning to treat PTSD using a virtual terrorist "bus bombing" scenario, in which participants are positioned in a cafe across the street from a city bus that stops and explodes (Josman et al. 2006). These various VRET scenarios may become a primary treatment of PTSD in the future, and VRET at least provides an additional modality for clinicians faced with patients who are resistant to other therapies or who have treatment-resistant PTSD.

Virtual Iraq

The University of Southern California's Institute for Creative Technologies has spearheaded the development of a highly sophisticated virtual reality environment, Virtual Iraq. The environment was based on Full Spectrum Warrior, a commercially successful Xbox game and U.S. Army–funded combat tactical simulation trainer. The virtual environment has undergone progressive evolution, with the application of both existing and novel art and technology assets in response to feedback from patients and therapists.

Virtual Iraq consists of Middle Eastern–themed city and desert road scenarios (Figure 9–1*A, B*) intended to resemble the environments most service members encounter during deployment to Iraq. An 18-square-block city setting includes a marketplace, desolate streets, old buildings, ramshackle apartments, warehouses, mosques, shops, and dirt lots strewn with junk. Access to building interiors and rooftops is available, and the backdrop creates the illusion of being immersed in a densely populated desert city. Virtual vehicles and animated pedestrians (civilian and military) can be inserted or removed from scenes, and helicopters can be made to take off, fly overhead, and land. A desert road scenario incorporates expansive sand dunes interspersed with palm trees and other vegetation, intact and broken-down structures, bridges, battle wreckage, a checkpoint, debris, and virtual human figures who create ambushes at various points. The patient can be positioned as the driver, as a passenger, or in the turret of a Humvee, traveling alone or within a convoy; fellow passengers may suffer visible wounds.

The therapist can adjust the time of day or night, level of illumination, and weather conditions (e.g., sandstorm, rain), and can insert a night vision perspective or ambient sounds (e.g., wind, motors, city noise, prayer call). The therapist can insert users anywhere within the virtual environment, based on his or her perception of the patient's needs at that point in time. Patients can drive the Humvee with a standard gamepad controller, and can walk through the city with either the gamepad or a "thumb-mouse" controller mounted on

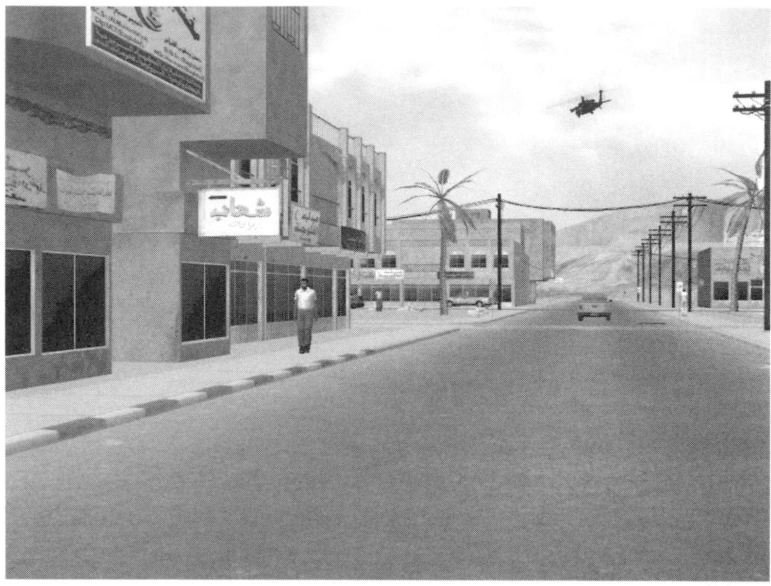

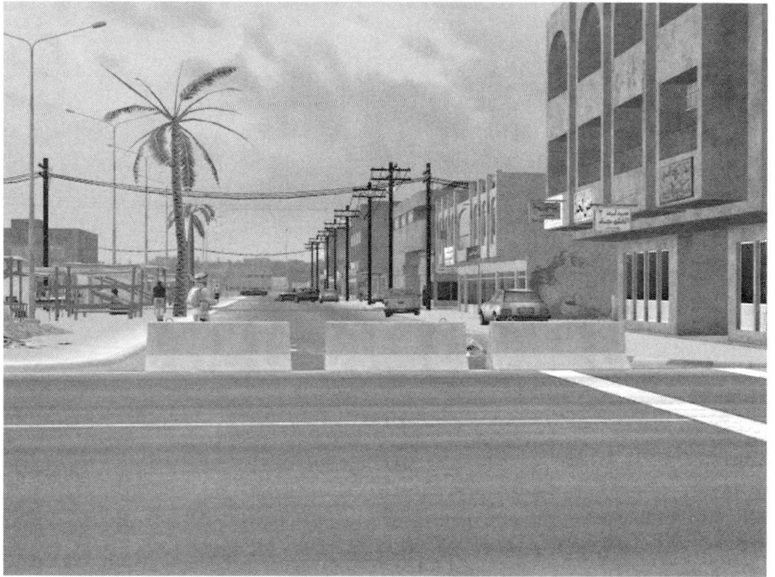

Figure 9–1. *A.* Middle Eastern city scenarios shown in Virtual Iraq.

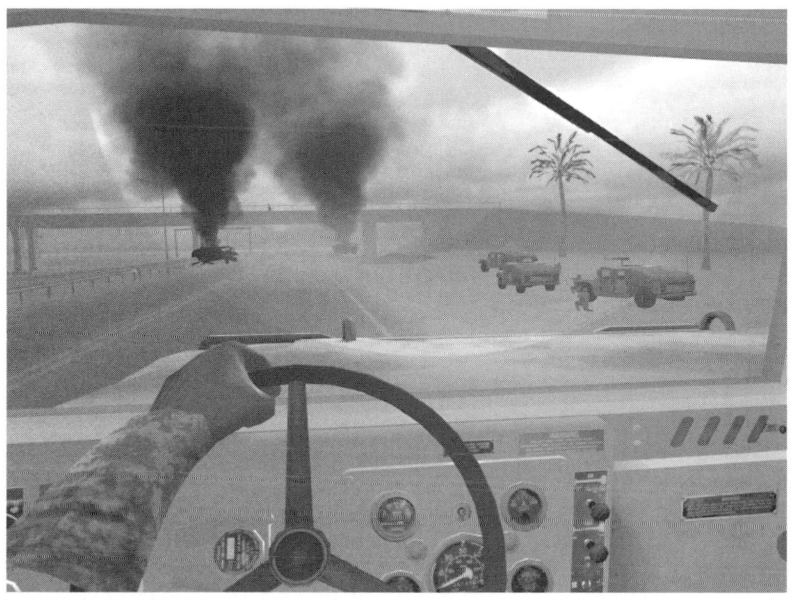

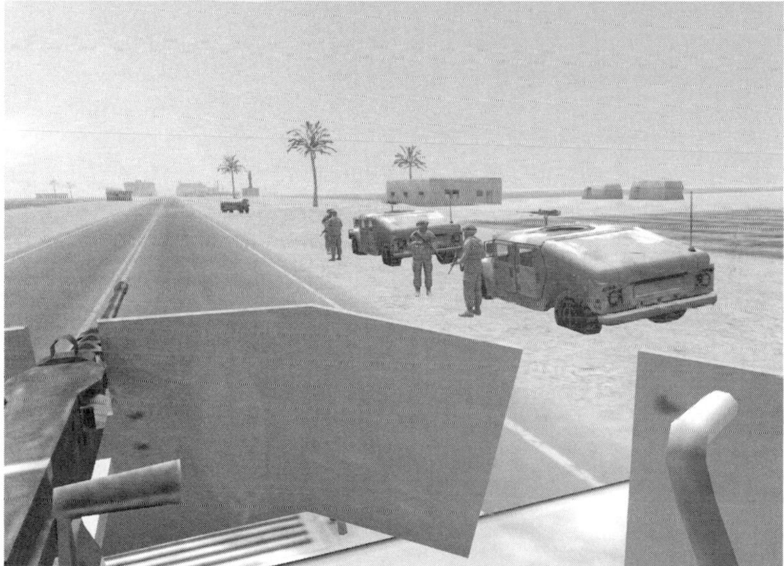

Figure 9–1. *B.* Middle Eastern desert road scenarios, Virtual Iraq.

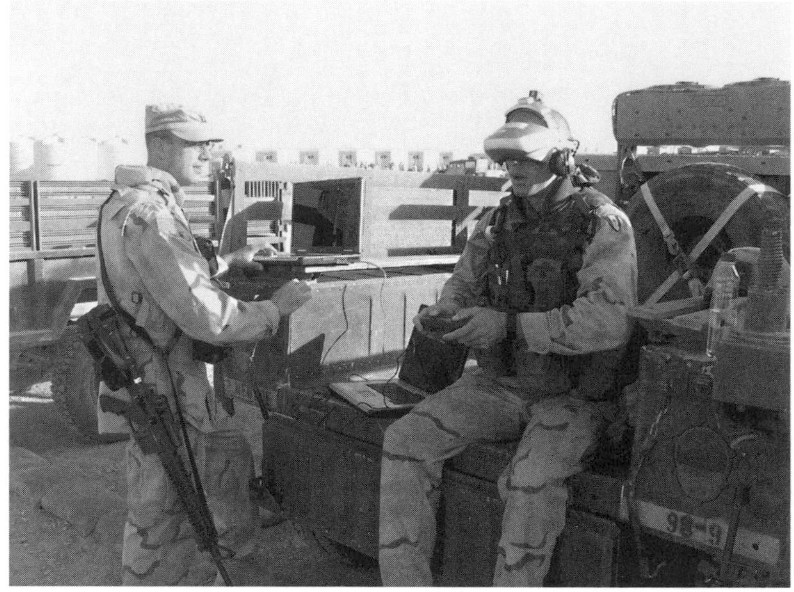

Figure 9–2. User testing with initial prototype of Virtual Iraq embedded within a combat stress control team in Iraq.

a replica of an M16 rifle. The visual stimuli presented via the head-mounted display can be supplemented by directional three-dimensional audio, vibrotactile, and olfactory stimuli. The therapist has the "Wizard of Oz" capability to introduce and remove each stimulus with the click of a mouse on a computer screen, while being in full audio contact with the patient. This enables an individually customized approach, taking into account the patient's past experience and treatment progress. The incorporation of new stimulus options based on patient and clinician feedback and the iterative creation of more complex events have been other vital features of the work to date. New supplemental options include terrain that is more characteristic of Afghanistan, with, for example, snow-capped mountains in the background, as well as the scent of roasting lamb.

The high prevalence of PTSD in service members returning from Iraq and Afghanistan, coupled with the relatively low cost of the system (less than $10,000 for the full system, including computers), has led to widespread use

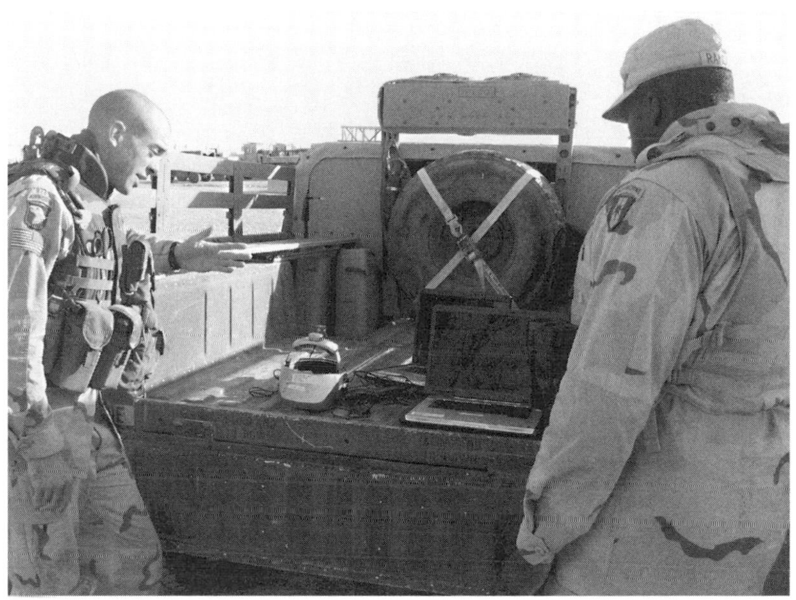

Figure 9–3. User giving feedback on experience with initial prototype of Virtual Iraq embedded within a combat stress control team in Iraq.

of Virtual Iraq as a research tool for the treatment of PTSD in studies across the United States (Parsons and Rizzo 2008). Virtual Iraq is currently in use for VRET research and a variety of other PTSD-related investigations with active-duty service members and veterans at Naval Medical Center–San Diego (NMCSD), Madigan Army Medical Center, Camp Pendleton, Emory University, Walter Reed Army Medical Center, the Weill Medical College of Cornell University, and 14 other Veterans Affairs, military, and university laboratory sites. User-centered tests with early prototypes of the Virtual Iraq application were conducted at NMCSD, as well as within an Army Combat Stress Control team in Iraq (see Figures 9–2 and 9–3). This informal feedback provided essential information on the content, realism, and usability of the initial "intuitively designed" system.

To date, both a case report and the results of an open trial have been published describing experience with the Virtual Iraq environment in the treatment of PTSD. The case report from Emory University documented a 56%

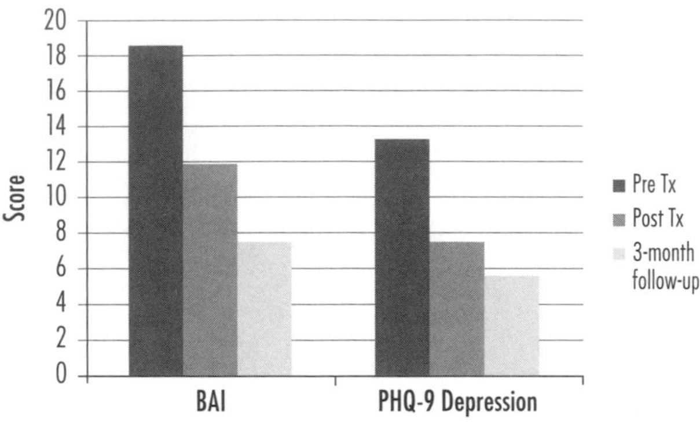

Figure 9–4. Beck Anxiety Inventory (BAI) and Patient Health Questionnaire (PHQ-9) Depression results for 20 service members recently returned from Iraq and diagnosed with PTSD at Naval Medical Center–San Diego and Camp Pendleton.

Tx=treatment. Average number of sessions <11.

reduction in the CAPS score for a veteran of Operation Iraqi Freedom with PTSD, representing a significant decrease in clinical severity (Gerardi et al. 2008).

The open clinical trial was conducted with active-duty service members recently returned from Iraq and diagnosed with PTSD at NMCSD and Camp Pendleton (Rizzo et al. 2009). Service members who had no benefit with conventional PTSD treatments, such as group counseling and SSRIs, consented to a protocol featuring an average of 90- to 120-minute sessions twice weekly for 5 weeks. The actual number and frequency of sessions were adjusted to meet individual needs. Analyses of the first 20 treatment completers (19 male, 1 female; mean age=28, age range 21–51) identified a significant decrease in mean PCL-M score, from a baseline of 54.4 (SD=9.7) to 35.6 (SD=17.4) after treatment (t=5.99, df=19, P<0.001). Symptoms declined more than 50%, correcting for the PCL-M no-symptom baseline of 17, and 16 of 20 completers no longer met DSM-IV criteria for PTSD at posttreatment. Scores on the Beck Anxiety Inventory decreased significantly, from 18.6 (SD=9.5) to 11.9 (SD=13.6) after treatment (t=3.37, df=19, P<0.003), and scores on the nine-item Patient Health Questionnaire (PHQ-9) for depression decreased

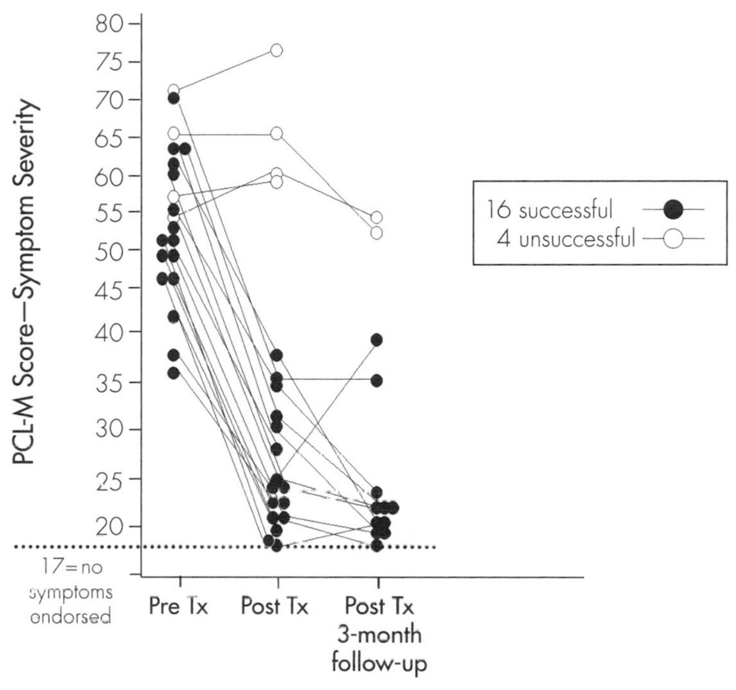

Figure 9–5. PTSD Checklist-Military (PCL-M) assessment over time of 20 service members recently returned from Iraq and diagnosed with PTSD at Naval Medical Center–San Diego and Camp Pendleton.

Tx = treatment. Average number of sessions < 11.

from 13.3 (SD = 5.4) to 7.1 (SD = 6.7) (t = 3.68, df = 19, P < 0.002). The average number of sessions for this sample was just under 11. Results are graphically displayed in Figures 9–4 and 9–5.

The study at NMCSD has been successful in establishing VRET as feasible for treatment of service members with PTSD. The Virtual Reality Therapy and Imaging in Combat Veterans trial, which is currently under way at Walter Reed Army Medical Center, is important to document efficacy: 44 service members are randomly assigned to VRET or to prolonged exposure, the best-evidenced form of imaginal exposure. Each arm features twelve

90-minute sessions over approximately 6 weeks, with half the time during VRET sessions 4–11 spent in the Virtual Iraq environment. The primary outcome measure is the score on the CAPS, administered at the end of treatment and at the end of a 12-week follow-up period, compared with the baseline CAPS score. Secondary measures include the PCL-M, the Beck Depression Inventory to assess depression, the Beck Anxiety Inventory to assess anxiety, and the 36-Item Short Form Health Survey (SF-36) and the World Health Organization Disability Assessment Schedule II to assess functional status. One of four VRET completers achieved the targeted 30% decrease in CAPS score at the end of treatment, compared with none of the participants in the prolonged exposure arm. The average decrease in the CAPS score of 13% for VRET, versus 6% for prolonged exposure, is much less robust than anticipated. However, subjects have also reported to their study therapists decreased avoidant behavior, such as using the subway and attending restaurants, sporting events, and movie theaters. There are some disincentives for service members to acknowledge the extent of improvement. If they remain on active duty, recovery might increase their risk for repeat deployment; also, if they have a medical board or disability assessment in progress, significant improvement might reduce or eliminate subsequent disability payments. More recent participants seem to be responding better, however, so the lack of anticipated improvement in some early subjects might also represent a learning curve for study therapists, or more successful identification of motivated participants over time. In any case, greater numbers of participants should be more revealing.

Optimism remains about the potential for VRET to attract service members who resist traditional approaches, and to achieve a higher response rate in at least a segment of this population. The well-documented reluctance of service members with mental disorders to seek mental health care (Hoge et al. 2004) is a significant concern, and recent efforts by the military to better prepare service members for combat need to be supplemented by efforts to persuade service members to get treatment. Use of VRET might help address this problem, especially by embedding it within "postcombat reset training" and thus decreasing the perceived stigma of seeking treatment by incorporating it into designated duties upon return from deployment. VRET may prove especially appealing to young military personnel, whose experience with digital gaming technology may render VRET more attractive and comfortable.

The virtual environment may also prove useful in prevention or screening. Individual or group virtual training before deployment could enable soldiers to practice their duties in a simulated, stressful war environment, providing greater preparation and confidence for performance under fire. Such training might help negate factors strongly associated with PTSD, such as perceived preparedness for duties and unit cohesion. In regard to screening, there is a known "honeymoon" period following return from deployment, when soldiers are relieved to be out of harm's way and less likely to acknowledge PTSD symptoms. These symptom reports increase markedly within 3–6 months after return. To help with identifying predictors of PTSD, soldiers could be exposed to the virtual environment shortly after return, monitored for physiological responses (blood pressure, heart rate, skin impedance, etc.), and followed for the development of PTSD. Identification of predictors could facilitate early interventions to prevent PTSD.

From the perspective of the clinician, virtual reality systems can serve as skill extenders, providing approaches that are most beneficial in the context of overall care delivered by a thoughtful professional cognizant of the complexity of PTSD. These systems are not intended for use as "self-help" or in an automated treatment protocol.

Other Emerging and Alternative Nonpharmacological Therapies

Eye Movement Desensitization and Reprocessing

Shapiro (1989) initially described eye movement desensitization and reprocessing (EMDR) as "eliciting… sequences of large-magnitude, rhythmic saccadic eye movements while holding in mind the most salient aspect of a traumatic memory" (p. 214). In that article, Shapiro provided a case report of a patient who had a marked improvement in anxiety, flashbacks, intrusive thoughts, and sleep disturbances after a single session. This case report and other anecdotal accounts of remarkable improvement of PTSD within a few sessions began to attract attention in the early 1990s. Shapiro has subsequently expanded the approach to incorporate eight phases, following an informational processing model seeking to correct maladaptive storage of perceptual information (Shapiro 2002). Elements of CBT and of psychodynamic, experiential, physiological, and interactional therapies are included to facilitate resolution of memories, desensitize stimuli currently inducing distress, and incorporate adaptive skills, attitudes, and behaviors to improve functional status. Shapiro described a standardized approach that includes methods of dual stimulation (eye movements are one method, with alternating taps and auditory tones also having been employed), cognitive reorganization, sequential targeting of information, and free association.

Systematic reviews of EMDR have drawn mixed conclusions. The more positive perspectives include a 1998 meta-analysis of psychotherapies, in which the greatest effect sizes were reported for CBT and EMDR, with EMDR appearing to confer benefit with a smaller number of sessions and in less time (Van Etten and Taylor 1998); a 2002 review finding that 12 of 12 randomized controlled trials (RCTs) supported the efficacy of EMDR (Maxfield and Hyer 2002); and a 2003 qualitative review reporting similar impact with exposure, CBT and/or stress inoculation training, and EMDR (Hembree and Foa 2003). However, two recent reviews raised methodological concerns: one meta-analysis found some evidence of efficacy when EMDR was compared with other therapies that did not include exposure, while noting that the quality of the methods was highly variable (P.R. Davidson and Parker 2001), and the other noted that although 15 of 16 RCTs reported positive findings for EMDR, most of the studies were small and unblinded, had high dropout rates, and were of inconsistent quality (Centre for Reviews and Dissemination 2007). Foa and Meadows (1997) were more explicit in their concerns, citing mixed evidence from studies "inundated with methodological flaws," a perspective later echoed by others (Harvey et al. 2003).

The Institute of Medicine's recent review of the evidence identified 10 RCTs that compared EMDR with other treatments plus a wait-list control or with a wait-list only (Berg et al. 2008). Six of 10 studies had major methodological limitations, such as high dropout rates, inadequate or absent treatment of missing values, and failure to perform independent, blinded assessment of outcomes. The other four studies had no or few major flaws; two showed no effect with EMDR, whereas the other two demonstrated that EMDR resulted in a statistically significant improvement in CAPS scores or remission of PTSD. Although Hembree and Foa (2003) suggested that eye movement may not be integral to the effect of EMDR, and Shapiro emphasized the reprocessing element more in recent writings (Shapiro 2002) than in earlier accounts, which highlighted the role of eye movement, the Institute of Medicine concluded that insufficient evidence is available to determine the added value of the eye movement component (Berg et al. 2008). Well-designed studies are needed to determine the overall merits of EMDR, as well as how valuable eye movement is in this approach.

Biofeedback

Biofeedback enables patients to observe what happens with their heart rate, blood pressure, body temperature, or other bodily functions when under stress conditions; the intent is to foster self-control over these reactions. Hickling et al. (1986) reported on an open trial utilizing 8–14 sessions of biofeedback and relaxation training, in addition to individual group therapy, for six patients with PTSD. Although some improvement was reported, the numbers were insufficient for statistical analysis, and the study had numerous methodological limitations, including a lack of controls; lack of blinded, independent assessment of subjects; and suboptimal outcome measures for PTSD (primary measures used were the Minnesota Multiphasic Personality Inventory, State-Trait Anxiety Inventory, and Beck Depression Inventory). A subsequent study found that biofeedback and relaxation training were less effective than EMDR (Silver et al. 1995), and a larger study involving 90 Vietnam veterans found little evidence supporting the efficacy of biofeedback, relaxation training, or deep breathing exercises (Watson et al. 1997). Another well-designed RCT confirmed that EMDR achieved better results than biofeedback-assisted relaxation at the end of treatment and at 3-month follow-up (Carlson et al. 1998). Biofeedback may still have an adjunctive role, but it does not appear to have significant merit as a stand-alone treatment.

Hypnosis

Despite its use for more than a century in the treatment of dissociative disorders and the aftermath of trauma, there has been no scientific assessment of hypnosis in the treatment of PTSD. However, hypnosis has been used as an adjunctive treatment, such as in association with EMDR. This may be a useful element of therapy for those individuals with PTSD who are easily hypnotized, but it should be appropriately evaluated in prospective, controlled studies.

Acupuncture

One small study has been reported comparing acupuncture with group CBT and with a wait-list control in the treatment of PTSD. Relatively large effect sizes were reported for both acupuncture (1.29) and group CBT (1.42) at the end of treatment, with the benefits sustained at 3-month follow-up (Hollifield et al. 2007). However, group CBT, as opposed to individual CBT, is not yet a proven therapy. In another recently reported (Engel et al. 2008) but not yet published trial, service members at Walter Reed Army Medical Center were randomly assigned to receive either eight 90-minute acupuncture sessions or usual care. This trial identified significantly greater reductions in PTSD symptoms with acupuncture. These studies show some promise for acupuncture, but additional methodologically rigorous trials are necessary, with a comparison to sham acupuncture or an evidence-based intervention.

Emerging and Alternative Pharmacological Therapies

An Institute of Medicine report assessing the evidence for various treatments of PTSD concluded that no pharmacological therapies have indisputable efficacy (Berg et al. 2008); therefore, all pharmacological approaches might still be considered emerging or alternative. In this section, we focus on several pharmacological agents that are considered promising by some researchers or clinicians, but as of yet have not been tested in well-designed, prospective clinical trials.

D-Cycloserine

D-cycloserine (DCS) was approved by the U.S. Food and Drug Administration more than 20 years ago for the treatment of tuberculosis and has documented safety in humans. More recently, DCS has been shown in animal studies to facilitate the extinction of learned fear and to produce generalized extinction (Davis et al. 2006). DCS is thought to act as a partial agonist at *N*-methyl-D-aspartate glutamate receptors believed to be important in short-term learning and memory. Thus, some researchers have begun to test DCS in conjunction with exposure therapy to synergistically enhance the action of glutamate released into synapses in response to psychotherapy.

The first clinical application was a randomized, double-blind, placebo-controlled trial of DCS in conjunction with VRET for 28 patients with acrophobia (Ressler et al. 2004). Those receiving DCS had significantly greater improvement on multiple outcome measures compared with those receiving placebo, both early in the course of treatment and 3 months later. Two studies found that compared with placebo, 50 mg of DCS administered 1 hour prior to exposure therapy sessions for treatment of social phobia induced a higher response rate (Guastella et al. 2008; Hofmann et al. 2006). Several studies have also assessed the efficacy of DCS in conjunction with exposure therapy for obsessive-compulsive disorder. The two studies with positive findings used 100 mg of DCS 1 hour prior to each of 10 exposure sessions (Wilhelm et al. 2008) and 125 mg 2 hours prior to 10 exposure sessions (Kushner et al. 2007). The only study to find no advantage to adjunctive DCS used 250 mg 4 hours before each of twelve 90-minute sessions (Storch et al. 2007). Rothbaum (2008) postulated several possible explanations for Storch et al.'s (2007) negative trial: 1) DCS may have been given too early; 2) the dose may have been too high, resulting in more antagonistic action, given that DCS is a partial agonist; and 3) because more and longer sessions were used in both arms, the response rate was so high in the comparison group that it made distinction between DCS and placebo difficult. Any or all of these may be factors necessitating additional studies to clarify the benefit of DCS for clinical practice. Several studies are in progress to assess the efficacy of DCS in enhancing the response to exposure therapy for PTSD. At this point, DCS has significant potential as a novel agent that can enhance the response to psychotherapy rather than as monotherapy.

St. John's Wort

Studies of St. John's wort (*Hypericum perforatum*) for mild to moderate depression have had mixed results; some initial studies with positive findings had methodological limitations, and subsequent larger, more rigorous trials or meta-analyses indicated less efficacy. Although no studies have been conducted in patients with PTSD to argue for or against the use of St. John's wort, its over-the-counter status means that some patients with PTSD may present after having initiated it on their own.

Kava Kava

No studies have been reported evaluating the efficacy of kava kava (*Piper methysticum*) for PTSD, but it is the most popular herbal remedy for anxiety, based on some initial, methodologically limited studies. More recent studies have failed to demonstrate benefit. For example, a meta-analysis of three placebo-controlled trials of kava kava for generalized anxiety disorder found no evidence of benefit, and in fact identified a significant effect in favor of placebo for patients who had higher baseline anxiety (Connor et al. 2006). A large Internet-based placebo-controlled trial of kava kava likewise found a trend, although not statistically significant, favoring placebo for the relief of anxiety (Jacobs et al. 2005). Based on another meta-analysis, in which kava kava and homeopathy were lumped together as complementary and alternative therapies for generalized anxiety disorder, Hidalgo et al. (2007) reported that study participants taking those alternatives fared worse than those receiving placebo. There seems little evidence that would support the use of kava kava in PTSD treatment, though further study is necessary to clarify this assertion.

Valerian Root

Valerian root (*Valeriana officinalis*) is a popular remedy for insomnia, although it has not been studied specifically for PTSD. One meta-analysis suggested some evidence of benefit for insomnia, with improved sleep quality identified in 6 of 16 studies; however, there was evidence of publication bias (Bent et al. 2006). A subsequent systematic review of 29 trials assessed both safety and efficacy (Taibi et al. 2007). Although valerian appears to be safe, most studies found no difference in efficacy between valerian and placebo; in particular, none of the most recent and most methodologically rigorous studies found any evidence of benefit for valerian. Current evidence does not indicate a need for further studies of valerian in PTSD treatment.

Inositol

Inositol is a building block in the lipid component of cell membranes. In the mid-1990s, Israeli researchers conducted small, methodologically limited studies of inositol for the treatment of both depression (Levine et al. 1995) and PTSD (Kaplan et al. 1996); findings suggested possible benefit in the former condition but not the latter. No further studies have been done with inositol for PTSD, but a Cochrane review reported no clear evidence of benefit from use of inositol in the treatment of depression in four trials with a total of 141 participants (Taylor et al. 2004). There does not appear to be reason to pursue additional work with inositol in the treatment of PTSD.

Conclusion

A large number of emerging and alternative treatments are being considered for PTSD. Currently, the most active research among nonpharmacological therapies is with virtual reality exposure. Preliminary evidence looks encouraging, although the studies are still ongoing. Among the emerging pharmacotherapy approaches, the use of D-cycloserine augmentation of exposure therapy remains quite promising, but again the results of current trials are essential to determine whether enthusiasm is justified.

Key Clinical Points

- Current therapeutic regimens are effective in a majority of patients, but many individuals continue to have persistent symptoms of PTSD despite conventional treatment.
- Virtual reality therapy is an immersive treatment that simulates the trauma-relevant environments with precise control of a variety of inputs and may provide another useful means of intervention.
- EMDR has produced marked improvement in some cases of PTSD, but it is not yet clear which elements of the therapy are necessary.
- Biofeedback therapy focuses individuals on monitoring their own body under stress conditions; on the basis of current evidence, biofeedback may have an adjunctive role in PTSD treatment, but not as a first-line intervention.
- Hypnosis and acupuncture may have potential for use in the treatment of PTSD, as suggested by findings in small studies, but further research is needed to determine the role of these therapies, and they cannot be recommended at this time based on current evidence.
- D-Cycloserine augmentation of exposure therapy appears promising, but further research will better determine the utility of this drug.
- St. John's wort, kava kava, inositol, and valerian root have been evaluated for the treatment of PTSD, but current scientific evidence does not support the use of these compounds.

References

Anderson P, Rothbaum BO, Hodges LF: Virtual reality exposure in the treatment of social anxiety: two case reports. Cogn Behav Pract 10:240–247, 2003

Aukstakalnis S, Blatner D: The Art and Science of Virtual Reality. Berkeley, CA, Peach Pit Press, 1992

Ballenger JC, Davidson JR, Lecrubier Y, et al: Consensus statement on posttraumatic stress disorder from the International Consensus Group on Depression and Anxiety. J Clin Psychiatry 61:60–66, 2000

Bent S, Padula A, Moore D, et al: Valerian for sleep: a systematic review and meta-analysis. Am J Med 119:1005–1012, 2006

Berg AO, Breslau N, Lezak MD, et al: Treatment of Posttraumatic Stress Disorder: An Assessment of the Evidence. Washington, DC, National Academies Press, 2008

Bordnick P, Graap K, Copp H, et al: Virtual reality cue reactivity assessment in cigarette smokers. Cyberpsychol Behav 8:487–492, 2005

Botella C, Baños RM, Perpiñá C, et al: Virtual reality treatment of claustrophobia: a case report. Behav Res Ther 36:239–246, 1998

Botella C, Baños RM, Villa H, et al: Virtual reality in the treatment of claustrophobic fear: a controlled, multiple-baseline design. Behav Ther 33:583–595, 2000

Botella C, Osma J, García-Palacios A, et al: Treatment of flying phobia using virtual reality: data from a 1-year follow-up using a multiple baseline design. Clin Psychol Psychother 11:311–323, 2004

Brady K, Pearlstein T, Asnis GM, et al: Efficacy and safety of sertraline treatment of posttraumatic stress disorder: a randomized controlled trial. JAMA 284:563–564, 2000

Britt TW: The stigma of psychological problems in a work environment: evidence from the screening of service members returning from Bosnia. J Appl Physiol 30:1599–1618, 2000

Cardena E, Spiegel D: Dissociative reactions to the San Francisco Bay Area earthquake of 1989. Am J Psychiatry 150:474–478, 1993

Carlin AS, Hoffman HG, Weghorst S: Virtual reality and tactile augmentation in the treatment of spider phobia: a case report. Behav Res Ther 35:153–158, 1997

Carlson JG, Chemtob CM, Rusnak K, et al: Eye movement desensitization and reprocessing (EMDR) treatment for combat-related posttraumatic stress disorder. J Trauma Stress 11:3–24, 1998

Centre for Reviews and Dissemination: Eye movement desensitization and reprocessing in the treatment of posttraumatic stress disorder: a review of an emerging therapy. Database of Abstracts of Reviews of Effects 2007

Connor KM, Payne V, Davidson JR: Kava in generalized anxiety disorder: three placebo-controlled trials. Int J Clin Psychopharmacol 21:49–53, 2006

Davidson JR, Rothbaum BO, van der Kolk BA, et al: Multicenter, double-blind comparison of sertraline and placebo in the treatment of posttraumatic stress disorder. Arch Gen Psychiatry 58:485–492, 2001

Davidson PR, Parker KC: Eye movement desensitization and reprocessing (EMDR): a meta-analysis. J Consult Clin Psychol 69:305–316, 2001

Davis M, Ressler K, Rothbaum BO, et al: Effects of D-cycloserine on extinction: translation from pre-clinical to clinical work. Biol Psychiatry 60:369–375, 2006

Difede J, Hoffman HG: Virtual reality exposure therapy for World Trade Center posttraumatic stress disorder: a case report. Cyberpsychol Behav 5:529–535, 2002

Difede J, Hoffman H, Jaysinghe N: Innovative use of virtual reality technology in the treatment of PTSD in the aftermath of September 11. Psychiatr Serv 53:1083–1085, 2002

Difede J, Cukor J, Patt I, et al: The application of virtual reality to the treatment of PTSD following the WTC attack. Ann N Y Acad Sci 1071:500–501, 2006

Difede J, Cukor J, Jayasinghe N, et al. Virtual reality exposure therapy for the treatment of posttraumatic stress disorder following September 11, 2001. J Clin Psychiatry 68:1639–1647, 2007

Emmelkamp PM, Bruynzeel M, Drost L, et al: Virtual reality treatment in acrophobia: a comparison with exposure in vivo. Cyberpsychol Behav 4:335–339, 2001

Engel CC, Harper Cordova E, Benedek D, et al: Acupuncture for posttraumatic stress disorder: a randomized trial in a military population. Engel CC, Principal Investigator. National Clinical Trials Identifier 00320138. Abstract no 196398. Paper presented at the 24th annual meeting, International Society for Traumatic Stress Studies, Chicago, IL, November 13–15, 2008

Foa EB, Kozak MJ: Emotional processing of fear: exposure to corrective information. Psychol Bull 99:20–35, 1986

Foa EB, Meadows EA: Psychosocial treatments for posttraumatic stress disorder: a critical review. Annu Rev Psychol 48:449–480, 1997

Foa EB, Riggs DS, Massie ED, et al: The impact of fear activation and anger on the efficacy of exposure treatment for PTSD. Behav Ther 26:487–499, 1995

Foa EB, Davidson RT, Frances A: The expert consensus guideline series: treatment of posttraumatic stress disorder. J Clin Psychiatry 60:5–76, 1999

Foa EB, Rothbaum BO, Furr A: Is the efficacy of exposure therapy for posttraumatic stress disorder augmented with the addition of other cognitive behavior therapy procedures? Psychiatr Ann 33:47–53, 2003

Gamito P, Oliveira J, Morais D, et al: War PTSD: a VR pre-trial case study. Annual Review of Cybertherapy and Telemedicine 4:191–198, 2007

Garcia-Palacios A, Hoffman H, Carlin A, et al: Virtual reality in the treatment of spider phobia: a controlled study. Behav Res Ther 40:983–993, 2002

Gerardi M, Rothbaum BO, Ressler K, et al: Virtual reality exposure therapy using a virtual Iraq: case report. J Trauma Stress 21:209–213, 2008

Glantz K, Rizzo AA, Graap K: Virtual reality for psychotherapy: current reality and future possibilities. Psychotherapy: Theory, Research, Practice, Training 40:55–67, 2003

Gold JI, Kim SH, Kant AJ, et al: Virtual anesthesia: the use of virtual reality for pain distraction during acute medical interventions. Seminars in Anesthesia, Perioperative Medicine and Pain 24:203–210, 2005

Guastella AJ, Richardson R, Lovibond PF, et al: A randomized controlled trial of D-cycloserine enhancement of exposure therapy for social anxiety disorder. Biol Psychiatry 63:544–549, 2008

Harvey AG, Bryant RA, Tarrier N: Cognitive behavior therapy for posttraumatic stress disorder. Clin Psychol Rev 23:501–522, 2003

Hembree EA, Foa EB: Interventions for trauma-related emotional disturbances in adult victims of crime. J Trauma Stress 16:187–199, 2003

Hickling EJ, Sison GF Jr, Vanderploeg RD: Treatment of posttraumatic stress disorder with relaxation and biofeedback training. Biofeedback Self Regul 11:125–134, 1986

Hidalgo RB, Tupler LA, Davidson JR: An effect-size analysis of pharmacologic treatments for generalized anxiety disorder. J Psychopharmacol 21:864–872, 2007

Hofmann SG, Meuret AE, Smits JA, et al: Augmentation of exposure therapy with D-cycloserine for social anxiety disorder. Arch Gen Psychiatry 63:298–304, 2006

Hoge CW, Castro CA, Messer SC, et al: Combat duty in Iraq and Afghanistan, mental health problems, and barriers to care. N Engl J Med 351:13–22, 2004

Hollifield M, Sinclair-Lian N, Warner TD, et al: Acupuncture for posttraumatic stress disorder: a randomized controlled pilot trial. J Nerv Ment Dis 195:504–513, 2007

Jacobs BP, Bent S, Tice JA, et al: An internet-based randomized, placebo-controlled trial of kava and valerian for anxiety and insomnia. Medicine (Baltimore) 84:197–207, 2005

Jaycox LH, Foa EB, Morral AR: Influence of emotional engagement and habituation on exposure therapy for PTSD. J Consult Clin Psychol 66:185–192, 1998

Jaycox LH, Zoellner L, Foa EB: Cognitive-behavior therapy for PTSD in rape survivors. J Clin Psychol 58:891–906, 2002

Josman N, Somer E, Reisberg A, et al: BusWorld: designing a virtual environment for PTSD in Israel: a protocol. Cyberpsychol Behav 9:241–244, 2006

Kaplan Z, Amir M, Swartz M, et al: Inositol treatment of post-traumatic stress disorder. Anxiety 2:51–52, 1996

Klinger E, Bouchard S, Légeron P, et al: Virtual reality therapy versus cognitive behavior therapy for social phobia: a preliminary controlled study. Cyberpsychol Behav 8:76–88, 2005

Koopman C, Classen C, Spiegel D: Predictors of posttraumatic stress symptoms among survivors of the Oakland/Berkeley, Calif., firestorm. Am J Psychiatry 151:888–894, 1994

Krijn M, Emmelkamp PM, Olafsson RP, et al: Virtual reality exposure therapy of anxiety disorders: a review. Clin Psychol Rev 24:259–281, 2004

Kushner MG, Kim SW, Donahue C, et al: D-cycloserine augmented exposure therapy for obsessive-compulsive disorder. Biol Psychiatry 62:835–838, 2007

Levine J, Barak Y, Kofman O, et al: Follow-up and relapse analysis of an inositol study of depression. Isr J Psychiatry Relat Sci 32:14–21, 1995

Maxfield L, Hyer L: The relationship between efficacy and methodology in studies investigating EMDR treatment of PTSD. J Clin Psychol 58:23–41, 2002

Morrow K, Docan C, Burdea G, et al: Low-cost virtual rehabilitation of the hand for patients post-stroke, in Proceedings of the 5th International Workshop on Virtual Rehabilitation. New York, August 2006, pp 6–10

Parsons TD, Rizzo AA: Initial validation of a virtual environment for assessment of memory functioning: Virtual Reality Cognitive Performance Assessment Test. Cyberpsychol Behav 11:16–24, 2008

Powers MB, Emmelkamp PM: Virtual reality exposure therapy for anxiety disorders: a meta-analysis. J Anxiety Disord 39:250–261, 2008

Ressler KJ, Rothbaum BO, Tannenbaum L, et al: Cognitive enhancers as adjuncts to psychotherapy: use of D-cycloserine in phobic individuals to facilitate extinction of fear. Arch Gen Psychiatry 61:1136–1144, 2004

Rizzo AA, Kim G: A SWOT analysis of the field of virtual rehabilitation and therapy. Presence: Teleoperators and Virtual Environments 14:1–28, 2005

Rizzo AA, Wiederhold M, Buckwalter JG: Basic issues in the use of virtual environments for mental health applications, in Virtual Reality in Clinical Psychology and Neuroscience. Edited by Riva G, Wiederhold B, Molinari E. Amsterdam, The Netherlands, IOS Press, 1998, pp 21–42

Rizzo AA, Schultheis MT, Kerns K, et al: Analysis of assets for virtual reality applications in neuropsychology. Neuropsychol Rehabil 14:207–239, 2004

Rizzo AA, Newman B, Parsons T, et al: Development and clinical results from the Virtual Iraq exposure therapy application for PTSD. Presented at International Workshop on Virtual Rehabilitation, July 2009. Available at: ftp://ftp.ict.usc.edu/arizzo/NATO2010

Rose FD, Brooks BM, Rizzo AA: Virtual reality in brain damage rehabilitation: review. Cyberpsychol Behav 8:241–262, 2005

Rothbaum BO: Critical parameters for D-cycloserine enhancement of cognitive-behavioral therapy for obsessive-compulsive disorder. Am J Psychiatry 165:293–296, 2008

Rothbaum BO, Hodges LF: The use of virtual reality exposure in the treatment of anxiety disorders. Behav Modif 23:507–525, 1999

Rothbaum BO, Hodges LF, Kooper R, et al: Effectiveness of virtual reality graded exposure in the treatment of acrophobia. Am J Psychiatry 152:626–628, 1995

Rothbaum BO, Hodges L, Watson BA, et al: Virtual reality exposure therapy in the treatment of fear of flying: a case report. Behav Res Ther 34:477–481, 1996

Rothbaum BO, Hodges L, Smith S, et al: A controlled study of virtual reality exposure therapy for the fear of flying. J Consult Clin Psychol 68:1020–1026, 2000a

Rothbaum BO, Meadows EA, Resick P, et al: Cognitive-behavioral treatment position paper summary for the ISTSS Treatment Guidelines Committee. J Trauma Stress 13:558–563, 2000b

Rothbaum BO, Hodges LF, Ready D, et al: Virtual reality exposure therapy for Vietnam veterans with posttraumatic stress disorder. J Clin Psychiatry 62:617–622, 2001

Rothbaum BO, Hodges L, Anderson PL, et al: Twelve-month follow-up of virtual reality and standard exposure therapies for the fear of flying. J Consult Clin Psychol 70:428–432, 2002

Rothbaum BO, Anderson P, Zimand E, et al: Virtual reality exposure therapy and standard (in vivo) exposure therapy in the treatment of fear of flying. Behav Ther 37:80–90, 2006

Shapiro F: Eye movement desensitization: a new treatment for post-traumatic stress disorder. J Behav Ther Exp Psychiatry 20:211–217, 1989

Shapiro F: EMDR 12 years after its introduction: past and future research. J Clin Psychol 58:1–22, 2002

Silver SM, Brooks A, Obenchain J: Treatment of Vietnam War veterans with PTSD: a comparison of eye movement desensitization and reprocessing, biofeedback, and relaxation training. J Trauma Stress 8:337–342, 1995

Smith SG, Rothbaum BO, Hodges L: Treatment of fear of flying using virtual reality exposure therapy: a single case study. Behavior Therapist 22:154–158, 1999

Stewart JC, Yeh SC, Jung Y, et al: Intervention to enhance skilled arm and hand movements after stroke: a feasibility study using a new virtual reality system. J Neuroeng Rehabil 4:1–18, 2007

Storch EA, Merlo LJ, Bengtson M, et al: D-cycloserine does not enhance exposure-response prevention therapy in obsessive-compulsive disorder. Int Clin Psychopharmacol 22:230–237, 2007

Taibi DM, Landis CA, Petry H, et al: A systematic review of valerian as a sleep aid: safe but not effective. Sleep Med Rev 11:209–230, 2007

Taylor MJ, Wilder H, Bhagwagar Z, et al: Inositol for depressive disorders. Cochrane Database Syst Rev CD004049, 2004

Van Etten ML, Taylor S: Comparative efficacy of treatments of posttraumatic stress disorder: an empirical review. JAMA 268:633–638, 1998

Walshe DG, Lewis EJ, Kim SI, et al: Exploring the use of computer games and virtual reality in exposure therapy for fear of driving following a motor vehicle accident. Cyberpsychol Behav 6:329–334, 2003

Warner CH, Appenzeller GN, Mullen K, et al: Soldier attitudes toward mental health screening and seeking care upon return from combat. Mil Med 173:563–569, 2008

Watson CG, Tuorila JR, Vickers KS, et al: The efficacies of three relaxation regimens in the treatment of PTSD in Vietnam War veterans. J Clin Psychol 53:917–923, 1997

Weathers FW, Litz BT, Herman DS, et al: The PTSD Checklist (PCL): reliability, validity, and diagnostic utility (abstract). International Society for Traumatic Stress Studies. October 1993. Available at: http://www.pdhealth.mil/library/downloads/pcl_sychometrics.doc. Accessed December 2, 2009.

Wiederhold BK, Wiederhold MD: Three-year follow-up for the treatment of fear of flying: a controlled investigation. J Consult Clin Psychol 70:1112–1118, 2002

Wilhelm S, Buhlman U, Tolin DF, et al: Augmentation of behavior therapy with D-cycloserine for obsessive-compulsive disorder. Am J Psychiatry 165:335–341, 2008

Wood DP, Murphy JA, Center KB, et al: Combat related post traumatic stress disorder: a multiple case report using virtual reality graded exposure therapy with physiological monitoring. Stud Health Technol Inform 132:556–561, 2008

Zohar J, Amital D, Miodowalk C, et al: Double-blind placebo-controlled pilot study of sertraline in military veterans with posttraumatic stress disorder. J Clin Psychopharmacol 22:190–195, 2002

10

Assessment of Functioning and Disability

Nina A. Sayer, Ph.D.

Kathleen F. Carlson, Ph.D.

Paula P. Schnurr, Ph.D.

Psychiatric evaluations are used to identify patients' needs, develop treatment plans, and monitor progress and outcomes. In this chapter, we focus on assessment of functioning and disability as part of the psychiatric evaluation of individuals with possible posttraumatic stress disorder (PTSD). Although the importance of assessing functional status among individuals with serious mental illness, including schizophrenia, has received considerable attention in the clinical and scientific literature, the value of incorporating such assessments into standard clinical evaluations of individuals with possible PTSD has received limited attention. We discuss the reasons clinicians should assess functioning and monitor treatment outcomes in patients with PTSD; present a conceptual framework to guide these evaluations; describe the domains that should be considered; and review different methods of assessment.

Rationale for Assessment of Functioning and Disability

There are at least five interrelated reasons for including assessment of functioning in standard psychiatric assessment of individuals with possible PTSD. First, functional assessment has been built into the diagnosis of PTSD in the *Diagnostic and Statistical Manual of Mental Disorders*, 4th Edition, Text Revision (DSM-IV-TR; American Psychiatric Association 2000). The DSM-IV-TR criteria for PTSD include Criterion F, which states that the symptoms cause significant psychological distress or impairment in functioning.

Second, many individuals with PTSD have significant functional impairments. Some findings suggest that people with PTSD have especially severe impairments compared with individuals who have mood and other anxiety disorders (Mendlowicz and Stein 2000; Rapaport et al. 2005). Table 10–1 lists those domains with identified functional impairment(s) in PTSD, along with examples of research identifying these impairments since DSM began including Criterion F for the diagnosis of PTSD. Emerging from this body of literature is a pattern of social and occupational impairments among individuals with PTSD. The occupational problems may, of course, be related to difficulties managing social interactions. Importantly, these functional problems have a significant impact on the individual with PTSD, the individual's family members, and society as a whole (Kessler 2000). The importance of assessing functioning is further underscored by the possibility that individuals with PTSD who have extreme functional disability may benefit from interventions focused on daily activities rather than from symptom-based approaches (see Penk and Flanner 2000 for a review of psychosocial rehabilitation for patients with PTSD). A functional assessment, therefore, should be an integral part of developing a treatment plan.

Third, although correlated, symptoms and functioning can vary separately (Miller at al. 2008) and may differentially respond to treatment (Shalev 1997). This is why two individuals with comparable PTSD severity may have different levels of functioning and different types of functional problems. We reviewed the randomized controlled trials included in Bisson et al.'s (2007) meta-analysis of psychotherapy for PTSD to see if changes in functioning accompanied changes in symptoms over the course of the trials. Thirteen of the 38 trials included in this meta-analysis used a functional or quality-of-life measure as an outcome. In most of these studies, significant improvements in functioning accompanied symptom reduction (Cloitre et al. 2002; Echeburua et al. 1997; Ehlers et al. 2005; Foa et al. 1999; Marcus et al. 1997; Marks et al. 1998; Neuner et al. 2004; Paunovic and Öst 2001; Power et al. 2002). However, in some studies, there was not a corresponding improvement in functioning (Keane et al. 1989; Schnurr et al. 2003), and in other studies, some functional areas improved significantly while others did not (Blanchard et al. 2003; Krakow et al. 2001). In light of these findings, treating clinicians should not make assumptions about functional status based solely on evaluation of psychiatric symptoms. In evaluating treatment response, clinicians need to determine whether meaningful functional impairments remain after symptom resolution or, conversely, functioning improved while PTSD symptoms persisted.

The fourth reason for assessing functioning involves patients' treatment preferences and subjective views of their problems. Some individuals with PTSD may experience some or all of their problems as functional and may value improvement in functional domains, such as relationships and work, as equal to or more important than improvement in core symptoms of PTSD (see, e.g., Johnson et al. 1996; Zatzick et al. 2007). Evaluation of functioning, therefore, is essential to identifying patients' perceived needs and treatment goals.

The fifth reason is to identify areas of intact functioning and environmental factors that could facilitate recovery. These positive factors can be leveraged over the course of treatment and may help a patient maintain hope in spite of his or her trauma history and current symptoms. The focus on strengths is integral to psychosocial rehabilitation and has been recommended for inclusion in assessment of PTSD (Meichenbaum 1994).

In summary, clinicians should assess functioning in addition to PTSD symptomatology to determine whether patients with possible PTSD could benefit from services or interventions geared toward improving day-to-day functioning. Such assessments can be used to evaluate the impact of interventions on functional outcomes that are important to patients, as well as to identify intact functional areas and resources within the individual or his or her environment that may facilitate treatment and recovery.

Table 10–1. Functional domains impaired in individuals with PTSD

Domain and reference	Key findings
Marriage and other intimate relationships	
Koenen et al. 2008	Vietnam veterans with severe PTSD symptoms 30 years after service reported lower levels of marital satisfaction, and were more frequently divorced, than veterans without severe PTSD symptoms.
Riggs et al. 1998	Significantly more Vietnam veterans with PTSD and their partners showed intimate relationship distress than those without PTSD (75% vs. 32%).
Sexual functioning	
Cosgrove et al. 2002	Male combat veterans with PTSD had lower overall sexual satisfaction and orgasmic function than those without PTSD. Significantly more veterans with PTSD than veterans without PTSD had erectile dysfunction (85% vs. 22%).
Green et al. 2005	Female college sophomores who had ever had PTSD were more likely than those who had never had PTSD to have a history of pregnancy, abortion, being tested for HIV, and high-risk sexual behavior.
Koenen et al. 2008	Vietnam veterans with severe PTSD symptoms 30 years after service reported poorer levels of sexual satisfaction than those without severe PTSD symptoms.
Riggs et al. 1998	Vietnam veterans with PTSD and their partners showed significantly greater fear of intimacy than those without PTSD.
Parenting	
Koenen et al. 2008	Vietnam veterans with severe PTSD symptoms 30 years after service reported higher levels of parenting difficulties than those without severe PTSD symptoms.
Ruscio et al. 2002	Perceived overall quality of relationships with children was significantly lower for Vietnam veterans with PTSD than for those without PTSD.

Table 10–1. Functional domains impaired in individuals with PTSD *(continued)*

Domain and reference	Key findings
Friendships	
Blanchard et al. 1995	Motor vehicle crash survivors with PTSD showed significantly more impairment in relations with friends than those without PTSD.
Recreation	
Kuhn et al. 2003	Motor vehicle accident survivors with PTSD showed significantly more impairment in recreation/use of leisure time than those without PTSD.
Homelessness	
O'Connell et al. 2008	Previously homeless veterans with PTSD had 85% increased risk of reduced housing tenure after intervention, compared with those without PTSD.
Violent behavior	
Freeman and Roca 2001	Vietnam veterans with PTSD reported higher levels of aggression and higher incidence of potentially dangerous firearm-related behaviors, and owned more handguns and combat-type knives than veterans without PTSD.
McFall et al. 1999	Vietnam combat veterans in inpatient psychiatric care for PTSD were 7.4 times more likely to report engagement in one or more acts of violence than psychiatric inpatients without PTSD.
Intimate partner violence	
Orcutt et al. 2003	PTSD symptom severity was directly related to perpetration of intimate partner violence by male Vietnam veterans.
Taft et al. 2008	PTSD symptoms were directly related to male-to-female perpetration of psychological and physical intimate relationship abuse in a community sample of intimate partners.

Table 10–1. Functional domains impaired in individuals with PTSD *(continued)*

Domain and reference	Key findings
General productive activity	
Blanchard et al. 1995	Motor vehicle accident survivors with PTSD showed significantly more impairment in work, school, or homemaking performance than those without PTSD.
Zatzick et al. 2008	Patients with PTSD were 2.5 times more likely than those without PTSD to not be engaged in productive activity (working, student, homemaking, caretaking, volunteering) 12 months after hospitalization for traumatic injury.
Gainful employment	
Magruder et al. 2004	Veterans who were not working due to disability had significantly higher PTSD symptom levels than those who were not working due to retirement or who were working.
Resnick and Rosenheck 2008	Veterans in Veterans Affairs (VA)–compensated work therapy program who had PTSD (~16%) were 19% less likely to be employed at discharge from the program than those without PTSD.
Savoca and Rosenheck 2000	Vietnam veterans with a lifetime diagnosis of PTSD were 8.5% less likely to be employed in the late 1980s than veterans without PTSD.
Zatzick et al. 1997a	Male Vietnam veterans with PTSD were 3.3 times more likely to be not working (including school and homemaking) than those without PTSD.
Zatzick et al. 1997b	Female Vietnam veterans with PTSD were 10 times more likely to be not working (including school and homemaking) than those without PTSD.
Zatzick et al. 2008	Patients with PTSD were 3.5 times more likely than those without PTSD to not be working 12 months after hospitalization for traumatic injury.

Table 10–1. Functional domains impaired in individuals with PTSD *(continued)*

Domain and reference	Key findings
Work productivity	
Boscarino et al. 2006	Among workers exposed to the World Trade Center disaster, PTSD (vs. no PTSD) was significantly associated with reports of three or more lower-quality workdays in the 4 weeks prior to the survey.
Hoge et al. 2007	Iraq war veterans with PTSD were more likely than those without PTSD to report missing 2 or more workdays in the month before the survey.
S.G. Resnick and Rosenheck 2008	Veterans in VA-compensated work therapy program with PTSD (~16%) worked significantly fewer days in the 90 days prior to discharge from the program than those without PTSD.
Wages/benefits	
Savoca and Rosenheck 2000	Employed Vietnam veterans with a lifetime diagnosis of PTSD earned, on average, $2.38 less per hour in the late 1980s than those without PTSD.

Conceptual Framework and Definitions

The World Health Organization's (2001) *International Classification of Functioning, Disability and Health*, commonly referred to as ICF, provides the conceptual framework for this chapter. The ICF was developed to assess the consequences of physical and mental health conditions (e.g., PTSD) in terms of an individual's ability to function in his or her environment (World Health Organization 2001). ICF was developed for use with the *International Statistical Classification of Diseases and Related Health Problems*, 10th Revision (ICD-10; World Health Organization [WHO] 1992) but conceivably is also compatible with other diagnostic classification systems, including DSM. In 2001, the 191 member states of the World Health Organization agreed to adopt ICF as the basis for scientific standardization of data on health and disability worldwide. ICF represents the most well-accepted and contemporary view of functioning and disability and is widely used in the rehabilitation medicine community.

The ICF is grounded in a biopsychosocial model that views functioning and disability as the outcome of interactions among a health condition, manifestations of that health condition at different levels, and contextual factors (Figure 10–1). The actual classification system is organized into two parts: Part 1 addresses functioning and disability, and Part 2 covers contextual factors, both personal and environmental, that facilitate or interfere with functioning. ICF and its development are described in detail elsewhere (Whiteneck 2006).

Components of Part 1 include 1) body structure and function, 2) activities, and 3) participation as a member of society. The ICF refers to the "body" as the human organism and includes not only physical aspects of the human body but also mental functions. The intrusive, avoidance, numbing, and hyperarousal symptoms of PTSD would be classified as impairments in mental functions. Activities are classified at the individual level and refer to "the execution of a task or action by an individual" (WHO 2002, p. 10). Participation is at the societal level and refers to "involvement in a life situation" (WHO 2002, p. 10), including social role functioning. For instance, difficulty leaving the house during the day would be an activity limitation, and unemployment or lack of social interactions would be classified as participation restrictions. *Disability* is an overarching term used to describe limitations or disturbance at any of these three levels (body, activity, or participation).

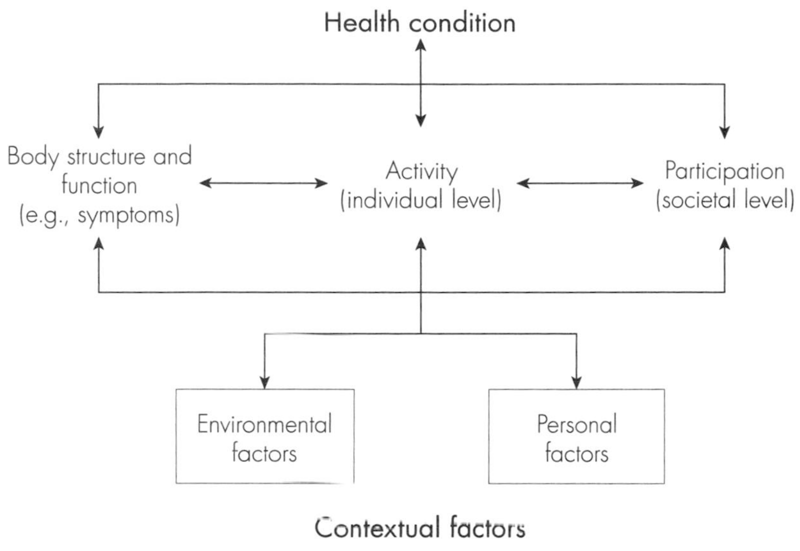

Figure 10–1. Model of disablement according to the *International Classification of Functioning, Disability and Health.*

Source. World Health Organization 2001.

According to the ICF, the ultimate level of disability people experience is a product of their own impairments in interaction with their physical and social environment. An important contribution of the ICF to the disability field is an explicit acknowledgment of the role of environment in undermining or facilitating individual performance (Whiteneck 2006).

We focus below on assessment of limitations in functioning as embodied by the ICF activity and participation domains. Limitations in body structure or function in individuals with psychiatric disorders are assessed using symptom or diagnostic measures. Secondarily, we discuss contextual factors that may be particularly relevant for adults with PTSD.

Selection of Domains for Assessment

Table 10–2 presents a list of the activity and participation domains included in the ICF, along with a description of each. As intended by the ICF developers, the scope is broad and, consequently, in many contexts it may not be feasible for clinicians to fully assess impairments and functioning in each of the nine activity and participation domains. Available research on functional problems in those diagnosed with PTSD, as outlined in Table 10–1, suggests that assessment of various aspects of a patient's social and occupational functioning should be prioritized (Domains 7 and 8 in Table 10–2).

An individual's ability to be gainfully employed and to contribute to society through meaningful work is inextricably linked to mental and physical health, as well as recovery trajectory (Agerbo 2005; Bjarnason and Sigurdardottir 2003; Crist et al. 2000; Ross and Mirowsky 1995; Vestling et al. 2003). Individuals with PTSD may need more substantial assistance for reentering the workplace (Strauser and Lustig 2001), especially if the trauma was work related (MacDonald et al. 2003; Strauser 2008). Although the discussion of occupational functioning often focuses on gainful employment, we encourage clinicians to include other types of productive activity in functional assessments. These activities can include school and educational activities, informal employment, housework, and volunteer work. Other types of civic and community participation should also be considered.

Individuals with PTSD may experience impairments in domains other than those of social and occupational functioning, particularly if they have co-occurring physical impairments or injuries. In particular, patients with physical limitations may have difficulties with self-care functions and performance of everyday tasks necessary for independent living, referred to as activities of daily living (ADLs) and instrumental activities of daily living (IADLs), respectively.

Measures of Global, Social, and Occupational Functioning

Despite the need for assessment of functioning in individuals with PTSD, relatively little expert consensus is available to aid clinicians in selecting measurement tools and methods for this patient population. As is the case with diagnostic assessments, clinicians can use unstructured, semistructured, or structured interviews, as well as questionnaires, to assess functioning and disability. In some instances, it may also be useful to obtain information from informants, such as family members or significant others, particularly when

Table 10–2. Activity and participation domains from the *International Classification of Functioning, Disability and Health*

Domain	Description
1. Learning and applying knowledge	Learning to read, solving problems
2. General tasks and demands	Carrying out daily routine
3. Communication	Speaking, conversation
4. Mobility	Getting around inside or outside home
5. Self-care	Washing oneself, dressing
6. Domestic life	Preparing meals, acquiring a place to live
7. Interpersonal interactions and relationships	Relating with strangers, formal relationships, family relationships
8. Major life areas	Work, employment, remunerative employment
9. Community, social, and civic life	Recreation and leisure, religion and spirituality

Source. World Health Organization 2001.

patients have difficulty describing their problems due to comorbidities that impair cognition (e.g., brain injury or psychosis) or when patients request family member involvement. The clinician should assess both current functional status and the patient's level of functioning before the onset of PTSD and related comorbidities. This "baseline" information will help the clinician understand any trauma-related alterations in the patient's life course and may inform goal setting.

In this section, we review eight of the most commonly used and promising interview and self-report measures of functioning appropriate for clinical and research application in working with adults with PTSD. Because no functional measures have been designed specifically for PTSD, we include generic rather than diagnosis-specific measures. Most of these measures were developed before ICF and hence do not use the same terminology or map perfectly onto this model of disability. However, we include these measures in this chapter because they examine activity and participation domains found to be impaired among patients with PTSD.

We do not review all types of functional measures. For instance, we do not include measures of ADLs and IADLs. Additionally, we do not focus on quality-of-life measures. Some investigators have proposed that quality of life is conceptually distinct from functioning because the former includes enjoyment and life satisfaction (Institute of Medicine 2007; Rapaport et al. 2005). However, because quality of life is a multidimensional construct that can include functioning, the distinction between quality of life and functioning is often blurred in mental health research. Of note, some instruments that we review as functional measures are described as quality-of-life measures in other publications. (For more information on quality-of-life measures, see Gladis et al. 1999 and Olatunji et al. 2007.)

Second, we do not review measures and methods to assess response bias. Response biases lead to the underreporting and overreporting of impairments and therefore are an important factor in any clinical evaluation that relies on a patient's self-report. It is particularly important to measure response biases in the context of forensic or disability evaluations. (For a review of techniques used to assess response bias in PTSD, see Arbisi 2005 and P.J. Resnick et al. 2008.)

The eight selected measures, including their format, psychometric properties, and domains assessed, are summarized in Table 10–3. One measure is used for assessment of global functioning only; another two are used only for evaluation of occupational functioning. The remaining measures examine multiple dimensions, as well as render a global functioning score.

Global Assessment of Functioning

The Global Assessment of Functioning (GAF) scale may be the most commonly used measure of functioning (Moos et al. 2002). It has been included as the fifth axis in a DSM multiaxial diagnosis since 1980. Since that time, it has changed from a 7-point scale in DSM-III (American Psychiatric Association 1980) to a 90-point scale in DSM-III-R (American Psychiatric Association 1987), and then to a 100-point scale in DSM-IV-TR (American Psychiatric Association 2000, p. 34). The current version of the GAF is based on the Global Assessment Scale developed by Endicott et al. (1976).

The GAF scale is organized into 10 bands (10 points each) that yield 100 possible points. GAF instructions recommend first finding the decile band that seems to best describe the patient's degree of symptomatology or functional severity. GAF scores, therefore, represent a mixture of symptom severity and occupational and social functional impairment ratings. This is problematic, given that symptoms and occupational and interpersonal functioning do not necessarily covary (Goldman et al. 1992).

The Social and Occupational Functioning Assessment Scale (SOFAS), included in DSM-IV-TR in Appendix B, "Criteria Sets and Axes Provided for Further Study," was designed to address this flaw in the GAF. It is also a 100-point single-item scale. The SOFAS differs from the GAF in its exclusive focus on the individual's level of social and occupational functioning (American Psychiatric Association 2000). The SOFAS is not widely used currently and psychometric studies have yielded mixed results (e.g., Hay et al. 2003). Furthermore, although it disentangles symptom ratings from functional ratings, the SOFAS confounds the rating of social with occupational functioning. Due to problems inherent in this approach, the Department of Veterans Affairs (VA) Mental Illness Research, Education and Clinical Center (MIRECC) developed a version of the GAF called the MIRECC GAF, which includes separate scales for social, occupational, and psychological (e.g., symptom severity) functioning (Niv et al. 2007). Initial reliability and validity data obtained in a sample of individuals with schizophrenia and schizoaffective disorder were promising (Niv et al. 2007).

DSM-IV-TR does not include information on the reliability and validity of the GAF. Research has shown, however, that in the absence of systematic training, reliability is generally poor (Söderberg et al. 2005). Without training, some raters may score average symptom occurrence or functionality over time, whereas others will rate the most recent episode or the lowest level of these two components. In disorders such as PTSD, in which symptom severity and functionality can fluctuate, these two approaches will yield very different GAF scores (Watson et al. 2002). Furthermore, it is difficult to make assessments using the GAF when multiple impairments are present, as is often the case with PTSD (Brown et al. 2001). We could identify only limited information about the scale's validity in the scientific literature.

GAF and SOFAS are copyrighted by the American Psychiatric Association (www.appi.org/permissions.cfx). The MIRECC GAF version is available through the MIRECC website (www. desertpacific.mirecc.va.gov/gaf/index .shtml).

Table 10–3. Measures of functioning appropriate for adults with PTSD

Scale and reference	Format	Alternative forms	Number of items	Domains	Advantages	Disadvantages
Global Assessment of Functioning (GAF; American Psychiatric Association 2000)	Interview	Yes	100-point single item, divided into deciles	Overall level of functioning, taking into account symptom severity and social and occupational functioning	Readily available, brief to administer	Score combines symptom severity and occupational and social functional impairment; reliability and validity are limited without systematic training.
Longitudinal Interval Follow-up Evaluation (LIFE; Keller et al. 1987)	Interview	No, but sections may be used separately	13; additional items for different familial relationships	Work status and functioning, household functioning, marital status, family relationships, friendships, sexual functioning, recreation, satisfaction, Global Social Adjustment and Global Assessment of Functioning	Broad coverage; rater takes into account context when rating impairment; designed for tracking changes over time and following treatment; no fees or license	Interviewer training is required; interview is time-consuming to administer.

Table 10–3. Measures of functioning appropriate for adults with PTSD *(continued)*

Scale and reference	Format	Alternative forms	Number of items	Domains	Advantages	Disadvantages
Social Adjustment Scale (SAS; Weissman and Bothwell 1976)	Interview; self-report	Yes	54	Work (as employee, homemaker, or student); social/leisure activities; relationships with extended family; roles as spouse, parent, and member of a family unit	Strong psychometric properties; commonly used with psychiatric patients; coverage of various social roles; norms available for abbreviated versions	Interview version is time-consuming; license and fees are required for self-report versions.
Sheehan Disability Scale (SDS; Sheehan 1983)	Interview; self-report	Yes	3 (visual analog scale with verbal anchors)	Rating of symptom-related dysfunction in work/school, social, and family life	Brief to administer; no scoring manual needed; sensitive to change; translations in many languages	Specific problems are not identified within broad areas assessed; symptoms are not disentangled from functioning.

Table 10–3. Measures of functioning appropriate for adults with PTSD *(continued)*

Scale and reference	Format	Alternative forms	Number of items	Domains	Advantages	Disadvantages
36-Item Short Form Health Survey (SF-36; Ware et al. 1993)	Self-report	Yes	36	Physical functioning, physical role functioning, bodily pain, general health, vitality, social functioning, emotional functioning, and mental health; also produces global physical and mental component scores	Strong psychometric properties; sensitive to change; translations in multiple languages; norms available	License and fees are required; scoring algorithm is relatively complex.
World Health Organization Disability Assessment Schedule–Second Version (WHODAS II; World Health Organization 2000)	Interview; self-report	Yes	36	Understanding and communicating; mobility; self-care; getting along with others; life activities; participation in society	Cross-culturally developed; linked to ICF; strong psychometric properties in international studies; sensitive to change; translations in multiple languages	Interview form requires training; scoring is somewhat complex; approval from WHO is required.

Table 10–3. Measures of functioning appropriate for adults with PTSD *(continued)*

Scale and reference	Format	Alternative forms	Number of items	Domains	Advantages	Disadvantages
Work Limitations Questionnaire (WLQ; Lerner et al. 2001)	Interview	Yes	25	Work-related time management, physical demands, interpersonal and mental demands; productivity demands	Brief to administer; strong psychometric properties; psychiatric samples included in scale development	License and fees are required; non-work-related productive activities are not assessed; missed time is not captured quantitatively.
Work Productivity and Activity Impairment (WPAI; Reilly et al. 1993)	Interview; self-report	Yes	6	Hours absent from work due to health problems; hours absent due to other reasons; hours actually worked; impact of health problems on productivity at work; impact of health problems on productivity in daily activities outside of work	Readily available; brief to administer; translation in Spanish; strong psychometric properties; nonspecific to occupation or health problem; includes assessment of non-work-related productivity; sensitive to change	Validity with interviewer-administered version may be stronger; psychometrics have not been tested in psychiatric samples.

Note. ICF = *International Classification of Functioning, Disability and Health* (World Health Organization 2001); WHO = World Health Organization.

Longitudinal Interval Follow-up Evaluation

The Longitudinal Interval Follow-up Evaluation (LIFE) is an integrated system for assessing the long-term course of psychiatric disorders (Keller et al. 1987). The most recent version is called LIFE: DSM-IV Version (Keller et al. 1997). The psychosocial functioning section of the most recent version of the LIFE interview assesses a wide range of functional domains, including work, relationships, sexual, household, recreation, and overall life satisfaction. The interviewer rates impairment in each domain such that higher values indicate greater impairment. Ratings of work functioning (outside and within the home and at school) reflect impairment due to psychopathology. For example, the rater would indicate "not applicable" to the work item if an individual is not working because he or she is caring for a sick parent. The interviewer also rates Global Social Adjustment and completes the GAF, discussed previously. Ratings are made for each month within a selected time period, with 6–12 months being the most typical period of time covered during a LIFE Interview. Although the psychosocial functioning section can be administered as a stand-alone measure, information gained through the other parts of the LIFE Interview (including course of Axis I disorders and treatments received) provides the context needed for rating impairment in the psychosocial domains. It takes approximately 30–45 minutes to administer the psychosocial section of the LIFE and up to several hours to administer the full interview.

The LIFE has acceptable to excellent reliability in clinical samples, including patients with anxiety disorders (Keller et al. 1987; Warshaw et al. 2001), and has been used in anxiety disorder and PTSD research (Blanchard et al. 1995; Kuhn et al. 2003). A 5-item version of the LIFE, called LIFE-RIFT, demonstrated good psychometric properties in a sample of patients with mood disorders (Leon et al. 1999). LIFE-RIFT takes only a few minutes to administer. The LIFE is available from Dr. Keller, and LIFE-RIFT is included in the appendix of the article by Leon et al. (1999).

Social Adjustment Scale

The Social Adjustment Scale (SAS; Weissman and Bothwell 1976) was developed as an outcome measure for drug treatment and psychotherapy trials in patients with depression and has since been used for studies involving a range of patients, including those with PTSD. Both the interview and the self-report

(SAS-SR) versions of SAS contain 54 questions covering role performance in six areas of role functioning: 1) work (as employee, homemaker, or student); 2) social and leisure activities; 3) relationships with extended family; and roles as a 4) spouse, 5) parent, and 6) member of a family unit. An advantage to the SAS is that it assesses a number of areas of social function, including parenting and marital functioning, that may be impaired among individuals with PTSD. Two scoring methods are used: a mean score for each domain and an overall score obtained by summing the item scores and dividing by the number of items checked. The self-report measure generally takes 15–20 minutes to complete, whereas the interview version takes up to an hour. Shorter and screening versions of the SAS-SR have also been developed, which consist of 24 and 12 items, respectively (Weissman 2007). All SAS scales are under copyright. Permission to use the SAS interview may be requested from Dr. Weissman, who developed the instrument. The full SAS-SR and its versions are available for purchase from Multi-Health Systems (www.mhs.com).

Sheehan Disability Scale

The Sheehan Disability Scale (SDS; Sheehan 1983) was developed to assess individuals with psychiatric symptoms for functional impairment in three areas: 1) work/school, 2) social life, and 3) family life. SDS has commonly been used in drug and psychotherapy studies of PTSD. The patient rates, on a 10-point visual analog scale, the extent to which he or she experiences problems in each of the three domains due to his or her symptoms. The patient can also be rated by an interviewer. The scale takes 1–2 minutes to complete. The numerical ratings of 0–10 can be translated into a percentage, if desired. The three items may be summed into a single-dimensional measure of global functional impairment that ranges from 0 (*unimpaired*) to 30 (*highly impaired*). Clinicians should pay special attention to patients who score 5 or higher on any of the three scales, because such high scores are associated with significant functional impairment. The scale has adequate reliability and validity in psychiatric samples and appears to be sensitive to change with treatment. The scale has been adapted for various purposes, although we are not aware of studies examining the psychometric properties of these versions. One version assesses several domains of work (Sheehan Work Disability Scale); another adds an item about balancing work, personal life, and career; and a third adds an item about religious or spiritual practice. Dr. Sheehan holds the copyright to the SDS, but the scale can be downloaded without charge from www.cqaimh.org/pdf/tool_lof_sds.pdf.

36-Item Short Form Health Survey

The 36-Item Short Form Health Survey (SF-36) is a highly reliable and valid survey developed as part of the Medical Outcomes Study (Ware et al. 1993). It has been widely used in PTSD clinical trials, is sensitive to change, and takes about 10 minutes to administer. It evaluates eight domains of health-related functioning that reflect perception of general symptoms or impairment; activity limitations; and participation (physical role functioning, emotional functioning, and social functioning). The SF-36 produces two composite scores: the physical component summary score and the mental component summary score. Scores range from 0 to 100, and a linear *t*-score transformation method is used so that summary scores have a mean of 50 and a standard deviation of 10. Scores above 50 are better and those below 50 are worse than the U.S. population mean. The most current version (SF-36 v2) was introduced to correct deficiencies identified in the original version (Ware 2003; Ware et al. 2000). Shorter, alternative versions of the SF-36, including the SF-12 and the more recent SF-12 v2, have undergone extensive testing (Ware et al. 2002). Anyone wishing to use a version of the SF, other than the versions developed by the VA for use with veterans (Veterans RAND 36-Item Health Survey [VR-36] and Veterans RAND 12-Item Health Survey [VR-12]; Kazis et al. 2006), needs to register and obtain a license through QualityMetric (www.qualitymetric.com). The VR-36, VR-12, and scoring algorithms are in the public domain and can be used free of charge. They can be obtained by agreeing to the stipulations listed on the RAND Corporation website (www.rand.org/health/surveys_tools/mos/mos_core_36item_terms.html) in a letter to Dr. Lewis Kazis (lek@bu.edu).

World Health Organization Disability Assessment Schedule II

The World Health Organization Disability Assessment Schedule II (WHODAS II; World Health Organization 2000) is a 36-item instrument assessing difficulty in six domains of life in the last 30 days. There are three versions: the self-report, structured interview, and proxy versions. The World Health Organization estimates that the self-report version requires about 20 minutes to complete. The subscales reflect limitations in activity (communication, physical mobility, self-care) and participation restrictions (interpersonal interactions, domestic responsibilities and work, participation in society). The instrument also provides a summary score, with higher scores indicating greater severity of disability (World Health Organization 2000). WHODAS II has been cross-culturally developed and field-tested in 16 languages in 14 countries. Available psychometric information from this international work is promising, although WHODAS II has not been used extensively in individuals with PTSD. Twelve-item interview and self-report versions of the WHODAS II may be useful to screen for problems or for use when domain-specific information regarding functioning is not required. The original self-report version of the WHODAS was designed to assess social adjustment problems specifically in individuals with psychiatric disorders (World Health Organization 1988). WHODAS II, in contrast, applies more broadly to the impact of any disorder on everyday functioning. The WHODAS II and scoring algorithms are available at www.who.int/icidh/whodas/index.html.

Work Limitations Questionnaire

The Work Limitations Questionnaire (WLQ) is a 25-item work-specific questionnaire shown to be reliable and valid for measuring the impact of health problems on work functioning (Lerner et al. 2001). An 8-item short-form version has also been created. The WLQ has been used in research based on psychiatric samples and also holds promise as an instrument that could be incorporated into clinical assessments. Questions address a 2-week period in four dimensions: time management, physical demands, interpersonal and mental demands, and productivity demands. Subscale scores range from 0 to 100, with higher scores reflecting greater difficulty. The WLQ assesses health impacts only on paid labor. Further information, including licensing and applicable fees, is available at the website for Tufts Medical Center's Institute for Clinical Research and Health Policy Studies (http://160.109.101.132/icrhps/resprog/thi/wlq.asp).

Work Productivity and Activity Impairment

The Work Productivity and Activity Impairment (WPAI) questionnaire assesses the impact of health problems on work productivity (Reilly et al. 1993). The WPAI is the most frequently used health-related work productivity research instrument, and is documented to have good psychometric properties, including test-retest reliability and construct validity (Prasad et al. 2004). The WPAI consists of six self- or interviewer-administered questions. Domains assessed include hours absent from work due to health problems, as well as the impact of health problems on productivity at work and in daily activities outside of work. The instrument has been used in mental health research (Chirban et al. 1997; Ettigi et al. 1997; Jacobs et al. 1997; Wittchen and Beloch 1996) and in studies involving individuals with PTSD (Zhang et al. 2004). There is a general health version (WPAI-GH), as well as a specific health problem version (WPAI-SHP). Printable versions of the instruments, their coding, and their scoring are available for use through the developer's website and may be used without permission (www.reillyassociates.net/Index.html).

Assessment of Contextual Factors

Personal contextual factors include gender, minority status, age, lifestyle, habits, upbringing, coping styles, education, profession, personality characteristics, marital status, and overall behavioral patterns (World Health Organization 2002). Environmental factors include the physical, social, and attitudinal environments, as well as informal and formal organizations and services related to work, medical care, communication, government, transportation, and the community (World Health Organization 2002). Table 10–4 describes the environmental factors listed in the ICF. These factors can inhibit or facilitate functioning.

Despite international consensus that environmental factors interact with individual health conditions to produce disability outcomes, methods for quantifying the effect of the environment on participation in society are limited. We identified only one tool in a peer-reviewed publication that assesses the frequency and magnitude of a broad range of environmental barriers; the Craig Hospital Inventory of Environmental Factors (CHIEF; Whiteneck et al. 2004) is a 25-item questionnaire with five factor-analytically derived subscales assessing attitude and support barriers, service and assistance barriers, physical and structural barriers, policy barriers, and work and school barriers. There is also a 12-item version called the CHIEF Short Form (CHIEF-SF). To the best of our knowledge, although initial reliability and validity data are promising,

Table 10–4. Environmental factors from the *International Classification of Functioning, Disability and Health*

Domain	Description
1. Products and technology	Food, drugs, technical aids
2. Natural environment and human-made changes to the environment	Landforms, local population, plants, animals, climate, light, sound, air quality
3. Support and relationships	Physical and emotional support from family, friends, peers, health professionals
4. Attitudes	Customs, ideologies, values, norms, stigma
5. Services, systems, and policies	Programs, systems, policies

Source. World Health Organization 2001.

CHIEF has not been tested or used with individuals who have primary psychiatric disabilities. This instrument has been copyrighted (for information, contact charrison-felix@craighospital.org or dmelick@craighospital.org).

The more common approach has been for researchers and clinicians to identify the areas of the environment of most relevance for a given purpose and to select a measure targeting that specific domain. Environmental factors that may be particularly relevant for individuals with PTSD include social support, stigma and discrimination, and disability compensation.

Social Support and Stigma

Domains 3 and 4 listed in Table 10–4 include social support and stigma, respectively. A large body of scientific literature demonstrates the protective function of social support and the detrimental effect of social stress on a range of health outcomes for individuals with mental health problems, including trauma survivors (e.g., Brewin et al. 2000). Similarly, we recommend evaluating the role of prejudicial attitudes and discrimination in patients' lives, because research consistently demonstrates that stigma impacts health and well-being as well as treatment behavior among individuals with psychiatric disorders, including PTSD (e.g., Corrigan 2004; Hoge et al. 2004; Sayer et al. 2009). Importantly, some social support barriers and manifestations of discrimination may be amenable to interventions. For example, the clinician may determine that the patient's family does not understand his or her PTSD and could benefit from family education. In another instance, the clinician may help the patient identify resources to help him or her counter discrimination at work or in housing. For a review of social support measures and interventions, we refer readers to a comprehensive book on this topic edited by Cohen et al. (2000). Measures of stigma are also reviewed elsewhere (e.g., Link et al. 2004).

Compensation and Disability Systems

Individuals with possible PTSD can seek benefits or compensation through various systems depending on the context in which the precipitating trauma occurred, including workers' compensation, personal injury litigation, the Social Security Administration, and the VA. Among individuals who seek these benefits, the relevant disability or compensation program becomes a contextual factor that may affect their symptoms, functional status, and participation in society. Features of the claims processes themselves may have deleterious effects on the individual with possible PTSD because the application or legal processes can be time-consuming, protracted, and, at least from the claimant's perspective, adversarial (Bryant et al. 1997). For individuals with PTSD, the claim or litigation process may also serve as a reminder of the precipitating trauma, particularly if it requires a PTSD examination or written documentation of trauma. Additionally, because disability and compensation systems provide benefits to individuals who can establish PTSD-related disability, "secondary-gain" incentives, whether conscious or unconscious, may result in more extreme levels of psychopathology or disability than would be expected (Frueh et al. 2000). On the other hand, involvement in a disability or compensation system may have positive correlates, including triggering participation in treatment and, for those who are awarded benefits, improved access to services, improved financial well-being, and validation or recognition of trauma and associated suffering (Sayer et al. 2004a, 2004b; Spoont et al. 2007). Research on the effect of compensation for PTSD and associated functional problems is limited and inconclusive (Sayer et al. 2007). Nevertheless, clinicians evaluating individuals with PTSD need to consider the complex ways in which involvement in a compensation or disability system may promote or impede their patients' recovery.

Conclusion

The effects of PTSD manifest themselves in ways that extend far beyond the core symptoms. A subset of individuals with PTSD may experience extreme functional impairment, and many more are likely to experience at least some functional difficulties in one or more domains. To fully capture the spectrum of trauma's impact, a PTSD assessment battery should include measures of functioning in addition to measures of core PTSD symptoms and psychiatric comorbidities. This information is essential for treatment planning and for monitoring response to treatment. To someone who has PTSD, functional difficulties may be more distressing than even the PTSD symptoms themselves.

The ICF provides an internationally accepted, comprehensive framework for assessing functioning and disability that can be applied easily to PTSD assessment. We recommend that clinicians become aware of all domains included in the ICF and prioritize evaluation of higher-order functional dimensions, including global, social, and occupational functioning. Other domains may be more relevant in certain contexts or with patients who have physical limitations. The specific measures that clinicians use should depend on the context of the evaluation, including the amount of time available and the patient's presenting problems and functional goals. In addition, clinicians should consider contextual factors that may also influence an individual's symptoms, functioning, and response to treatment. Contextual factors that may be of particular relevance in PTSD include social networks, stigma and discrimination, and disability compensation. Understanding the impact of contextual factors will allow the clinician to better understand the factors outside the clinical setting that may facilitate or impede a patient's recovery, as well as to determine whether there is a need for interventions targeting treatment and recovery barriers.

For example, consider two veterans of the war in Afghanistan, both of whom have PTSD. One veteran has a rich social network, including a supportive spouse, and the other is divorced with few friends. In the first case, treatment may involve mobilizing the veteran's social network and perhaps even providing couples therapy. In the second case, treatment instead may involve helping the veteran develop skills to build or repair the social network—for example, with the provision of social skills training. Imagine further that the stigma of receiving mental health care is a significant barrier to treatment for both veterans. Although the social network may be one channel for helping the first veteran to overcome this stigma, a different strategy is necessary to help the second patient (e.g., challenging cognitions, care management, peer support).

Clinicians undoubtedly are familiar with such scenarios and the need to incorporate the inherent differences into case formulation and treatment planning. We recommend grounding these activities in the ICF framework and using standardized assessments of functioning. Doing so can enrich the clinician's understanding of a patient's needs and facilitate application of this understanding in developing an optimal and patient-centered treatment strategy. In short, careful assessment of functioning can help the clinician treat the whole person.

Key Clinical Points

- Functional assessments are integral to developing an effective treatment plan for individuals with PTSD. Because many individuals struggling with PTSD have significant functional impairments, a diagnosis of PTSD alone does not provide sufficient information about service needs, and some individuals may value improvement in functional domains, such as relationships and work, as equal to or more important than core symptoms of PTSD.
- Functional assessments also allow clinicians to identify areas of intact functioning and environmental supports that can be leveraged to facilitate treatment participation and recovery.
- The ultimate level of disability people experience is a product of their own impairments in interaction with their physical and social environment.
- Generally, clinicians assessing functioning in individuals with possible PTSD should prioritize assessment of social and occupational functioning. The assessment of occupational functioning could include assessment of educational activities, informal employment, housework, and volunteer work as well as gainful employment. Clinicians should select psychometrically sound measures to assess functioning that fit the context of the evaluation, including the amount of time available and the patient's presenting problems and functional goals.
- Social support is often protective for individuals with PTSD, and such support, or lack thereof, should be evaluated and addressed in a global treatment plan.

- Clinicians evaluating individuals with PTSD will need to consider the complex ways in which involvement in a compensation or disability system may promote or impede their patients' recovery.

References

Agerbo E: Effect of psychiatric illness and labour market status on suicide: a healthy worker effect? J Epidemiol Community Health 59:598–602, 2005

American Psychiatric Association: Diagnostic and Statistical Manual of Mental Disorders, 4th Edition, Text Revision. Washington, DC, American Psychiatric Association, 2000

Arbisi PA: Use of the MMPI-2 in personal injury and disability evaluations, in MMPI-2: A Practitioner's Guide. Edited by Butcher JN. Washington, DC, American Psychological Association, 2005, pp 407–441

Bisson JI, Ehlers A, Matthews R, et al: Psychological treatments for chronic posttraumatic stress disorder: systematic review and meta-analysis. Br J Psychiatry 190:97–104, 2007

Bjarnason T, Sigurdardottir TJ: Psychological distress during unemployment and beyond: social support and material deprivation among youth in six northern European countries. Soc Sci Med 56:973–985, 2003

Blanchard EB, Hickling EJ, Taylor AE, et al: Psychiatric morbidity associated with motor vehicle accidents. J Nerv Ment Dis 183:495–504, 1995

Blanchard EB, Hickling EJ, Devineni T, et al: A controlled evaluation of cognitive behavioural therapy for posttraumatic stress in motor vehicle accident survivors. Behav Res Ther 41:79–96, 2003

Boscarino JA, Adams RE, Figley CR: Worker productivity and outpatient service use after the September 11th attacks: results from the New York City terrorism outcome study. Am J Ind Med 49:670–682, 2006

Brewin CR, Andrews B, Valentine JD: Meta-analysis of risk factors for posttraumatic stress disorder in trauma-exposed adults. J Consult Clin Psychol 68:748–766, 2000

Brown TA, Campbell LA, Lehman CL: Current and lifetime comorbidity of the DSM-IV anxiety and mood disorders in a large clinical sample. J Abnorm Psychol 110:588–599, 2001

Bryant B, Mayou R, Lloyd-Bostock S: Compensation claims following road accidents: a six-year follow-up study. Med Sci Law 37:326–336, 1997

Chirban JT, Jacobs RJ, Warren J, et al: The 36-Item Short Form Health Survey (SF-36) and the Work Productivity and Activity Impairment (WPAI) Questionnaire in panic disorder. Disease Management and Health Outcomes 1:154–164, 1997

Cloitre M, Koenen KC, Cohen LR, et al: Skills training in affective and interpersonal regulation followed by exposure: a phase-based treatment for PTSD related to childhood abuse. J Consult Clin Psychol 70:1067–1074, 2002

Cohen S, Underwood LG, Gottlieb BH: Social Support Measurement and Intervention: A Guide for Health and Social Scientists. New York, Oxford University Press, 2000

Corrigan P: How stigma interferes with mental health care. Am Psychol 59:614–625, 2004

Cosgrove DJ, Gordon Z, Bernie JE, et al: Sexual dysfunction in combat veterans with post-traumatic stress disorder. Urology 60:881–884, 2002

Crist P, Rangos JG, Davis CG, et al: The effects of employment and mental health status on the balance of work, play/leisure, self-care, and rest. Occupational Therapy in Mental Health 15:27–42, 2000

Echeburua E, de Corral P, Zubizarreta I, et al: Psychological treatment of chronic posttraumatic stress disorder in victims of sexual aggression. Behav Modif 21:433–456, 1997

Ehlers A, Clark D, Hackmann A, et al: Cognitive therapy for posttraumatic stress disorder: development and evaluation. Behav Res Ther 43:413–431, 2005

Endicott J, Spitzer RL, Fleiss JS, et al: The Global Assessment Scale: a procedure for measuring overall severity of psychiatric disturbance. Arch Gen Psychiatry 33:766–771, 1976

Ettigi P, Meyerhoff AS, Chirban JT, et al: The quality of life and employment in panic disorder. J Nerv Ment Dis 185:368–372, 1997

Foa EB, Dancu CV, Hembree EA, et al: A comparison of exposure therapy, stress inoculation training, and their combination for reducing posttraumatic stress disorder in female assault victims. J Consult Clin Psychol 67:194–200, 1999

Freeman TW, Roca V: Gun use, attitudes towards violence, and aggression among combat veterans with chronic posttraumatic stress disorder. J Nerv Ment Dis 189:317–320, 2001

Frueh BC, Hamner MB, Cahill SP, et al: Apparent symptom overreporting in combat veterans evaluated for PTSD. Clin Psychol Rev 20:853–885, 2000

Gladis MM, Gosch EA, Dishuk NM, et al: Quality of life: expanding the scope of clinical significance. J Consult Clin Psychol 67:320–331, 1999

Goldman HH, Skodol AE, Lave TR: Revising axis V for DSM-IV: a review of measures of social functioning. Am J Psychiatry 149:1148–1156, 1992

Green BL, Krupnick JL, Stockton P, et al: Effects of adolescent trauma exposure on risky behavior in college women. Psychiatry 68:363–378, 2005

Hay P, Katsikitis M, Begg J, et al: A two year follow-up study and prospective evaluation of the DSM-IV axis V. Psychiatr Serv 54:1028–1030, 2003

Hoge CW, Castro CA, Messer SC, et al: Combat duty in Iraq and Afghanistan, mental health problems and barriers to care. N Engl J Med 351:13–22, 2004

Hoge CW, Terhakopian A, Castro CA, et al: Association of posttraumatic stress disorder with somatic symptoms, health care visits, and absenteeism among Iraq war veterans. Am J Psychiatry 164:150–153, 2007

Institute of Medicine: A 21st Century System for Evaluating Veterans for Disability Benefits. Washington, DC, Institute of Medicine of the National Academies, 2007

Jacobs RJ, Davidson JRT, Gupta S: The effects of clonazepam on quality of life and work productivity in panic disorder. Am J Manag Care 3:1187–1196, 1997

Johnson DR, Rosenheck R, Fontana A, et al: Outcome of intensive inpatient treatment for combat-related posttraumatic stress disorder. Am J Psychiatry 153:771–777, 1996

Kazis LE, Miller DR, Skinner KM, et al: Dissemination of methods and results from the Veterans Health Study. J Ambul Care Manage 29:310–319, 2006

Keane TM, Fairbank JA, Caddell JM, et al: Implosive (flooding) therapy reduces symptoms of PTSD in Vietnam combat veterans. Behav Ther 20:245–260, 1989

Keller MB, Lavori PW, Friedman B, et al: The Longitudinal Interval Follow-up Evaluation: a comprehensive method for assessing outcome in prospective longitudinal studies. Arch Gen Psychiatry 44:540–548, 1987

Keller MB, Warshaw MG, Dyck I, et al: LIFE-IV: The Longitudinal Interval Follow-up Evaluation for DSM IV. Providence, RI, Brown University, Department of Psychiatry and Human Behavior, 1997

Kessler RC: Posttraumatic stress disorder: the burden to the individual and to society. J Clin Psychiatry 61:4–12, 2000

Koenen KC, Stellman SD, Sommer JF Jr: Persisting posttraumatic stress disorder symptoms and their relationship to functioning in Vietnam veterans: a 14-year follow-up. J Trauma Stress 21:49–57, 2008

Krakow B, Hollifield M, Johnston L, et al: Imagery rehearsal therapy for chronic nightmares in sexual assault survivors with posttraumatic stress disorder: a randomized controlled trial. JAMA 286:537–545, 2001

Kuhn E, Blanchard EB, Hickling EJ: Posttraumatic stress disorder and psychosocial functioning within two samples of MVA survivors. Behav Res Ther 41:1105–1112, 2003

Leon AC, Solomon DA, Mueller TI, et al: The Range of Impaired Functioning Tool (LIFE-RIFT): a brief measure of functional impairment. Psychol Med 29:869–878, 1999

Lerner D, Amick BC, Rogers WH, et al: The Work Limitations Questionnaire. Med Care 39:72–85, 2001

Link BG, Yang LH, Phelan JC, et al: Measuring mental illness stigma. Schizophr Bull 30:511–541, 2004

MacDonald HA, Colotla V, Flamer S, et al: Posttraumatic stress disorder (PTSD) in the workplace: a descriptive study of workers experiencing PTSD resulting from work injury. J Occup Rehabil 13:63–77, 2003

Magruder KM, Frueh BC, Knapp RG, et al: PTSD symptoms, demographic characteristics, and functional status among veterans treated in VA primary care clinics. J Trauma Stress 17:293–301, 2004

Marcus S, Marquis P, Sakai C: Controlled study of treatment of PTSD using EMDR in an HMO setting. Psychotherapy 34:307–315, 1997

Marks I, Lovell K, Noshirvani H, et al: Treatment of posttraumatic stress disorder by exposure and/or cognitive restructuring: a controlled study. Arch Gen Psychiatry 55:317–325, 1998

McFall M, Fontana A, Raskind M, et al: Analysis of violent behavior in Vietnam combat veteran psychiatric inpatients with posttraumatic stress disorder. J Trauma Stress 12:501–517, 1999

Meichenbaum D: Clinical Handbook/Practical Therapist Manual for Assessing and Treating Adults With Posttraumatic Stress Disorder (PTSD). Waterloo, Canada, Institute Press, 1994

Mendlowicz MV, Stein MB: Quality of life in individuals with anxiety disorders. Am J Psychiatry 157:669–682, 2000

Miller MW, Wolf EJ, Martin E, et al: Structural equation modeling of associations among combat exposure, PTSD symptom factors, and Global Assessment of Functioning. J Rehabil Res Dev 45:359–369, 2008

Moos RH, Nichol AC, Moos BS: Global Assessment of Functioning ratings and the allocation and outcomes of mental health services. Psychiatr Serv 53:730–737, 2002

Neuner F, Schauner M, Klaschik C, et al: A comparison of narrative exposure therapy, supportive counseling and psychoeducation for treating posttraumatic stress disorder in an African refugee settlement. J Consult Clin Psychol 72:579–587, 2004

Niv N, Cohen AN, Sullivan G, et al: The MIRECC version of the Global Assessment of Functioning scale: reliability and validity. Psychiatr Serv 58:529–535, 2007

O'Connell MJ, Kasprow W, Rosenheck RA: Rates and risk factors for homelessness after successful housing in a sample of formerly homeless veterans. Psychiatr Serv 59:268–275, 2008

Olatunji BO, Cisler JM, Tolin DF: Quality of life in anxiety disorders: a meta-analytic review. Clin Psychol Rev 27:572–581, 2007

Orcutt HK, King LA, King DW: Male-perpetrated violence among Vietnam veteran couples: relationships with veteran's early life characteristics, trauma history, and PTSD symptomatology. J Trauma Stress 16:381–390, 2003

Paunovic N, Öst LG: Cognitive-behavior therapy versus exposure therapy in the treatment of PTSD in refugees. Behav Res Ther 39:1183–1197, 2001

Penk W, Flanner RB: Psychosocial rehabilitation, in Effective Treatments for PTSD: Practice Guidelines From the International Society for Traumatic Stress Studies. New York, Guilford, 2000, pp 224–246

Power K, McGoldrick T, Brown K, et al: A controlled comparison of eye movement desensitization and reprocessing versus exposure plus cognitive restructuring versus waiting list in the treatment of posttraumatic stress disorder. Clin Psychol Psychother 9:299–318, 2002

Prasad M , Wahlqvist P , Shikiar R, et al: A review of self-report instruments measuring health-related work productivity: a patient-reported outcomes perspective. Pharmacoeconomics 22:225–244, 2004

Rapaport MH, Clary C, Fayyad R, et al: Quality-of-life impairment in depressive and anxiety disorders. Am J Psychiatry 162:1171–1178, 2005

Reilly MC, Zbrozek AS, Dukes EM: The validity and reproducibility of work productivity and activity impairment instrument. Pharmacoeconomics 4:353–365, 1993

Resnick PJ, West S, Payne JW: Malingering of posttraumatic disorders, in Clinical Assessment of Malingering and Deception, 3rd Edition. Edited by Rogers R, Resnick PJ. New York, Guilford, 2008, pp 109–127

Riggs DS, Byrne CA, Weathers FW, et al: The quality of the intimate relationships of male Vietnam veterans: problems associated with posttraumatic stress disorder. J Trauma Stress 11:87–101, 1998

Ross CE, Mirowsky J: Does employment affect health? J Health Soc Behav 36:230–243, 1995

Ruscio AM, Weathers FM, King LA, et al: Male war-zone veterans' perceived relationships with their children: the importance of emotional numbing. J Trauma Stress 15:351–357, 2002

Savoca E, Rosenheck R: The civilian labor market experiences of Vietnam-era veterans: the influence of psychiatric disorders. J Ment Health Policy Econ 3:199–207, 2000

Sayer NA, Spoont M, Nelson D: Disability compensation for PTSD and use of VA mental health care (letter). Psychiatr Serv 55:589, 2004a

Sayer NA, Spoont M, Nelson D: Veterans seeking disability benefits for posttraumatic stress disorder: who applies and the self-reported meaning of disability compensation. Soc Sci Med 58:2133–2143, 2004b

Sayer NA, Murdoch M, Carlson KF: Compensation and PTSD: consequences for symptoms and treatment. PTSD Research Quarterly 18:1–8, 2007

Sayer NA, Friedemann-Sanchez G, Spoont M, et al: A qualitative study of determinants of PTSD treatment initiation in veterans. Psychiatry 72:238–255, 2009

Schnurr PP, Friedman MJ, Foy DW, et al: Randomized trial of trauma-focused group therapy for posttraumatic stress disorder: results from a Department of Veterans Affairs cooperative study. Arch Gen Psychiatry 60:481–489, 2003

Shalev AY: Discussion: treatment of prolonged posttraumatic stress disorder—learning from experience. J Trauma Stress 10:415–423, 1997

Sheehan DV: The Anxiety Disease. New York, Scibners, 1983

Söderberg P, Tungström S, Armelius BA: Reliability of Global Assessment of Functioning ratings made by clinical psychiatric staff. Psychiatr Serv 56:434–438, 2005

Spoont M, Sayer NA, Nelson D, et al: Does filing a PTSD disability claim promote mental health care participation among veterans? Mil Med 172:572–575, 2007

Strauser DR: Trauma symptomatology: implications for return to work. Work 31:245–252, 2008

Strauser DR, Lustig DC: The implications of posttraumatic stress disorder on vocational behavior and rehabilitation planning. J Rehabil 67:26–30, 2001

Taft CT, Schumm JA, Marshall AD, et al: Family-of-origin maltreatment, posttraumatic stress disorder symptoms, social information processing deficits, and relationship abuse perpetration. J Abnorm Psychol 117:637–646, 2008

Vestling M, Tufvesson B, Iwarsson S: Indicators of return to work after stroke and the importance of work for subjective well-being and life satisfaction. J Rehabil Med 35:127–131, 2003

Ware JE: Conceptualization and measurement of health-related quality of life: comments on an evolving field. Arch Phys Med Rehabil 84 (suppl 2):S43–S51, 2003

Ware JE, Snow KK, Kosinski M, et al: SF-36 Health Survey: Manual and Interpretation Guide. Boston, MA, Health Institute, New England Medical Center, 1993

Ware JE, Kosinski M, Dewey JE: How to Score Version Two of the SF-36 Health Survey. Lincoln, RI, Quality Metric, 2000

Ware JE, Kosinski M, Turner-Bowker DM: User's Manual for the SF-12v2TM Health Survey With a Supplement Documenting the SF-12 Health Survey. Lincoln, RI, Quality Metric, 2002

Warshaw MG, Dyck I, Allsworth J, et al: Maintaining reliability in a long-term psychiatric study: an ongoing inter-rater reliability monitoring program using the Longitudinal Interval Follow-up Evaluation. J Psychiatr Res 35:297–305, 2001

Watson P, McFall M, McBrin C, et al: Best practice manual for posttraumatic stress disorder (PTSD) compensation and pension examinations. 2002. Available at: http://www.avapl.org/pub/PTSD%20Manual%20final%206.pdf. Accessed November 30, 2009.

Weissman M: SAS-SR Short and Screener Technical Manual. Toronto, ON, Canada, Multi-Health Systems, 2007

Weissman MM, Bothwell S: Assessment of social adjustment by patient self-report. Arch Gen Psychiatry 33:1111–1115, 1976

Whiteneck G: Conceptual models of disability: past, present, and future, in Workshop on Disability in America, A New Look: Summary and Background Papers: Based on a Workshop of the Committee on Disability in America: a New Look, Board on Health Sciences Policy. Edited by Field MJ, Jette AM, Martin LG. Washington, DC, National Academies Press, 2006, pp 50–66

Whiteneck G, Harrison-Felix CL, Mellick DC, et al: Quantifying environmental factors: a measure of physical, attitudinal, service, productivity and policy barriers. Arch Phys Med Rehabil 85:1324–1335, 2004

Wittchen HU, Beloch E: The impact of social phobia on quality of life. Int Clin Psychopharmacol 11 (suppl 3):15–23, 1996

World Health Organization: WHO Psychiatric Disability Assessment Schedule (WHO/DAS: With a Guide to Its Use). Geneva, World Health Organization, 1988

World Health Organization: International Statistical Classification of Diseases and Related Health Problems, 10th Revision. Geneva, World Health Organization, 1992

World Health Organization: Disability Assessment Schedule II (WHODAS II). Geneva, World Health Organization, 2000

World Health Organization: International Classification of Functioning, Disability and Health. Geneva, World Health Organization, 2001

World Health Organization: Towards a Common Language for Functioning, Disability and Health: ICF: The International Classification of Functioning, Disability and Health. Geneva, World Health Organization, 2002

Zatzick DF, Marmar CR, Weiss DS, et al: Posttraumatic stress disorder and functioning and quality of life outcomes in a nationally representative sample of male Vietnam veterans. Am J Psychiatry 154:1690–1695, 1997a

Zatzick DF, Weiss DS, Marmar CR, et al: Post-traumatic stress disorder and functioning and quality of life outcomes in female Vietnam veterans. Mil Med 162:661–665, 1997b

Zatzick DF, Russo J, Rajotte E, et al: Strengthening the patient-provider relationship in the aftermath of physical trauma through an understanding of the nature and severity of posttraumatic concerns. Psychiatry 70:260–273, 2007

Zatzick DF, Jurkovich GJ, Rivara FP, et al: A national U.S. study of posttraumatic stress disorder, depression, and work and functional outcomes after hospitalization for traumatic injury. Ann Surg 248:429–437, 2008

Zhang W, Ross J, Davidson JR: Posttraumatic stress disorder in callers to the Anxiety Disorders Association of America. Depress Anxiety 19:96–104, 2004

PART III

Special Topics

11

Children and Adolescents

Stephen J. Cozza, M.D.
Jennifer M. Guimond, Ph.D.

The scientific understanding of posttraumatic stress disorder (PTSD) in children is a relatively recent development. Previous assumptions about children's resilience led to the belief that although children might be exposed to stressful situations, they would have no long-term psychiatric sequelae from those experiences. Early child trauma work by Terr (1979, 1983) with children of the Chowchilla kidnapping and by Pynoos et al. (1987) with children exposed to a fatal sniper attack brought new evidence to the scientific community that children and adolescents can and do develop posttraumatic symptoms consistent with PTSD. Over the past 25 years, a robust literature has emerged linking traumatic exposures to the development of PTSD in children. Although PTSD can be reliably identified, diagnosed, and treated in children, clinicians need to be mindful of the unique developmental considerations of the disorder in the pediatric population.

Developmental Considerations of PTSD

Although PTSD was introduced as a distinct clinical disorder in the *Diagnostic and Statistical Manual of Mental Disorders*, Third Edition (DSM-III; American Psychiatric Association 1980), the classification system did not formally recognize that pediatric patients may present with a different clinical manifestation until the fourth edition (DSM-IV; American Psychiatric Association 1994). The developmental differences between infants, young children, schoolchildren, teens, and adults have been shown to affect the nature and expression of posttraumatic sequelae (De Bellis and Van Dillen 2005). The lack of understanding of these differences and the inadequacy of early diagnostic symptoms may explain why some studies using DSM-III criteria yielded very low prevalence rates in younger populations (Lavigne et al. 1996). Young children are less likely to evidence emotional numbing, may have fewer avoidant symptoms (or are incapable of describing them), and may present with a wider range of behavioral changes (e.g., aggression) as a result of traumatic exposure (Dyregrov and Yule 2006). DSM-IV-TR (American Psychiatric Association 2000) requires that to receive a PTSD diagnosis, children and adolescents must meet the same diagnostic criteria as adults (reexperiencing, avoidance or numbing, and hyperarousal), but recognizes that children, particularly younger children, may express symptoms in ways more characteristic of their age. Table 11–1 illustrates current modifications in DSM-IV-TR criteria that better account for child-specific posttraumatic responses.

Scheeringa et al. (1995; Scheeringa 2008) have recommended further revision of the DSM PTSD diagnostic criteria for younger children. These recommended changes would rely less on children's limited verbal capacity and substitute more developmentally attuned observable Criterion C items (e.g., constriction of play, social withdrawal). Additionally, the changes would not require that intrusive recollection be distressing (Criterion B) and would call for only one (rather than three) of seven Criterion C avoidance or numbing symptoms to qualify for diagnosis (Scheeringa 2008). When Scheeringa et al. (2003) used age-modified criteria to evaluate a group of preschool children who had witnessed violence, they found a PTSD prevalence rate of 26%, which is comparable to rates typically cited in the literature for other trauma-exposed groups. In comparison, when the study group used DSM-IV diag-

Table 11–1. DSM-IV-TR PTSD criteria modifications for children

	Adult criteria	Child modifications
Criterion A (2)	The person's response involved intense fear, helplessness, or horror.	In children, this may be expressed by disorganized or agitated behavior.
Criterion B (1)	Recurrent and intrusive distressing recollections of the event, including images, thoughts, or perceptions.	In young children, repetitive play may occur in which themes or aspects of the trauma are expressed.
Criterion B (2)	Recurrent distressing dreams of the event.	In children, there may be frightening dreams without recognizable content.
Criterion B (3)	Acting or feeling as if the traumatic event were recurring (includes a sense of reliving the experience, illusions, hallucinations and dissociative flashback episodes, including those that occur on awakening or when intoxicated).	In young children, trauma-specific reenactment may occur.

Source. Adapted from *Diagnostic and Statistical Manual of Mental Disorders,* 4th Edition, Text Revision, pp. 467–468. Washington, DC, American Psychiatric Association, 2000. Copyright 2000, American Psychiatric Association. Used with permission.

nostic criteria to screen the same population of young children, no PTSD was found (Scheeringa et al. 2003).

Children may exhibit subthreshold posttraumatic stress symptoms and still be profoundly affected. Carrion et al. (2002) reported that of 59 traumatized children (ages 7–14 years), those who met DSM-IV criteria for two of the three PTSD symptom clusters showed impairment and distress similar to those of the children who met criteria in all three symptom areas. Older subjects in this group evidenced symptom clustering more consistent with adult clinical presentations (Carrion et al. 2002).

Together, these findings suggest a need to adequately identify developmental variants of posttraumatic psychopathology in younger children, because symptom levels that may not meet DSM-IV-TR criteria can still result in significant distress and dysfunction, requiring treatment. Further study is necessary, and further modification to existing diagnostic criteria may be appropriate. Given the manifestations of traumatic response in children, clinicians are encouraged to collect information from multiple sources, including children, parents, teachers, day care providers, or other involved adults, in an effort to form a complete clinical picture.

Comorbidity

As with adults, traumatic sequelae in children can lead to a range of comorbid conditions. Those reported in the literature include multiple developmental problems (Famularo and Fenton 1994); additional psychiatric problems, such as anxiety, attention-deficit/hyperactivity disorder, psychosis, depression, substance abuse/dependence, and suicidal ideation (Famularo et al. 1996; Kilpatrick et al. 2003); teen health risk behaviors (Danielson et al. 2006; Seng et al. 2005); and various medical disorders (Seng et al. 2005). Although PTSD is the focus of this chapter, clinicians should be prepared to address a broad range of posttraumatic health conditions so that all of a child's problems can be adequately identified and treated.

Childhood Traumatic Grief: A Unique Clinical Condition

Childhood traumatic grief (CTG) is a relatively new and developing construct intended to highlight the potential impact on children of a sudden, unexpected, and traumatic death of a loved one. CTG complicates a child's ability to mourn the loss of a loved one due to problematic trauma symptoms (hyperarousal, psychological distress, and avoidance) (Pynoos 1992). Because memories can become traumatic triggers to these upsetting symptoms, children will avoid memories of the deceased, even pleasant or positive memories, to avoid recurring traumatic symptoms. Children may also avoid identification with their loved ones in an attempt to protect themselves from a similar fate, especially when deaths were violent or painful (Pynoos 1992). Although many symptoms of CTG and PTSD overlap, scientists distinguish between these two conditions (Cohen et al. 2002). A child may experience PTSD and uncomplicated bereavement without CTG. By definition, CTG is marked by the presence of partial or fully developed PTSD that specifically complicates a child's capacity to mourn the death. A study evaluating the construct of CTG found that although highly correlated with PTSD and depression in a cohort of 132 bereaved children and adolescents, CTG is a distinct clinical entity (Brown et al. 2008). These authors also identified relationships between CTG severity and the level of trauma associated with the death, as well as between CTG and the emotional reaction of important adults to the death. Results of this developing literature underscore the importance of recognizing CTG as a distinct condition requiring unique clinical intervention.

Childhood Trauma Exposures

Children and adolescents are exposed to a variety of traumatic exposures. The National Child Traumatic Stress Network (NCTSN) identifies 11 categories of childhood trauma on its website (www.nctsn.org). These are listed in Table 11–2, along with brief descriptions.

Complex Trauma

Complex trauma is different from other individual traumatic experiences listed in Table 11–2. Complex trauma occurs when children experience multiple and caustic traumatic stressors (e.g., child physical abuse, sexual abuse, neglect, domestic violence) early in life and over a prolonged period of time, resulting in a pattern of developmental deviations distinct from PTSD (van der Kolk 2005). Sequelae include patterns of emotional, behavioral, and cognitive dysregulation; diminished interpersonal trust and relatedness; and functional impairment (van der Kolk 2005). Given mounting evidence of the devastating consequences of complex trauma and the inadequacy of the PTSD diagnosis to adequately describe the clinical experience, the Complex Trauma Task Force of NCTSN and other experts have proposed that a new diagnosis, developmental trauma disorder, be used to better describe these sequelae (van der Kolk 2005).

Prevalence of Childhood Trauma Exposure

Several large epidemiological studies have described elevated rates of traumatic exposure in the U.S. pediatric population. Finkelhor et al. (2005) reported rates of victimization experiences in the Developmental Victimization Study,

Table 11–2. NCTSN trauma types

Trauma type	Description
Community and school violence	Participation in or victimization from predatory, criminal, or interpersonal violence (to include rape or murder) within the community or school setting
Complex trauma	Exposure to chronic and typically multiple forms of abuse and neglect, often occurring within the home setting, with consequences of emotional dysregulation and misperception of and vulnerability to future traumatic events
Domestic violence	Actual or threatened physical or sexual violence or emotional abuse between adults in an intimate relationship
Medical trauma	Exposure of children and their families to pain, injury, illness, or medical procedures
Natural disasters	A result of natural catastrophes, such as earthquakes, hurricanes, fires, or floods
Neglect	Inadequate supervision, protection, or provision of resources, emotional support, education, or medical care that is required based on a child's developmental age and individual circumstances
Physical abuse	A single act or a pattern of continuous acts of imposing physical pain or injury on children; may occur as a result of punishment that is inappropriate for a child's developmental age or condition
Refugee and war-zone trauma	Exposure to war, political violence, torture, war crimes, genocide, displacement, or child soldiering
Sexual abuse	Developmentally inappropriate or coercive sexual activity between children or with an older person that may include physical contact or not (e.g., exhibitionism, pornography)
Terrorism	The intended use of threats of violence or actual violence to incite fear, coerce, or intimidate
Traumatic grief	A pathological response to the death of a loved one that typically is traumatic in nature and results in an inability to effectively grieve the loss; in such circumstances, a child's memory of the deceased serves as a traumatic reminder leading to terrifying thoughts, images, or memories

Note. NCTSN=National Child Traumatic Stress Network.

Source. Adapted from National Child Traumatic Stress Network: "Types of Traumatic Stress." Available at: http://www.nctsnet.org/nccts/nav.do?pid=typ_main. Accessed December 27, 2009. Used with permission.

using a national sample of over 2,000 children ages 2–17 years. The authors found that 71% of the study sample endorsed exposure to a variety of traumatic experiences, including personal assault and property theft, within the previous year, with many subjects endorsing multiple lifetime exposures. Based on a telephone survey of 4,000 adolescents, Kilpatrick and Saunders (1997) reported subject exposure rates of 17.4%, 8.1%, and 39.4% for physical assault, sexual assault, or witnessing interpersonal violence, respectively. Copeland et al. (2007) reported on a rural North Carolina sample of 1,420 pediatric subjects, concluding that by age 16 years, two-thirds of the group had been exposed to at least one significant trauma. Similarly, Breslau et al. (2004) reported elevated rates of trauma exposure in a large sample of urban youth; 62.6% of males and 33.7% of females reported a history of assaultive violence, with 82.5% of the sample endorsing some traumatic exposure during their lifetime.

Prevalence of Childhood PTSD

PTSD prevalence rates for children and adolescents have been studied in both community and trauma-exposed samples. In most studies, lifetime prevalence rates of PTSD in children and adolescents are similar to, if not higher than, rates for adults. Rates of PTSD are typically higher in girls than boys in similarly sampled populations. The National Comorbidity Survey (Kessler et al. 1995) of U.S. teenagers and adults reported a lifetime prevalence of PTSD of 7.8% in the younger cohort (ages 15–24 years), with greater prevalence reported by female (10.4%) than by male (5.0%) respondents. The findings suggested that this younger age group had higher relative risk for PTSD than older cohorts in this large sample. Giaconia et al. (1995) reported lifetime PTSD prevalence of 6.3% in their longitudinal study of 384 adolescents who had been followed since age 5 years. In this sample, 43% of the population reported at least one significant trauma, and these participants had higher reported PTSD lifetime prevalence (14.5%) when compared with the total sample (6.3%). In their large community-based nationally representative survey of U.S. adolescents, Kilpatrick and Saunders (1997) reported 5% prevalence rates in teenagers under age 18 years.

PTSD prevalence has also been examined in groups that have been exposed to natural disasters, terrorism, medical trauma, physical and sexual abuse, domestic violence, and war. Prevalence rates have been variable, but they are uniformly elevated in all trauma-exposed groups when compared with community samples. A few examples are displayed in Table 11–3.

As shown in Table 11–3, studies of child responses in natural disasters have included high rates of PTSD, along with comorbid depression, that persist long after the traumatic event. Such findings are evident across age groups. These and other studies have uncovered various risk factors that contribute to the development of pediatric posttraumatic disorders. Among natural disasters, rates of PTSD varied by proximity to the event (Goenjian et al. 1995), child characteristics, access to social support, and children's coping (Vernberg et al. 1996). In addition, among school-age children involved in an Australian bushfire, McFarlane (1987) found that mothers' responses to the disaster (including their experience of intrusive memories or a change in parenting) better predicted child outcomes than did the level of child exposure.

Regarding terrorism and war, both the number of potential exposures and the intensity of individual traumas (e.g., war atrocities) can have powerful and long-lasting consequences for children (Barenbaum et al. 2004). Pfefferbaum et al. (1999) reported the results of a survey of over 3,000 students conducted 7 weeks after the Oklahoma City bombing, finding that bereaved youth were noted to have significantly elevated posttraumatic symptom scores when compared with nonbereaved subjects, with mean symptom scores of those who lost an immediate family member being highest. The authors highlighted the important role of personal loss in the development of posttraumatic symptoms in this pediatric cohort.

De Bellis and Van Dillen (2005) grouped childhood PTSD risk factors into three categories: those risk factors that precede the traumatic event, those risk factors related to the traumatic event, and those factors or conditions that contribute after the trauma. Table 11–4 summarizes the authors' findings.

Therapeutic Interventions

Studies examining the utility of treatments for children and adolescents with PTSD, as with many psychiatric conditions, are relatively recent and are limited in comparison to studies on adult populations. As recently as 1995, no empirically studied treatments for traumatized children were published in the literature (Cohen 2008). Within the past 15 years, considerable work has been accomplished to provide treatment alternatives, particularly in the area of psychosocial interventions. The study of medication effects on pediatric PTSD populations remains far more limited.

Psychosocial Interventions

All psychosocial treatments discussed in the following sections 1) are based in theory; 2) are generally accepted in clinical practice; 3) have a book, manual, or other writings that specify the treatment protocol; and 4) do not constitute a substantial risk of harm. Certain psychosocial modalities may be used in clinical practice; however, they are not discussed here unless they meet these requirements. For example, although play therapy is often used in the treatment of childhood trauma, no empirical evidence supports its independent use. However, play techniques are incorporated in many evidence-based interventions as a means of enhancing communication (Cohen et al. 2003). A summary of available evidence-based psychosocial interventions, their mode of engagement, subject target ages, and NCTSN level of supportive evidence is provided in Table 11–5.

Cognitive-Behavioral Therapy

There are several adaptations of cognitive-behavioral therapy (CBT) for trauma, referred to as trauma-specific CBT. Core components of trauma-specific CBT include psychoeducation, relaxation training, coping skill development, exposure, and cognitive restructuring (Cohen et al. 2003; Perrin et al. 2000; Taylor and Chemtob 2004). Several trauma-specific CBT interventions have been tested. These interventions differ mostly in the balance between and emphasis on cognitive and behavioral components (Stallard 2006). Compared with other interventions, trauma-specific CBT has the most evidence for efficacy in treating PTSD; it also has been shown to be superior to wait-list conditions and other treatments in preschoolers, children, and adolescents (Nikulina et al. 2008; Silverman et al. 2008). In addition, the treatment studies supporting trauma-specific CBT have included a wide range of ethnicities, greater effect size, and greater effect on comorbid conditions compared with other treatments (Silverman et al. 2008).

Trauma-Focused Cognitive-Behavioral Therapy

Trauma-focused CBT (TF-CBT; Cohen et al. 2006b) was originally developed for use with sexually abused children, but has been adapted for children

Table 11–3. Prevalence of PTSD and other trauma-related disorders for different types of trauma

Sample	Exposure	Time since event	Prevalence rates
Natural disasters			
808 children ages 5–12 years (McFarlane 1987)	Australian bushfire	8 months/ 26 months	PTSD symptoms: 53%/57%
218 children ages 8–16 years (Goenjian et al. 1995; Pynoos et al. 1993)	Armenian earthquake	1.5 years	PTSD symptoms: 26%–95%[a] Comorbid depression: 13%–75%[a]
568 students in grades 3–5 (Vernberg et al. 1996)	Hurricane Andrew	3 months	PTSD symptoms: 56% moderate to severe
323 children ages 12–14 years (Hsu et al. 2002)	Taiwanese earthquake	6 weeks	PTSD diagnosis: 22%
167 children ages 7–14 years (Thienkrua et al. 2006)	Thailand tsunami	8 weeks	PTSD diagnosis: 6%–11%[a]
70 children ages 3–6 years (Scheeringa and Zeanah 2008)	Hurricane Katrina	>5 months	PTSD diagnosis: 50% using alternate criteria for young children Major depressive disorder: 43%
War and terrorism			
234 children ages 7–12 years (Thabet and Vostanis 2000)	Gaza Strip: long-standing military conflict	6 months/ 18 months	PTSD symptoms: 40%/10% moderate to severe
2,976 children ages 9–14 years (Smith et al. 2002)	Bosnia-Herzegovina war	2 years	PTSD symptoms: 52%

Table 11–3. Prevalence of PTSD and other trauma-related disorders for different types of trauma *(continued)*

Sample	Exposure	Time since event	Prevalence rates
8,236 students ages 9–21 years (Hoven et al. 2005)	World Trade Center attacks	6 months	Probable PTSD: 11% Any anxiety/depressive disorder: 29%
Medical procedures			
104 adolescents ages 12–20 years (Mintzer et al. 2005)	Organ transplant recipients	1–14 years	PTSD symptoms: 31% Probable PTSD diagnosis: 14%
309 children ages <1–19 years (Schrag et al. 2008)	Cancer	<1–8 years	Stress-related mental disorder (i.e., PTSD, acute stress disorder, or adjustment disorders): 19%
Victimization and exposure to violence			
326 adolescents ages 12–17 years (Kilpatrick and Saunders 1997)	Sexual abuse/assault	Variable	PTSD: 19%–41%[b] (male) 27%–34%[b] (female)
701 adolescents ages 12–17 years (Kilpatrick and Saunders 1997)	Physical abuse/assault	Variable	PTSD: 12%–20%[b] (male) 21%–40%[b] (female)
1,585 adolescents ages 12–17 years (Kilpatrick and Saunders 1997)	Witnessed serious violence	Variable	PTSD: 8%–20%[b] (male) 21%–27%[b] (female)
373 children ages 8–14 years (McCrae et al. 2006)	Alleged child sexual abuse	Average of 5–6 months	PTSD symptoms: 8% Depression symptoms: 20%

[a]Varied by proximity to event.
[b]Varied by number of experiences.

Table 11–4. Risk factors for pediatric PTSD

Preexisting risk factors	Trauma-related risk factors	Posttraumatic risk factors
Poor social support	Degree of trauma exposure	Lack of social support
Adverse life events	Parent/child sense of danger	Continued negative life events
Poverty	Trauma-specific factors (e.g., traumatic loss, death of loved ones, loss of home)	Negative parental reactions
Child maltreatment		Lack of intervention/ treatment
Poor family functioning		
Family psychiatric history		
Behavioral inhibition		
Female gender		
Previous mental illness		
Poor physical health		

Source. Adapted from De Bellis and Van Dillen 2005.

exposed to a wide range of traumas. The standard treatment has been used with children ages 3–17 years from multiple ethnic backgrounds, and versions have also been adapted for use with Latino children (M.A. De Arellano, C.K. Danielson, "Culturally Modified Trauma Focused Treatment," unpublished manuscript, Medical University of South Carolina, Charleston, SC, 2005) and with Native American children (Bigfoot and Schmidt 2007). TF-CBT is a relatively short-term treatment (12–20 weeks) effective for PTSD in a child-only format. When the child has comorbid depressive symptoms or disruptive behaviors, TF-CBT works best with caregiver involvement.

TF-CBT uses cognitive-behavioral, interpersonal, and family therapy principles to address trauma-related symptoms, including PTSD, depression, trauma-related shame, and trauma-related cognitions. It incorporates a non-offending caregiver component that is designed to enhance caregiver support of the child, decrease the caregiver's distress related to the child's trauma, and increase positive parenting behaviors. Treatment components include parenting skills, psychoeducation, relaxation skills training, affective modulation skills training, cognitive processing, trauma narration, in vivo desensitization, conjoint caregiver-child sessions, and enhancement of safety and future development. These components, summarized by the acronym PRACTICE, are described briefly in Table 11–6. Therapeutic approaches, session guides, and intervention techniques are detailed in the TF-CBT clinician's guide (Cohen et al. 2006b).

In six randomized controlled trials, TF-CBT for child sexual abuse has been favorably compared with other treatments, including nondirective supportive therapy (Cohen and Mannarino 1996, 1997, 1998; Cohen et al. 2005) and child-centered therapy (Cohen et al. 2004). Nondirective supportive therapy groups had higher dropout rates than TF-CBT groups, suggesting that TF-CBT may be better accepted by families. Children in child-centered therapy (though not those in nondirective supportive therapy) were specifically invited to talk about the abuse; given superior results with TF-CBT, this suggests that simply talking about trauma is not sufficient for treatment. Rather, these studies imply that the trauma-specific processing and directed skill building are important aspects of effective PTSD treatment in children.

Deblinger et al. (1996) compared the efficacy of child-only, parent-only, and combined parent-child TF-CBT interventions with that of community treatment as usual in children ages 7–13 years who had been sexually abused. Children in the child-only and combined parent-child groups experienced a greater reduction in PTSD symptoms than those in the parent-only and community treatment groups at posttreatment and 2-year follow-up. In contrast, children in the parent-only and combined parent-child groups demonstrated greater reduction in externalizing behaviors and depressive symptoms, compared with child-only and community treatment groups, at posttreatment and 2-year follow-up. Thus, the child components of TF-CBT appear to be essential for reducing trauma symptoms, whereas the parent components appear to be important in reducing depression and behavior problems that may accompany PTSD.

In summary, TF-CBT has been shown effective in the treatment of sexually abused children and has been adapted for use in the treatment of multiple types of childhood trauma. In addition to effectively treating PTSD, TF-CBT has been shown to reduce other trauma-related symptoms, including behavior problems and depressive symptoms. Finally, when caregivers were assessed, those in TF-CBT groups demonstrated reductions in their own abuse-specific

Table 11–5. Psychosocial interventions

Treatment	Modality	Age range (years)	NCTSN level of evidence	Other considerations
Trauma-focused cognitive-behavioral therapy	Individual with parent sessions	3–17	Well supported and efficacious[a]	Also reduces behavioral problems and depression
Multimodality trauma treatment	Group	9–14	Supported and acceptable[b]	Designed for children who experienced a single-incident stressor Also reduces depression
Cognitive-behavioral intervention for trauma in schools	Group	10–15	Supported and probably efficacious[c]	Incorporates a component for teachers Parental involvement not necessary Also reduces behavioral problems and depression
Child-parent psychotherapy	Parent-child	0–6	Well supported and efficacious[a]	Long-term intervention Can be used in home-based settings Also reduces behavior problems
Trauma systems therapy	Family	6–19	Supported and acceptable[b]	Requires significant caregiver involvement and case management Also reduces behavior problems
Eye movement desensitization and reprocessing	Individual	6–17	Well supported and efficacious[d]	Requires specialized clinician training

Table 11–5. Psychosocial interventions *(continued)*

Note. NCTSN = National Child Traumatic Stress Network.

[a]At least two randomized controlled treatment outcome studies.

[b]At least one group study (controlled or uncontrolled) or a series of single-subject case studies.

[c]At least two studies utilizing some form of control without randomization.

[d]Not evaluated by NCTSN. Level of evidence rating given by the authors based on published research.

Source. Adapted from National Child Traumatic Stress Network: "National Child Traumatic Stress Network Empirically Supported Treatments and Promising Practices." March 22, 2005. Available at: http://www.nctsnet.org/nccts/nav.do?pid=ctr_top_trmnt_prom. Updated information on these treatments available at: http://nctsn.org/nccts/asset.do?id=650. Accessed December 1, 2009. Used with permission.

Table 11–6. Treatment components of trauma-focused cognitive-behavioral therapy

Treatment components (PRACTICE)	Description
Parenting skills	Increasing the caregiver's use of selective attention, effective discipline, and praise and reinforcement for appropriate behavior
Psychoeducation	Providing information to the child and caregiver about the type of trauma the child experienced and common reactions to trauma in order to validate and normalize the child's and caregiver's emotional responses
Relaxation skills	Teaching strategies for decreasing physiological hyperarousal, such as focused breathing and progressive muscle relaxation
Affective modulation skills	Enhancing the child's identification and expression of feelings, cognitive coping skills (e.g., thought stopping, positive self-talk), problem-solving abilities, and social skills
Cognitive processing	Improving understanding of the relationship between thoughts, feelings, and behaviors; teaching the child to change thoughts to be more accurate and helpful
Trauma narration	Helping the child develop a detailed narrative of the traumatic experience(s) as a form of exposure; identifying and processing any cognitive distortions related to the trauma
In vivo desensitization	Decreasing anxiety and generalized avoidance of trauma reminders
Conjoint child-caregiver sessions	Facilitating the child's sharing of the narrative with the caregiver to promote open communication and assist the caregiver in providing appropriate support
Enhancement of safety and future development	Developing concrete skills to address current and future safety issues for the child and caregiver

Source. Adapted from Cohen et al. 2006.

distress (Cohen et al. 2004; Deblinger et al. 1996, 1999, 2001), a useful finding given that parental adjustment following trauma can significantly impact child adjustment.

Multimodality Trauma Treatment

Multimodality trauma treatment (MMTT; Amaya-Jackson et al. 2003; March et al. 1998) is a CBT intervention based on social learning theory that is designed to address PTSD symptoms related to a single-incident trauma. The intervention uses storybooks, narrative exposure, cognitive games, and peer modeling to teach anxiety management training, promote interpersonal problem solving for anger control, induce gradual exposure, replace maladaptive trauma-related cognitive schemas with more helpful thought patterns, improve coping skills, and reduce concurrent depression and grief. The treatment is delivered in 11–13 group sessions, with one mid-treatment individual session to introduce narrative exposure and correct trauma-related misattributions and distortions.

MMTT is indicated for children ages 9–14 years (National Child Traumatic Stress Network 2008a) who are experiencing PTSD related to a single-incident stressor. It is a structured protocol that can be applied in a school or office-based setting. MMTT has been used with multiply traumatized children, with children who have comorbid behavior problems, and in an individual therapy format (Amaya-Jackson et al. 2003). It has also been adapted for individual therapy with preschool-age children. However, no empirical studies have been published for these populations, and no published data have addressed issues of diversity.

March et al. (1998) examined MMTT in students with PTSD, ages 10–15 years, in two elementary and two middle schools. The study used a pretreatment to posttreatment design, with intervention start dates staggered by 4 weeks to assess for time effects, and excluded children with abuse-related trauma and significant disruptive behavior issues. Symptoms of PTSD, general anxiety, depression, and trait anger significantly decreased from pretreatment to posttreatment. The pattern of symptom reduction was consistent across both the early- and late-start groups, as well as across elementary and middle school groups, and treatment gains were maintained at 6 months posttreatment. No symptom reduction was observed during the 4-week wait period for the late-start group, suggesting a treatment rather than time effect.

Cognitive-Behavioral Intervention for Trauma in Schools

Cognitive-behavioral intervention for trauma in schools (CBITS; Jaycox 2004) is a 10-session group intervention designed for use in an inner-city school mental health clinic with a culturally diverse population. It targets symptoms of PTSD, anxiety, and depression related to exposure to violence. CBITS components include psychoeducation, relaxation training, cognitive coping, social problem solving, and a trauma narrative, and uses didactics, age-appropriate stories and cartoons, games, and worksheets. Like MMTT, CBITS also incorporates an individual session to introduce imaginal exposure. It also offers optional multifamily group sessions that provide psychoeducation, treatment information, support, and parenting skills (Kataoka et al. 2003). CBITS uses many of the same components as TF-CBT, but the parent component is often attenuated or not included (Cohen et al. 2006b). CBITS incorporates a brief teacher psychoeducation component, making it unique among other evidence-based interventions.

Stein et al. (2003) compared CBITS to a wait-list control group in a sample of sixth-grade middle school students who had clinically significant community violence–related PTSD. Results indicated that the CBITS group, compared with the wait-list control, evidenced fewer self-reported PTSD and depression symptoms and fewer parent-reported emotional and behavior problems at posttreatment. No differences were found for teacher-reported behavior problems. The wait-list group had similar symptom improvement following CBITS treatment. Similarly, Kataoka et al. (2003) found CBITS to be effective, compared with a wait-list control, in reducing PTSD and depression symptoms in a sample of Latino immigrants in grades 3–8.

CBITS is indicated for children ages 10–15 years whose treatment needs can be met in a group setting and without significant parental involvement. It can be applied to a wide range of trauma events (Cohen et al. 2006b) and within a multicultural context. Clinicians are encouraged to use culturally relevant figures, materials, and concepts during group sessions (Ngo et al. 2008). In addition, CBITS has been adapted for use with Native American adolescents (Morsette et al. 2009).

Other Trauma-Specific Cognitive-Behavioral Therapy Interventions

Other reports have outlined the utility, flexibility, and adaptability of trauma-specific CBT. Giannopoulou et al. (2006) applied six group sessions of trauma-specific CBT with children ages 8–12 years who had survived an earthquake in Greece. They found treatment to be effective in reducing PTSD, depression, and general anxiety symptoms, and noted that treatment gains were maintained at 4-year follow-up. Shooshtary et al. (2008) applied four group sessions of trauma-specific CBT to earthquake survivors, ages 12–20 years, in Iran and found treatment to be superior to the wait-list control condition in reducing PTSD symptoms. Finally, Smith et al. (2007) examined individual trauma-specific CBT in children ages 8–18 years who had PTSD related to a single-incident trauma (mostly motor vehicle accidents or physical assaults). Results indicated that rates of PTSD, depression, and anxiety decreased more in the trauma-specific CBT group than in the wait-list control group.

Summary

Trauma-specific CBT is applicable to 1) children ages 3–17 years; 2) single- and multiple-incident traumas; 3) diverse cultural and ethnic groups; 4) individual, family, and group modalities; and 5) school and office settings. It is structured yet flexible and can be considered a first-line treatment in most cases of child and adolescent PTSD.

Other Psychosocial Treatments

Child-Parent Psychotherapy

Child-parent psychotherapy (CPP; Lieberman and Van Horn 2005) is a trauma-specific, relationship-based model of treatment developed for young children exposed to interpersonal violence; it incorporates psychodynamic, attachment-based, cognitive-behavioral, and social learning components (Lieberman et al. 2005, 2006). It is the only trauma-specific treatment designed for young children. CPP is based on the premise that mental health concerns in young children can be best addressed through the child's relationship with the primary caregiver. It works within the context of free play during joint parent-child sessions and incorporates parent-only sessions as indicated. During joint sessions, the child is provided with developmentally appropriate toys selected to elicit trauma play and foster social interaction. Specific interventions are directed at child maladaptive behaviors, by supporting developmentally appropriate interactions and creating a joint child-parent trauma narrative. CPP techniques are designed to address sensorimotor disorganization; disruption of biological rhythms; fearfulness; reckless, self-endangering, and accident-prone behavior; aggression; and punitive and critical parenting.

Lieberman et al. (2005) studied CPP in ethnically diverse children (ages 3–5 years) and their mothers who had been exposed to intimate partner violence. Almost one-half of the children had also been exposed to community violence, and one-third had experienced physical and/or sexual abuse. Results indicated that the CPP group showed greater improvement in trauma symptoms, behavior problems, and rates of trauma spectrum disorders than a comparison group receiving case management with nonsystematic individual therapy. Interestingly, mothers participating in CPP showed decreased avoidance symptoms. Attrition was limited to 14% in the CPP group and 12% in the comparison group, which is particularly impressive, because the treatment was conducted over the course of 50 weeks.

CPP is indicated for children up to age 6 years who have a stable caregiver and who have been exposed to interpersonal violence. It is applicable across multiple ethnic groups, including recent immigrants, because it incorporates discussions of cultural values and culturally related experiences. CPP is flexible in application and may be used in home-based sessions as well as office-based sessions. However, CPP is a long-term treatment and requires significant caregiver participation.

Trauma Systems Therapy

Trauma systems therapy (TST; Saxe et al. 2007) is a systems-based intervention designed to address trauma-related symptoms as well as factors in the surrounding social environment that perpetuate these symptoms. Using a social-ecological perspective, TST targets the "trauma system," because unsafe and/or unstable environments can repeatedly trigger reexperiencing states in traumatized children. The goals of TST are to help the child learn to regulate emotions in the face of trauma reminders and other stressful events and to create an environment that helps the child regulate emotions and behaviors by decreasing trauma reminders as well as facilitating healthy coping strategies.

The initial TST assessment categorizes children and families, based on the stability of the environment and the child's degree of dysregulation, into one of five phases of treatment: surviving, stabilizing, enduring, understanding, and transcending. Based on the child's phase of treatment, the clinician selects appropriate treatment interventions that are provided within seven treatment modules, each of which can be used across different phases of treatment. The treatment modules consist of 1) Ready-Set-Go, which addresses family engagement in treatment and barriers to care; 2) Stabilization on Site, which addresses safety and stability within the environment; 3) Services Advocacy; 4) Psychopharmacology; 5) Emotion Regulation; 6) Cognitive Processing; and 7) Meaning Making. All children and families begin with the Ready-Set-Go module, and additional modules are selected as indicated.

Although the components of TST are evidence based, research on the treatment as a whole is limited to only one published study to date. The developers of TST conducted an open trial of TST with multiply traumatized children ages 5–20 years (Saxe et al. 2005). The study found a reduction in trauma symptoms, emotional dysregulation, behavioral dysregulation, and environmental instability following 3 months of treatment. The attrition rate was 28%; however, high attrition is to be expected in less stable families.

TST is indicated for children ages 6–19 years from families with multiple problems, including interpersonal violence, substance abuse, poverty, child protective services involvement, and refugee status (National Child Traumatic Stress Network 2008b). It has been implemented with a variety of ethnic groups, including recent immigrants and refugees from African and Central American countries. Specific attention to cultural perspectives and barriers to care makes it appropriate for diverse families. Length of treatment varies, depending on each family's specific needs, but can be as long as 12 months. Caregiver engagement and an infrastructure that supports significant case management are vital for effective treatment implementation.

Eye Movement Desensitization and Reprocessing

Eye movement desensitization and reprocessing (EMDR) (Greenwald 1993; Shapiro 2001) is a structured treatment approach designed to alleviate distress related to traumatic memories and problematic cognitions related to trauma. EMDR is hypothesized to work by facilitating the processing of memories and promoting more adaptive cognitions regarding the trauma. The procedure involves using back-and-forth eye movements combined with recall of an image, focus on a related cognition, and awareness of physical sensations.

EMDR has been studied in children ranging from 6 to 17 years. In a study of Swedish children ages 6–16 years, Ahmad et al. (2007) found eight sessions of EMDR to be superior to a wait-list control in decreasing posttraumatic stress symptoms related to a variety of traumas. Chemtob et al. (2002) found similar results in a group of ethnically diverse Hawaiian children, ages 6–12 years, who were survivors of a disaster and continued to meet criteria for PTSD 1 year after receiving a school-based trauma-specific CBT. A 6-month follow-up assessment conducted after the wait-list group had received treatment revealed that 56% of the children no longer met PTSD diagnostic criteria. Jaberghaderi et al. (2004) compared EMDR to CBT in a group of sexually abused Iranian girls, ages 12–13 years. Both treatments were equally effective in reducing parent- and child-reported posttraumatic stress symptom scores. However, EMDR required fewer sessions (mean = 6 sessions) than CBT (mean = 11 sessions) to meet the termination criteria, and 3 girls in the CBT group had not met termination criteria after the study ended at 12 sessions. Finally, Puffer et al. (1998) reported greater improvement in PTSD symptoms among U.S. children ages 8–17 years, compared with a wait-list control group, after only a single session of EMDR.

Taken together, these studies suggest that EMDR can be an efficient treatment for PTSD in children and adolescents of varying cultural groups who are exposed to varying traumas. Younger children may require modifications to the standard EMDR protocol. Although EMDR is generally described as an individual therapy, parents may be present during the sessions. EMDR requires more specialized training than other trauma treatments.

Treatment of Childhood Traumatic Grief

Unique therapeutic efforts are required to treat those with childhood traumatic grief. Cohen et al. (2006a; Cohen and Mannarino 2004) adapted TF-CBT for child traumatic grief (TG-CBT). In addition to trauma components, TG-CBT provides psychoeducation about death, addresses ambivalent feelings about the deceased, facilitates mourning the loss and redefining the relationship with the deceased, seeks to preserve positive memories, encourages commitment to present and new relationships, and promotes making meaning of the traumatic loss. Like TF-CBT, TG-CBT includes a significant parent component. Results from open trials suggest that it is effective in reducing symptoms of PTSD and CTG (Cohen et al. 2006b, 2006c). TG-CBT is designed to address cultural beliefs and can be used with traumatic grief related to any type of trauma. It is indicated for children ages 6–18 years experiencing CTG from any type of event.

Trauma and grief component therapy (TGCT) (Layne et al. 2002; Saltzman et al. 2001a, 2001b) is designed as a group intervention for trauma-exposed or traumatically bereaved adolescents. TGCT addresses the complexity of traumatic experience, the interplay between trauma and grief, the influence of life adversities, and the importance of restoring developmental progression. It encourages use of social support, enhances problem solving and coping with secondary adversities, and supports maintenance of adaptive routines. TGCT has been shown effective in the treatment of traumatic grief of teenage earthquake survivors (Goenjian et al. 1997) and war-exposed teenagers (Layne et al. 2008).

Project Loss and Survival Team (Project LAST) is a group intervention that uses CBT and narrative techniques originally developed for survivors of homicide and for children exposed to violence (Salloum 2008). In an open trial with Hurricane Katrina child survivors ages 7–12 years who were experiencing grief or moderate to severe PTSD symptoms, Project LAST evidenced some initial encouraging results on PTSD symptoms, depression, and traumatic grief (Salloum and Overstreet 2008). However, more study is required.

Psychopharmacology

Although at least one national survey suggests that child psychiatrists routinely use pharmacotherapy in treating traumatized children (Cohen 2001), little scientific support exists for this practice. To date, only two randomized controlled trials of medication use have been reported, and neither provides significant assistance in day-to-day clinical decision making. Robert et al. (1999) found that imipramine was superior to chloral hydrate in the treatment of acute stress symptoms in 25 hospitalized burn patients ages 2–19 years. Imipramine was dosed at 1 mg/kg to a maximum dosage of 100 mg/day. No medication side effects were reported in either the imipramine or the chloral hydrate group. Notably, since this study was published, the use of imipramine in the pediatric population has been discouraged due to potentially serious cardiovascular side effects and the availability of newer and safer medications.

In the second randomized controlled trial, Cohen et al. (2007) compared TF-CBT with sertraline (approved by the U.S. Food and Drug Administration for adult PTSD) and TF-CBT with placebo in treating 24 sexually abused girls (ages 10–17 years) with PTSD symptoms. Although a small statistically significant improvement in Child Global Assessment Scale ratings for the

TF-CBT with sertraline group over the TF-CBT with placebo group was found, the authors concluded there was no clear benefit of adding sertraline to TF-CBT. Both study groups showed improvement, suggesting that the treatment effect was due to TF-CBT rather than the addition of medication. The lack of medication effect in this study may also have been related to the small sample size. On a positive note, no adverse medication effects were described in this group of children, who received a mean maximum dosage of 150 mg/day.

Two open-label trials of citalopram use in the pediatric population have been published. Seedat et al. (2001) reported the results of a 12-week open-label study of citalopram with eight adolescents diagnosed with moderate to severe PTSD. The subjects were treated with a fixed dosage of 20 mg/day. Core PTSD symptom scores showed significant improvement, but depressive symptoms were not improved. Citalopram was generally well tolerated, and adverse effects were mild (nausea, headache, tiredness, and moderate akathisia) and remitted without intervention. One teenager was withdrawn from the study due to nosebleeds, which did not appear associated with the citalopram. In an 8-week follow-up open-label study, Seedat et al. (2002) examined the effect of citalopram on PTSD in 24 children and adolescents compared with that in 14 adults. Study subjects started citalopram 20 mg/day and, if tolerated, were titrated to a dosage of 40 mg/day. The authors identified 67% of the child and adolescent group and 64% of the adult group as treatment responders. The authors concluded that the effects of citalopram were similar for both groups, with no significant medication adverse effects.

Two open-label reports describe the potential benefit of antiadrenergic medications in treating pediatric posttraumatic stress. Famularo et al. (1988) reported the effect of propranolol (initially dosed three times daily at 0.8 mg/kg/day and increased over a 2-week period to a maximum of 2.5 mg/kg/day) on 11 physically or sexually abused children (ages 6–12 years) with a diagnosis of PTSD. In this B-A-B pilot trial, the authors found that patients exhibited fewer hyperarousal and agitation symptoms when taking medication. In an uncontrolled study, Harmon and Riggs (1996) described the use of clonidine (0.05–0.20 mg/day) in the treatment of seven preschool children (ages 3–6 years) who had PTSD symptoms that had not improved using psychotherapy, and found reduction in aggression, hyperarousal, and sleep difficulties.

In summary, the rational use of medication in the treatment of children and adolescents diagnosed with PTSD is challenged by the lack of scientific evidence clearly demonstrating benefit. No particular medication can be recommended for use at this time. Therefore, certain guidelines should be considered in the choice of medication in any individual case. Given the established benefit of psychosocial interventions for pediatric PTSD, these treatments should be considered as first-line. Pharmacotherapy should be considered when psychosocial interventions are ineffective or only partially effective. Because comorbid conditions are commonly present in populations with PTSD, clinicians should consider the appropriate use of medications to target disorders (e.g., depression and anxiety) for which benefit has been established in the treatment of pediatric patients or in cases in which severity of symptoms or dangerousness requires a more urgent response (Cohen 2001). Medications can also be used rationally and safely to address symptoms associated with PTSD, such as insomnia or hyperarousal (Donnelly 2003). Clinicians should consider developmental age in making decisions about medication treatment and exercise greater caution with preschoolers (Gleason et al. 2007). When used, medications should be integrated into a multimodal treatment plan and continuously monitored for both clinical benefit and adverse effects. Finally, given the lack of scientific evidence for specific medication selection, clinicians should consider the following factors in choosing appropriate medications for children: the neurobiological underpinnings of PTSD, established safety profiles of medications in the pediatric population, and effective pharmacotherapy practice in adult PTSD treatment (Donnelly 2003).

Conclusion

Children and adolescents are exposed to a broad range of traumas. Epidemiological studies have shown the effect of these stressful experiences and the higher prevalence of PTSD in exposed populations. Clinicians must be mindful that posttraumatic symptoms in children may be different from those in adults and can vary with developmental level. Younger children exposed to traumatic events may develop symptoms not necessarily meeting DSM-IV-TR criteria for PTSD but still have profound distress or dysfunction. Adolescents are more likely to resemble adults in their posttraumatic symptoms. Other disorders and health problems are often comorbid with pediatric PTSD and must be recognized and considered as part of an overall treatment approach. Several established psychosocial treatments have been shown to be efficacious in the pediatric population. Although little rigorous scientific evaluation of the use of medications in pediatric PTSD exists, pharmacotherapy can be effectively integrated into an overall treatment plan when thoughtfully and judiciously approached.

Key Clinical Points

- Children and adolescents can develop symptoms consistent with PTSD, and providers should be aware of the unique aspects of PTSD within this population.
- Young children are less likely to have emotional numbing or avoidance symptoms and often present with a wider range of behavioral disturbances compared with older children, teens, and adults.
- Children and adolescents with posttraumatic symptoms often do not meet the current full criteria for PTSD.
- Children and adolescents with PTSD frequently have comorbid disorders, including developmental problems, attention-deficit/hyperactivity disorder, anxiety, and depression.
- Childhood traumatic grief is a relatively new construct that highlights the impact of the sudden, unexpected, and traumatic loss of a loved one interfering with the child's ability to mourn the loss.
- Complex trauma, occurring when a child is exposed to multiple traumatic stressors, can have a severe impact on multiple domains of function.
- Trauma-specific cognitive-behavioral therapies such as TF-CBT, MMTT, and CBITS are best supported by evidence for efficacy in treating PTSD in preschoolers, children, and adolescents.
- Child-parent psychotherapy, a trauma-specific relationship intervention developed for young children exposed to interpersonal violence, has shown efficacy in children up to age 6 years in reducing trauma symptoms and behavioral problems.
- Trauma systems therapy addresses trauma-related symptoms as well as the social environment perpetuating these symptoms, in order to help the child regulate emotional responses to these triggers.

- EMDR appears to be an effective intervention among children and adolescents, although the standard protocol may have to be altered depending on the age of the child.
- Although a few studies of pharmacological treatments for children and adolescents with PTSD have been completed, clear scientific evidence of benefit from such interventions is lacking. Pharmacotherapy for PTSD should be considered in children and adolescents only when psychosocial interventions have been ineffective and, when used, should be integrated into a multimodal treatment plan.
- As in all diagnoses, particular caution should be exercised in using medications with preschool-aged children.

References

Ahmad A, Larsson B, Sundelin-Wahlsten V: EMDR treatment for children with PTSD: results of a randomized controlled trial. Nord J Psychiatry 61:349–354, 2007

Amaya-Jackson L, Reynolds V, Murray MC, et al: Cognitive-behavioral treatment for pediatric posttraumatic stress disorder: protocol and application in school and community settings. Cogn Behav Pract 10:204–213, 2003

American Psychiatric Association: Diagnostic and Statistical Manual of Mental Disorders, 3rd Edition. Washington, DC, American Psychiatric Association, 1980

American Psychiatric Association: Diagnostic and Statistical Manual of Mental Disorders, 4th Edition. Washington, DC, American Psychiatric Association, 1994

American Psychiatric Association: Diagnostic and Statistical Manual of Mental Disorders, 4th Edition, Text Revision. Washington, DC, American Psychiatric Association, 2000

Barenbaum J, Ruchkin V, Schwab-Stone M: The psychosocial aspects of children exposed to war: practice and policy initiatives. J Child Psychol Psychiatry 45:41–62, 2004

Bigfoot DS, Schmidt SR: Honoring children, mending the circle. Paper presented at the 25th Annual Conference on Child Abuse and Neglect, Oklahoma City, OK, April 2007

Breslau N, Wilcox HC, Storr CL, et al: Trauma exposure and posttraumatic stress disorder: a study of youths in urban America. J Urban Health 81:530–543, 2004

Brown EJ, Amaya-Jackson L, Cohen J, et al: Childhood traumatic grief: a multi-site empirical examination of the construct and its correlates. Death Stud 32:899–923, 2008

Carrion VG, Weems CF, Ray R, et al: Toward an empirical definition of pediatric PTSD: the phenomenology of PTSD symptoms in youth. J Am Acad Child Adolesc Psychiatry 41:166–173, 2002

Chemtob CM, Nakashima J, Carlson JG: Brief treatment for elementary school children with disaster-related posttraumatic stress disorder: a field study. J Clin Psychol 58:99–112, 2002

Cohen JA: Pharmacologic treatment of traumatized children. Trauma Violence Abuse 2:155–171, 2001

Cohen JA: Treating PTSD and related symptoms in children: research highlights. PTSD Research Quarterly 19:1–7, 2008

Cohen JA, Mannarino AP: Factors that mediate treatment outcome of sexually abused preschool children. J Am Acad Child Adolesc Psychiatry 35:1402–1410, 1996

Cohen JA, Mannarino AP: A treatment study for sexually abused preschool children: outcome during a one-year follow-up. J Am Acad Child Adolesc Psychiatry 36:1228–1235, 1997

Cohen JA, Mannarino AP: Interventions for sexually abused children: initial treatment outcome findings. Child Maltreat 3:17–26, 1998

Cohen JA, Mannarino AP: Treatment of childhood traumatic grief. J Clin Child Adolesc Psychol 33:819–831, 2004

Cohen JA, Mannarino AP, Greenberg T, et al: Childhood traumatic grief: concepts and controversies. Trauma Violence Abuse 3:307–327, 2002

Cohen JA, Berliner L, Mannarino AP: Psychosocial and pharmacological interventions for child crime victims. J Trauma Stress 16:175–186, 2003

Cohen JA, Deblinger E, Mannarino AP, et al: A multisite, randomized controlled trial for children with sexual abuse-related PTSD symptoms. J Am Acad Child Adolesc Psychiatry 43:393–402, 2004

Cohen JA, Mannarino AP, Knudsen K: Treating sexually abused children: 1 year follow-up of a randomized controlled trial. Child Abuse Negl 25:135–145, 2005

Cohen JA, Mannarino AP, Deblinger E: Treating Trauma and Traumatic Grief in Children and Adolescents: A Clinician's Guide. New York, Guilford, 2006a

Cohen JA, Mannarino AP, Murray LK, et al: Psychosocial interventions for maltreated and violence-exposed children. J Soc Issues 62:737–766, 2006b

Cohen JA, Mannarino AP, Staron VR: A pilot study of modified cognitive-behavioral therapy for childhood traumatic grief (CBT-CTG). J Am Acad Child Adolesc Psychiatry 45:1465–1467, 2006c

Cohen JA, Mannarino AP, Perel JM, et al: A pilot randomized controlled trial of combined trauma-focused CBT and sertraline for childhood PTSD symptoms. J Am Acad Child Adolesc Psychiatry 46:811–819, 2007

Copeland WE, Keeler G, Angold A, et al: Traumatic events and posttraumatic stress in childhood. Arch Gen Psychiatry 64:577–584, 2007

Danielson CK, DeArellano MA, Ehrenreich JT, et al: Identification of high-risk behaviors among victimized adolescents and implications for empirically supported psychosocial treatment. J Psychiatr Pract 12:364–383, 2006

De Bellis MD, Van Dillen T: Childhood post-traumatic stress disorder: an overview. Child Adolesc Psychiatr Clin N Am 15:745–772, 2005

Deblinger E, Lippmann J, Steer R: Sexually abused children suffering posttraumatic stress symptoms: initial treatment outcome findings. Child Maltreat 1:310–321, 1996

Deblinger E, Steer RA, Lippmann J: Two-year follow-up study of cognitive behavioral therapy for sexually abused children suffering post-traumatic stress symptoms. Child Abuse Negl 23:1371–1378, 1999

Deblinger E, Stauffer LB, Steer RA: Comparative efficacies of supportive and cognitive behavioral group therapies for young children who have been sexually abused and their nonoffending mothers. Child Maltreat 6:332–343, 2001

Donnelly CL: Pharmacologic treatment approaches for children and adolescents with posttraumatic stress disorder. Child Adolesc Psychiatr Clin N Am 12:251–269, 2003

Dyregrov A, Yule W: A review of PTSD in children. Child Adolesc Ment Health 11:176–184, 2006

Famularo R, Fenton T: Early developmental history and pediatric posttraumatic stress disorder. Arch Pediatr Adolesc Med 148:1032–1038, 1994

Famularo R, Kinscherff R, Fenton T: Propranolol treatment for childhood posttraumatic stress disorder, acute type: a pilot study. Am J Dis Child 142:1244–1247, 1988

Famularo R, Fenton T, Kinscherff R, et al: Psychiatric comorbidity in childhood post traumatic stress disorder. Child Abuse Negl 20:953–961, 1996

Finkelhor D, Ormrod R, Turner R, et al: The victimization of children and youth: a comprehensive, national survey. Child Maltreat 10:5–25, 2005

Giaconia RM, Reinherz HZ, Silverman AB, et al: Traumas and posttraumatic stress disorder in a community population of older adolescents. J Am Acad Child Adolesc Psychiatry 34:1369–1380, 1995

Giannopoulou I, Dikaiakou A, Yule W: Cognitive-behavioural group intervention for PTSD symptoms in children following the Athens 1999 earthquake: a pilot study. Clin Child Psychol Psychiatry 11:543–553, 2006

Gleason MM, Egger HL, Emslie GJ: Psychopharmacological treatment for very young children: contexts and guidelines. J Am Acad Child Adolesc Psychiatry 46:1532–1572, 2007

Goenjian AK, Pynoos RS, Steinberg AM, et al: Psychiatric comorbidity in children after the 1988 earthquake in Armenia. J Am Acad Child Adolesc Psychiatry 34:1174–1184, 1995

Goenjian AK, Karayan I, Pynoos RS, et al: Outcome of psychotherapy among early adolescents after trauma. Am J Psychiatry 154:536–542, 1997

Greenwald R: Using EMDR With Children. Pacific Grove, CA, EMDR Institute, 1993

Harmon RJ, Riggs PD: Clonidine for posttraumatic stress disorder in preschool children. J Am Acad Child Adolesc Psychiatry 35:1247–1249, 1996

Hoven CW, Duarte CS, Lucas CP, et al: Psychopathology among New York City public school children 6 months after September 11. Arch Gen Psychiatry 62:545–552, 2005

Hsu CC, Chong MY, Yang P, et al: Posttraumatic stress disorder among adolescent earthquake victims in Taiwan. J Am Acad Child Adolesc Psychiatry 41:875–881, 2002

Jaberghaderi N, Greenwald R, Rubin A, et al: A comparison of CBT and EMDR for sexually abused Iranian girls. Clin Psychol Psychother 11:358–368, 2004

Jaycox L: Cognitive-Behavioral Intervention for Trauma in Schools. Longmont, CO, Sopris West, 2004

Kataoka SH, Stein BD, Jaycox LH, et al: A school-based mental health program for traumatized Latino immigrant children. J Am Acad Child Adolesc Psychiatry 42:311–318, 2003

Kessler RC, Sonnega A, Bromet E, et al: Posttraumatic stress disorder in the National Comorbidity Survey. Arch Gen Psychiatry 52:1048–1060, 1995

Kilpatrick DG, Saunders BE: Prevalence and consequences of child victimization: results from the National Survey of Adolescents: final report. Medical University of South Carolina National Crime Victims Research and Treatment Center. 1997. Available at: http://www.ncjrs.gov/pdffiles1/nij/grants/181028.pdf . Accessed December 1, 2009.

Kilpatrick DG, Ruggiero KJ, Acierno R, et al: Violence and risk of PTSD, major depression, substance abuse/dependence, and comorbidity: results from the National Survey of Adolescents. J Consult Clin Psychol 71:692–700, 2003

Lavigne JV, Gibbons RD, Christoffel KK, et al: Prevalence rates and correlates of psychiatric disorders among preschool children. J Am Acad Child Adolesc Psychiatry 35:204–214, 1996

Layne CM, Saltzman WR, Pynoos RS, et al: Trauma and Grief Component Therapy. New York, New York State Office of Mental Health, 2002

Layne CM, Saltzman WR, Poppleton L, et al: Effectiveness of a school-based group psychotherapy program for war-exposed adolescents: a randomized controlled trial. J Am Acad Child Adolesc Psychiatry 47:1048–1062, 2008

Lieberman AF, Van Horn P: "Don't Hit My Mommy!" A Manual for Child-Parent Psychotherapy With Young Witnesses of Family Violence. Washington, DC, Zero to Three Press, 2005

Lieberman AF, Van Horn P, Ghosh Ippen C: Toward evidence-based treatment: child-parent psychotherapy with preschoolers exposed to marital violence. J Am Acad Child Adolesc Psychiatry 44:1241–1248, 2005

Lieberman AF, Ghosh Ippen C, Van Horn P: Child-parent psychotherapy: 6-month follow-up of a randomized controlled trial. J Am Acad Child Adolesc Psychiatry 45:913–918, 2006

March JS, Amaya-Jackson L, Murray MC, et al: Cognitive-behavioral psychotherapy for children and adolescents with posttraumatic stress disorder after a single-incident stressor. J Am Acad Child Adolesc Psychiatry 37:585–593, 1998

McCrae JS, Chapman MV, Christ SL: Profile of children investigated for sexual abuse: association with psychopathology symptoms and services. Am J Orthopsychiatry 76:468–481, 2006

McFarlane AC: Posttraumatic phenomena in a longitudinal study of children following a natural disaster. J Am Acad Child Adolesc Psychiatry 26:764–769, 1987

Mintzer LL, Stuber ML, Seacord D, et al: Traumatic stress symptoms in adolescent organ transplant recipients. Pediatrics 115:1640–1644, 2005

Morsette A, Swaney G, Stolle D, et al: Cognitive Behavioral Intervention for Trauma in Schools (CBITS): school-based treatment on a rural American Indian reservation. J Behav Ther Exp Psychiatry 40:169–178, 2009

National Child Traumatic Stress Network: National Child Traumatic Stress Network empirically supported treatments and promising practices. March 22, 2005. Available at: http://www.nctsnet.org/nccts/nav.do?pid=ctr_top_trmnt_prom. Accessed December 1, 2009.

National Child Traumatic Stress Network: MMTT: multimodality trauma treatment (aka trauma-focused coping in schools)—culture-specific information. 2008a. Available at: http://www.nctsnet.org/nctsn_assets/pdfs/promising_practices/mmtt_cultural.pdf. Accessed December 1, 2009.

National Child Traumatic Stress Network: TST: trauma systems therapy. 2008b. Available at: http://www.nctsnet.org/nctsn_assets/pdfs/promising_practices/tst_general.pdf. Accessed December 1, 2009.

National Child Traumatic Stress Network: Types of traumatic stress. December 15, 2009. Available at: http://www.nctsnet.org/nccts/nav.do?pid=typ_main. Accessed December 27, 2009.

Ngo V, Langley A, Kataoka SH, et al: Providing evidence-based practice to ethnically diverse youth: examples from the Cognitive Behavioral Intervention for Trauma in Schools (CBITS) program. J Am Acad Child Adolesc Psychiatry 47:858–862, 2008

Nikulina V, Hergenrother JM, Brown EJ, et al: From efficacy to effectiveness: the trajectory of the treatment literature for children with PTSD. Expert Rev Neurother 8:1233–1246, 2008

Perrin S, Smith P, Yule W: Practitioner review: the assessment and treatment of post-traumatic stress disorder in children and adolescents. J. Child Psychol Psychiatry 41:277–289, 2000

Pfefferbaum B, Nixon SJ, Tucker PM, et al: Posttraumatic stress responses in bereaved children after the Oklahoma City bombing. J Am Acad Child Adolesc Psychiatry 38:1372–1379, 1999

Puffer MK, Greenwald R, Elrod DE: A single session EMDR study with twenty traumatized children and adolescents. International Electronic Journal of Innovations in the Study of the Traumatization Process and Methods for Reducing or Eliminating Related Human Suffering 3:2 Article 6, 1998. Available at: http://www.fsu.edu/~trauma/v3i2art6.html. Accessed December 1, 2009.

Pynoos RS: Grief and trauma in children and adolescents. Bereavement Care 11:2–10, 1992

Pynoos RS, Frederick C, Nader K, et al: Life threat and posttraumatic stress in school-age children. Arch Gen Psychiatry 44:1057–1063, 1987

Pynoos RS, Goenjian A, Tashjian M, et al: Post-traumatic stress reactions in children after the 1988 Armenian earthquake. Br J Psychiatry 163:239–247, 1993

Robert R, Blakeney P, Villarreal C, et al: Imipramine treatment in pediatric burn patients with symptoms of acute stress disorder: a pilot study. J Am Acad Child Adolesc Psychiatry 38:873–882, 1999

Salloum A: Group therapy for children after homicide and violence: a pilot study. Res Soc Work Pract 18:198–211, 2008

Salloum A, Overstreet S: Evaluation of individual and group grief and trauma interventions for children post disaster. J Clin Child Adolesc Psychol 37:495–507, 2008

Saltzman WR, Pynoos RS, Layne C, et al: Trauma/grief-focused intervention for adolescents exposed to community violence: results of a school-based screening and group treatment protocol. Group Dyn 5:291–303, 2001a

Saltzman WR, Steinberg RS, Layne CM, et al: A developmental approach to trauma/grief focused group psychotherapy for youth exposed to community violence. Journal of Child and Adolescent Group Therapy 11:43–56, 2001b

Saxe GN, Ellis BH, Fogler J, et al: Comprehensive care for traumatized children. Psychiatr Ann 35:443–448, 2005

Saxe GN, Ellis BH, Kaplow J: Collaborative Care for Traumatized Children and Teens: A Trauma Systems Therapy Approach. New York, Guilford, 2007

Scheeringa MS: Developmental considerations for diagnosing PTSD and acute stress disorder in preschool and school-age children. Am J Psychiatry 165:1237–1239, 2008

Scheeringa MS, Zeanah CH: Reconsideration of harm's way: onsets and comorbidity patterns of disorders in preschool children and their caregivers following Hurricane Katrina. J Clin Child Adolesc Psychol 37:508–518, 2008

Scheeringa MS, Zeanah CH, Drell MJ, et al: Two approaches to the diagnosis of posttraumatic stress disorder in infancy and early childhood. Am J Child Adolesc Psychiatry 34:191–200, 1995

Scheeringa MS, Zeanah CH, Myers L, et al: New findings on alternative criteria for PTSD in preschool children. J Am Acad Child Adolesc Psychiatry 42:561–570, 2003

Schrag NM, McKeown RE, Jackson KL, et al: Stress-related mental disorders in childhood cancer survivors. Pediatr Blood Cancer 50:98–103, 2008

Seedat S, Lockhat R, Kaminer D, et al: Open trial of citalopram for adolescents with PTSD. Int Clin Psychopharmacol 16:21–26, 2001

Seedat S, Stein DJ, Ziervogel C, et al: Comparison of response to a selective serotonin reuptake inhibitor in children, adolescents, and adults with posttraumatic stress disorder. J Child Adolesc Psychopharmacol 12:37–46, 2002

Seng JS, Graham-Bermann SA, Clark MK, et al: Posttraumatic stress disorder and physical comorbidity among female children and adolescents: results from service-use data. Pediatrics 116:767–776, 2005

Shapiro F: Eye Movement Desensitization and Reprocessing: Basic Principles, Protocols and Procedures, 2nd Edition. New York, Guilford, 2001

Shooshtary MH, Panaghi L, Moghadam JA: Outcome of cognitive behavioral therapy in adolescents after natural disaster. J Adolesc Health 42:466–472, 2008

Silverman WK , Ortiz CD, Viswesvaran C, et al: Evidence-based psychosocial treatments for children and adolescents exposed to traumatic events. J Clin Child Adolesc Psychol 37:156–183, 2008

Smith P, Perrin S, Yule W, et al: War exposure among children from Bosnia-Hercegovina: psychological adjustment in a community sample. J Trauma Stress 15:147–156, 2002

Smith P, Yule W, Perrin S, et al: Cognitive-behavioral therapy for PTSD in children and adolescents: a preliminary randomized controlled trial. J Am Acad Child Adolesc Psychiatry 46:1051–1061, 2007

Stallard P: Psychological interventions for post-traumatic reactions in children and young people: a review of randomised controlled trials. Clin Psychol Rev 26:895–911, 2006

Stein BD, Jaycox LH, Kataoka SH, et al: A mental health intervention for schoolchildren exposed to violence: a randomized controlled trial. JAMA 290:603–611, 2003

Taylor TL, Chemtob CM: Efficacy of treatment for child and adolescent traumatic stress. Arch Pediatr Adolesc Med 158:786–791, 2004

Terr LC: Children of Chowchilla: a study of psychic terror. Psychoanal Study Child 34:547–623, 1979

Terr LC: Chowchilla revisited: the effect of psychic trauma four years after a school-bus kidnapping. Am J Psychiatry 140:1543–1550, 1983

Thabet AA, Vostanis P: Posttraumatic stress disorder reactions in children of war: a longitudinal study. Child Abuse Negl 24:291–298, 2000

Thienkrua W, Cardozo BL, Chakkraband ML, et al: Symptoms of posttraumatic stress disorder and depression among children in tsunami-affected areas in southern Thailand. JAMA 296:549–559, 2006

van der Kolk BA: Developmental trauma disorder: toward a rational diagnosis for children with complex trauma histories. Psychiatr Ann 35:401–408, 2005

Vernberg EM, LaGreca AM, Silverman WK, et al: Prediction of posttraumatic stress symptoms in children after Hurricane Andrew. J Abnorm Psychol 105:237–248, 1996

12

Sexual Assault

Amy E. Street, Ph.D.
Margret E. Bell, Ph.D.
C. Beth Ready

Compared with some legal definitions of sexual assault that focus exclusively on the experience of forced rape, the term *sexual assault* tends to be used more broadly in the field of mental health, in recognition that a wide range of sexually coercive experiences and behaviors can negatively affect a victim's well-being. Specific to this book's topic of posttraumatic stress disorder (PTSD), any situation that takes away a victim's choice about whether to engage in sexual activity may foster feelings of helplessness, fear, and threat, thus leaving him or her vulnerable to traumatic stress reactions. Physical force is only one way that this choice may be taken away; sexual victimization also occurs when an individual is pressured to engage in unwanted sexual contact using psychological or social strategies, including coercion, threats of harm, and abuse of authority or power, or in situations in which the person is unable to give consent (e.g., due to intoxication or cognitive limitations). The nature of the sexual contact may range from touching, fondling, and petting to any degree of vaginal, anal, or oral penetration using a penis, finger, or object.

Although women are more likely to experience sexual assault than men, men can be victimized as well. Across recent decades, the prevalence of completed sexual assault, including forced vaginal, oral, or anal penetration by penis, finger, or object, has been around 12.9% in women and 3.3% in men. Attempted sexual assault (18.3% women, 5.6% men), sexual coercion (24.9% women, 23.2% men), and unsolicited sexual contact (24% women, 7.9% men) are even more common (Spitzberg 1999). Unfortunately, individuals who are sexually assaulted are more likely to experience future victimizations, with up to 39% of women sexually victimized at least twice in their lifetime (Kilpatrick et al. 1992). Experiencing childhood sexual abuse is a consistent and significant predictor of future sexual victimization for both men and women (Messman and Long 1996), although this effect may be more extreme in men (Elliott et al. 2004).

Race/ethnicity and age are important additional factors to consider when examining the distribution of sexual assault across the general population. Similar rates of victimization hold across Caucasian (17.7%) and African American (18.8%) women, but some racial groups, such as Native American women (34.1%), have a much higher prevalence of sexual victimization, whereas other groups, such as Asian (6.8%) and Hispanic (14.6%) women, appear less likely to experience sexual assault (Tjaden and Thoennes 1998, 2000). Little information exists regarding sexual assault across race/ethnicity in men. In terms of age, most sexual assaults in women occur during adolescence and young adulthood (Tjaden and Thoennes 1998), whereas a limited body of information suggests that on average, men may be even younger at the time of their first sexual assault (Elliott et al. 2004).

Despite public perception that the majority of sexual assaults are perpetrated by a stranger, most sexual assaults are perpetrated by someone known by the victim, such as a parent or relative (27%) or a husband or boyfriend (19%). In fact, assaults by a stranger account for only about one-quarter to one-third of sexual victimizations in the United States (Kilpatrick et al. 1992; U.S. Department of Justice 2008). Most sexual assaults go undetected by authorities or formal sources of help. For example, from 1992 to 2000, an estimated 31% of sexual assaults were reported to police, a relatively low percentage compared with crimes such as robbery (57%) and aggravated assault (55%). Recent trends reveal that sexual assaults committed by a stranger are more likely to be reported (41%) than those perpetrated by an intimate partner (24%), friend or acquaintance (27%), or other nonstranger (27%) (Hart and Rennison 2003). Low rates of reporting and help seeking are particularly unfortunate given the severe negative consequences that sexual victimization can have on a victim's mental health.

Sexual Assault and PTSD

Addressing sexual assault is critical in any volume on the treatment of PTSD, both because of the high prevalence of sexual assault and because sexual assault is an event that is highly predictive of a later PTSD diagnosis. Completed rape has been shown to be more highly associated with the development of PTSD than other violent crimes (Kilpatrick et al. 1989), with some estimates suggesting that 46% of female and 65% of male sexual assault survivors develop PTSD following the assault. Although many sexually victimized individuals do not develop chronic psychological symptoms, these rates are notable when compared with the prevalence of PTSD in other trauma populations, such as combat (38.8% of men), physical attack (26.5% of women, 1.8% of men), and life-threatening accidents (8.8% of women, 6.3% of men) (Kessler et al. 1995).

Given the intensity of the event, it is not surprising that almost all sexual assault victims report experiencing symptoms of reexperiencing, avoidance and numbing, and increased arousal characteristic of PTSD in the immediate aftermath of the assault. However, many victims are remarkably resilient, experiencing a sharp decrease in symptoms within a month after the assault and continuing to show additional improvements over time (Rothbaum et al. 1992). Three months after the assault, approximately half of victims no longer meet diagnostic criteria for PTSD, whereas half of victims, despite an initial decrease in the intensity of symptoms, will continue to report symptoms consistent with a PTSD diagnosis (Kilpatrick et al. 1992; Rothbaum et al. 1992). Both in the immediate aftermath of an assault and in the longer term, victims may suffer from a host of comorbid conditions in addition to PTSD, including depression, alcohol and drug abuse, and suicidal behaviors (Dickinson et al. 1999; Kilpatrick et al. 1997; Ullman and Brecklin 2002, 2003).

Social Reactions to Sexual Assault

The prevalence of PTSD following sexual assault raises this question: Why is sexual assault so predictive of subsequent psychopathology? One factor that may play a role is the social reactions encountered by victims of sexual assault (Ullman 1999). For example, it is not uncommon for family, friends, and other potential sources of social support to endorse "rape myths" that blame the victim or rationalize the perpetrator's actions (see Table 12–1). Similarly, victims may encounter minimization and questions about their credibility when interacting with formal sources of help, such as police, courts, and health care providers (Campbell 2008; Filipas and Ullman 2001). A host of research has linked such invalidating responses to more severe mental and physical symptomatology, including increased symptoms of PTSD (Andrews et al. 2003; Filipas and Ullman 2001; Koss et al. 2002; Ullman 1996; Ullman and Filipas 2001). Fear of negative reactions to disclosure may not only deprive victims of emotional support from others, but also prevent them from accessing services and treatment needed to prevent initial symptoms from becoming more chronic over time. Victims' internalization of victim-blaming societal messages about sexual assault may further compound feelings of self-blame, shame, and guilt. Given the acute sensitivity many victims have about negative reactions from others, the importance of therapists remaining aware of their own beliefs and monitoring their reactions to their work with sexual assault survivors cannot be overstated.

Assessment of Sexual Assault Survivors

Screening for Experiences of Sexual Assault

Asking all patients seeking mental health care about experiences of sexual assault is particularly important given its prevalence, the negative consequences for mental health, and victim reluctance to spontaneously disclose (Crowell and Burgess 1996; Fisher et al. 2003; Kimerling et al. 2008). Identifying a history of sexual assault early in treatment is important given that such a history can affect both treatment planning and the dynamics of treatment over time. All patients should be asked a series of brief screening questions during intake or the first few sessions of treatment. This can be done as part of an initial

Table 12–1. Common myths about sexual assault

Rape myths	Rape facts
The victim deserved to be raped because she was promiscuous or had a bad reputation.	Nobody deserves to be sexually assaulted. Victims are often targeted based on accessibility and vulnerability, not personal characteristics.
The victim could have prevented the rape if he or she really wanted to.	It is the assailant's choice to commit assault, not the victim's. Sexual assault is an act of control, and assailants use a variety of techniques to overpower their victims.
The victim is lying to "get back" at someone.	False reports of sexual assault are rare and no more likely than false reports of other crimes.
The victim just wanted attention.	Nothing justifies sexually assaulting someone.
The victim "was asking for it."	No one asks to be raped.
It is not sexual assault if the victim and/or perpetrator were drunk or using drugs.	Inability to consent does not qualify as consent. Sexual contact with an individual who is unable to consent is considered sexual assault. Assailants are responsible for their actions, even those committed under the influence of alcohol or drugs.
If the victim did not report the rape right away, he or she is lying.	Sexual assault is significantly underreported to authorities. There are many reasons a victim may not report the assault, including fear of social stigma and perpetrator retaliation.
The assailant acted in a moment of passion.	Sexual assault is an act of power and control. Most assaults are planned.
Men are not sexually assaulted.	Men can be victims of sexual assault. Men of all sexual orientations can be victimized.

psychosocial interview or in a written format as part of a self-report questionnaire. Before beginning the screening process, the clinician might choose to normalize the screening questions by saying, for example, "Experiences like these are unfortunately so common that I ask these questions of all my patients." Clinicians should avoid technical language or emotionally charged words such as *sexual assault* or *rape,* and instead use simple, behavioral language. Sample screening questions are provided in Table 12–2. If a patient

Table 12–2. Sample sexual assault screening questions

Has anyone ever touched you in a sexual way or had you touch them in a sexual way that made you uncomfortable?
Have you ever been touched sexually against your will or without your consent?
Have you ever had a sexual experience that made you uncomfortable?
Has anyone ever tried to make you have sex when you did not want to?
Have you ever been forced or pressured into having sex?

responds affirmatively to questions about sexual assault, it is important to provide immediate validation, such as by saying, "I'm very sorry you had that experience, but I'm glad you felt like you could tell me about it today."

Conducting Follow-Up Assessments

If a patient discloses that she[1] has been assaulted, the next step is to conduct a more detailed assessment to gather information about relevant psychosocial factors, the assault and its aftermath, and the victim's current psychological symptoms and functioning. Such information is critical for establishing an appropriate treatment plan. An assessment can best be performed through a combination of a clinical interview, perhaps including structured diagnostic interviews (see Table 12–3 for suggested content areas), and standardized assessment instruments (see Table 12–4 for suggestions). Because issues of PTSD assessment are covered extensively elsewhere in this volume (see Chapter 4, "Assessment and Diagnosis of PTSD"), we focus in this chapter on information with unique relevance for the assessment of sexual assault survivors.

Certain details of the patient's psychosocial history will be valuable in helping to detect factors that may impact short- and long-term reactions to the assault, to identify psychological vulnerabilities, and to provide guidance for treatment (Resnick and Newton 1992). Important content areas to address as part of the psychosocial history assessment include demographic information, including ethnicity/cultural identity, lifetime history of traumatic experiences, predominant coping strategies, social history, and current social

[1]Although victims of sexual assault can be male or female, for simplicity and clarity, feminine personal pronouns will be used in this chapter from this point forward.

Table 12–3. Content areas to assess during a clinical interview

Psychosocial history
Information about family of origin, including family's psychiatric history
Ethnicity/cultural identity
Lifetime history of potentially traumatic events
Occupational history, including current occupational functioning
Social history, including current levels of social support
Current daily activities
Existing coping strategies
The sexual assault
Extent of memory for assault
Time and location of assault
Type of assaultive event
Information about perpetrators (e.g., number of perpetrators, preexisting relationships)
Extent of violence during assault
Extent of physical injuries
Perception of life threat
Coping strategies used during assault (e.g., dissociation, distraction)
Emotional and cognitive reactions at time of assault
Medical or mental health care seeking at time of assault
Involvement with the criminal justice system
Disclosure of assault to others, including others' reactions
Extent to which victim currently labels event as sexual assault or rape
Psychological functioning
Current psychological symptoms and diagnostic status
Course and timeline of current psychological symptoms
Previous mental health care usage
History of psychological symptoms and mental health care prior to assault
Degree of guilt, shame, and self-blame
Any ongoing safety fears
Concerns about medical well-being and physical health

Table 12–4. Standardized assessment instruments specific to sexual assault

Measure	Authors	Description
Sexual assault experiences		
Sexual Experiences Survey	Koss et al. 1987	Brief self-report measure assessing sexual victimization experiences; separate male and female versions
Symptoms following assault		
Rape Aftermath Symptom Test	Kilpatrick 1988	Measure of rape-related fears and general anxiety
Rape Trauma Rating Scale	DiVasto 1985	Brief measure of symptoms common to sexual assault survivors following the assault, including sleep disorders, somatic reactions, self-blame, and anxiety
Sexual Assault Symptom Scale II	Ruch and Wang 2006	Self-report measure of symptoms often present in the aftermath of a sexual assault, including safety fears, self-blame, depression, anger/emotional lability, health fears, anger at the criminal justice system, and fears about the criminal justice system
Other postassault reactions		
Rape Attributions Questionnaire	Frazier 2003	Measure assessing victims' beliefs about why the sexual assault occurred as well as beliefs about control over sexual assaults
Social Reactions Questionnaire	Ullman 2000	Measure of victims' experiences of social support and negative social reactions following disclosure of sexual assault

and occupational functioning. A detailed psychosocial history can provide contextual information about the assault and its aftermath that will be important for treatment, such as the client's attributions of the event and the social reactions she may receive. Assessing clients' lifetime history of traumatic experiences will provide insight into potential issues that could guide the course of treatment and affect the therapeutic alliance. For example, sexual assault victims with previous experiences of interpersonal traumatic events, especially childhood sexual abuse, may be more vulnerable to problems such as emotion dysregulation, difficulties with assertiveness in interpersonal relationships, and maladaptive coping strategies (Classen et al. 2001; van der Kolk et al. 1996). Furthermore, social history and changes in social and occupational functioning following the assault can provide information regarding the magnitude of the client's current distress and identify additional issues related to the assault that should be targeted during treatment.

Although information about the sexual assault itself must be collected with particular sensitivity, details of the assault and its aftermath will help identify potential vulnerabilities for the development of PTSD. For example, completed rape (instead of, for example, attempted rape or fondling), a perception that one's life was in danger, and/or substantial physical injury incurred during the assault are predictive of the development of PTSD (Kilpatrick et al. 1989). Cognitive attributions of responsibility for the assault are common among sexual assault survivors and are also significant contributing factors in the development of PTSD. Social support, a protective factor in the onset of PTSD, is especially important to assess in working with sexual assault survivors, given that they are often hesitant to disclose and may receive negative reactions from others if they do (Koss et al. 2002; Ullman et al. 2007b).

Diagnostic assessment of psychological symptoms, including those of PTSD and common comorbid conditions such as depression and substance abuse, is also a central piece of the follow-up assessment after a patient discloses experiences of sexual assault. In addition, following sexual assault, individuals are more likely to experience impairments in sexual functioning and satisfaction relative to other trauma populations; therefore, these conditions should always be included as a part of formal diagnostic assessments with this population.

Unique Issues in the Assessment of Sexual Assault Survivors

While the psychological assessment of any trauma survivor must be handled sensitively, the assessment of sexual assault survivors presents some unique issues. Sexual assault survivors often experience significant feelings of shame or self-blame about their traumatic experiences. Survivors may be sensitive to perceptions of being judged when discussing the details of their sexual assault. Accordingly, if the sexual assault survivor has disclosed her experience at all, she has likely disclosed it to only a small number of close others. She herself is likely still confused about the experience. Given these issues, sexual assault survivors may find the assessment process, particularly assessment of the sexual assault event itself, emotionally difficult. A sexual assault survivor may experience distress during the assessment process, evidenced by intense emotion, including crying, shaking, or visible anxiety. Alternatively, she may demonstrate significant affective avoidance, evidenced by a robotic or monotonous recitation of details of the assault coupled with an affect that is flat or inconsistent with the content of the discussion. Assessment of details of the sexual assault experience may be further complicated if the survivor does not have a clear memory of the sexual assault event due to peritraumatic dissociation, psychogenic amnesia, alcohol or drug use at the time of the assault, or head trauma sustained during the assault.

A comprehensive assessment lays the groundwork for effective therapeutic intervention. The assessment itself, however, can include substantial therapeutic content. The assessment process provides the first opportunities for the therapist to express regret about the patient's experiences, validate the patient's distress, and normalize the patient's reactions. Accordingly, although the primary goal of the assessment is to gather information, it is important for the therapist to balance information gathering with rapport building. Given the nature of interpersonal victimization, sexual assault survivors may find establishing trust with a therapist to be particularly difficult. As such, attending to the therapeutic relationship will almost certainly lead to a more efficient and more accurate assessment. One potentially effective tool is to normalize the patient's reactions during the assessment process (e.g., "These kinds of questions can be very upsetting for people who have had extremely stressful experiences like the one you've had"). Another potentially effective tool is to allow the sexual assault survivor some control over the course and pacing of the assessment (e.g., "We can take a break from these questions whenever you feel you need one"). Continually updating a sexual assault survivor about the course of the assessment, including information about the timeline and assessment content still to be covered, can also provide her with a sense of control.

At times, the most appropriate action may be for the clinician to gather only general information about the sexual assault during this initial assessment phase, typically just enough detail to establish the assault as a Criterion A event and thus confirm the applicability of a PTSD diagnosis, based on the *Diagnostic and Statistical Manual of Mental Disorders*, 4th Edition, Text Revision (American Psychiatric Association 2000). This strategy may be useful for patients who have particular difficulty discussing the specifics of their experience or who are reluctant to disclose detailed information until a stronger therapeutic relationship has formed. In these situations, it is critical that the clinician balance respect for the patient's need to limit discussion of an extremely distressing topic, with a therapeutic stance that conveys it is always acceptable to talk about difficult, upsetting, or shameful topics in the therapy room. Without such a stance, the patient may incorrectly attribute the lack of detailed discussion to the therapist's lack of interest, reticence to discuss sexual assault, or perceived negative judgments about the patient.

Treatment Approaches for Sexual Assault Survivors With PTSD

Because psychotherapeutic approaches to the treatment of PTSD have been covered extensively elsewhere in this volume (see Chapter 7, "Psychosocial Treatments"), our focus in this chapter is exclusively on treatment approaches specifically investigated among survivors of sexual assault or having particular relevance for survivors of sexual assault. Recently, the Institute of Medicine convened a committee on the treatment of PTSD that undertook a systematic review of the PTSD literature (Institute of Medicine 2008). One of the primary findings of the committee's review was that exposure-based cognitive-behavioral therapies were the only psychotherapeutic treatments with a sufficient evidence base to conclude that they have efficacy in the treatment of PTSD. This information has particular relevance for patients who have experienced sexual assault. Exposure-based cognitive-behavioral therapies (often referred to as "trauma-processing therapies") were initially developed for and have been rigorously tested among sexual assault victims with PTSD.

One such therapy, prolonged exposure, requires a client to repeatedly confront anxiety-provoking memories (imaginal exposure) and situations and other stimuli reminiscent of her sexual assault (behavioral exposures) while in an objectively safe situation until the associated fear and anxiety decrease (Foa and Rothbaum 1998). Prolonged exposure has demonstrated effectiveness in several methodologically rigorous randomized controlled trials with sexual assault victims. Prolonged exposure has been shown to be superior to no treatment (Foa et al. 1991, 1999; Resick et al. 2002; Rothbaum et al. 2005; supportive counseling (Foa et al. 1991), and stress inoculation training (Foa et al. 1999) in reducing PTSD symptoms and comorbid symptoms of depression and anxiety among this population (Foa et al. 1991; Resick et al. 2002; Rothbaum et al. 2005).

Another exposure-based cognitive-behavioral therapy, Cognitive Processing Therapy, combines written exercises in which the traumatic event is recounted with cognitive restructuring strategies to challenge distorted thoughts related to the traumatic experience. The inclusion of cognitive therapy techniques allows the patient to address emotional reactions other than fear, including anger, humiliation, shame, and sadness, during therapy (Resick and Schnicke 1996). Cognitive processing therapy has demonstrated effectiveness in reducing symptoms of PTSD and associated depression, anxiety, anger, guilt, and shame among rape victims (Resick et al. 2002, 2008).

Given the evidence base, these trauma-processing therapies should be considered as a first-choice therapy for sexual assault victims when appropriate. However, therapeutic approaches that have not yet been subjected to extensive empirical study may also play an important role. For example, psychoeducation about sexual assault and about short- and long-term reactions common to sexual assault victims, including PTSD, can be extremely helpful. Because victims are often confused about their own behaviors, efforts by the clinician to help victims understand the function of some of these behaviors, validate underlying needs, and consider alternative ways to meet these needs can be a powerful way to help victims feel less "crazy" and out of control.

Although the Institute of Medicine's Committee on Treatment of Posttraumatic Stress Disorder concluded that coping skills training does not yet have a sufficient evidence base to definitively establish its efficacy in the treatment of PTSD (Institute of Medicine 2008), for some victims of sexual assault, this type of training represents an important adjunctive treatment. Skills-based protocols can be useful precursors for clients whose use of adaptive coping strategies should be strengthened before beginning a course of trauma-processing therapy, given that this work can be emotionally demanding and strain the resources of clients with more poorly developed strategies for coping with emotional distress. Alternatively, following a trial of trauma-processing therapy, some clients continue to report residual symptoms that can best be addressed by a skills-focused therapy protocol. One skills-based treatment protocol modified specifically for use with rape survivors, stress inoculation training, combines stress management strategies, such as muscle relaxation, breathing retraining, and cognitive coping strategies (e.g., self-dialogue), to allow victims of sexual assault to learn to manage their anxiety and fear reactions (Kilpatrick et al. 1982). Skills Training in Affect and Interpersonal Regulation, a treatment protocol developed for and tested among adult survivors of child sexual abuse (Cloitre et al. 2002), targets skills to regulate negative affect and interpersonal interactions. Although this protocol has not been tested specifically among victims of adult sexual assault, preliminary evidence of its effectiveness among child sexual abuse survivors suggests some utility, particularly among adult assault victims who could benefit from improved affect regulation skills.

Common Treatment Themes

Treatment of PTSD in sexual assault survivors focuses primarily on addressing symptoms of reexperiencing, avoidance, numbing, and hypervigilance, much as it would with PTSD secondary to other types of traumatic experiences. However, certain treatment complexities may arise more frequently or be more intractable when working with victims of sexual assault. Although these issues may be more common within the population of victims of sexual assault, the degree to which any given victim struggles with these issues will vary. More complex presentations may be particularly likely for survivors who were young at the time of the assault or who have had multiple experiences of sexual victimization over the course of their lifetime (Briere et al. 2008; Fergusson et al. 2008; Ullman et al. 2007a). Table 12–5 provides examples of behaviors that are indicative of some common treatment themes.

Table 12–5. Examples of common treatment themes

Trust
Avoidance of relationships
Suspiciousness
Indecisiveness or tendency to second-guess decisions
Excessive caution in relatively safe situations
Contradictory behavior, such as asking for but then rejecting help
Tendency to develop emotionally intimate relationships very quickly
Pattern of unstable relationships
Strong reactions to imperfections in own or others' behavior
No-shows for therapy appointments
Repeatedly beginning but then dropping out of therapy
Sexuality and sexual functioning
Avoidance of sex or physical intimacy
Hypersexuality
Strong reaction to even nonsexual touch
Sexual dysfunction or inability to perform sexually
Guilt about engaging in sex
Dissociation or numbness during sex
Asexual appearance or behavior
Engaging in sexually injurious behavior
Difficulties saying "no" to sex
Control
Repeatedly breaking rules or "pushing the limits"
Passivity
Submissiveness or excessive need to please others
Engaging in power struggles about trivial issues
Strong reactions to authorities or when in subordinate roles
Difficulties with employment
Tendency to "cut off one's nose to spite one's face"
Difficulty working with health care providers who adopt an expert role or are directive
Strong reactions when providers do not agree to requests

Table 12–5. Examples of common treatment themes *(continued)*

Self-blame, guilt, and shame
Poor self-image
Inability to accept praise or acknowledge accomplishments
Strong emotional reaction to engaging in nurturing self-care activities
Self-injurious or self-punishing behavior
Remaining in abusive relationships
Feeling "dirty" or like "damaged goods"
Denying that the sexual assault occurred
Delay between time of assault and disclosure or care seeking
Delay in disclosing experiences even once engaged in care
Leaving out particular details when discussing sexual assault
Interpersonal boundaries
Disclosure of intimate personal information in inappropriate settings
Sharing of only extremely limited personal information with others
Encroaching on others' personal space, such as by standing or sitting in overly close physical proximity to others
"Hard to read" emotionally, or emotionally sealed off
Constantly taking on others' problems as if they were one's own
Repeated requests for personal information about providers
Need for repeated contact with health care providers between sessions
Attempts to extend the length or frequency of sessions when not clinically necessary
Refusal to allow physical examination by medical providers
Safety and revictimization
Hypervigilance even in relatively safe situations
Reluctance to leave home or travel in unfamiliar areas
Limited social contact
Excessive risk taking
Engaging in unsafe sex
Self-injurious behavior
Abusive relationships
Insensitivity to signs of potentially dangerous situations
Strong reaction to missteps by health care providers

Trust

In working with sexual assault survivors, clinicians should keep in mind that sexual assault is an interpersonal trauma. Therefore, resolving issues about relating to others, including health care providers, is likely to be a significant component of therapy. For example, a victim may exhibit significant difficulties with trusting others, particularly if the perpetrator was someone she knew or even a close friend or intimate partner, as is often the case. In these situations, the sense of betrayal and confusion can be intense and lead victims to draw negative conclusions about the trustworthiness of others as well as the reliability of their own judgment.

Mistrust is one way a victim may attempt to protect herself from revictimization. That is, a victim may fear that trusting others will result in being assaulted again. This fear may be particularly salient if she believes errors in her own judgment led to the original assault. Rather than take the risk of being reassaulted, some victims isolate themselves, effectively avoiding relationships entirely. Others may engage in extensive approach-avoidance behaviors, reflecting indecisiveness about how to balance needs for intimacy and interpersonal connection with concerns about safety and self-protection.

Sexuality and Sexual Functioning

Like intimate relationships more generally, sex can take on complicated meanings for sexual assault survivors. Many victims come to associate sex with the pain and fear they experienced at the time of the assault. For some, sexual sensations or touch in general may trigger flashbacks or dissociative experiences, contributing to a feeling of being out of control during sex. Victims who became involuntarily sexually aroused or experienced physical pleasure in response to sexual stimulation during the assault may wonder if they really enjoyed the experience. As a result, they may experience tremendous guilt and view themselves as "dirty" or perverted. In response to these feelings, some victims may seek to become asexual in behavior and appearance. Some may be able to engage in sexual activity only when under the influence of drugs or alcohol. Still others may become hypersexual in an attempt to assert their sexual dominance or feel more in control sexually.

Control

As with other traumatic events, sexual assault typically involves an overwhelming sense of helplessness and loss of power and control. The internal disorientation, cognitive confusion, and emotional flooding typical during the aftermath of victimization may only compound these feelings. Thus, trauma survivors often experience strong emotional reactions to situations they see as threatening to their sense of control over themselves or their environments. Victims of sexual assault may, in particular, evidence strong reactions to situations where one individual has power over another, such as in employee-employer or patient–health care provider relationships. Racism, sexism, poverty, and other reflections of societal inequities may be emotional triggers as well. When encountering these sorts of situations, sexual assault victims may react with anger and "fight back" or, oppositely, feel helpless and exhibit excessively passive behavior.

Self-Blame, Guilt, and Shame

Relatedly, the intense self-blame and guilt often seen in sexual assault victims can be understood in part as an effort to reestablish control. Some victims may find it more palatable to believe they are to blame for the sexual assault rather than to accept inherent limitations on the ability to keep oneself safe. Self-blame may also be a mechanism to avoid confronting the notion that the perpetrator had intent, something that may be particularly difficult to accept if the perpetrator was previously a trusted person. Self-blame may be especially intractable if the victim "froze" at the time of the assault, had a sexual response during the assault, or in her opinion did not fight back adequately. Societal "just-world" beliefs about bad things only happening to bad people can exacerbate these feelings, particularly if the victim received negative responses from others when disclosing details of her assault.

Interpersonal Boundaries

Sexual assault survivors may struggle with interpersonal boundaries more than do individuals who have experienced other types of trauma. The profound violation of personal boundaries involved in sexual assault can create confusion about what is reasonable behavior in relationships, particularly for young victims or those who have experienced multiple instances of sexual trauma across their lifespan. As a result, victims may have difficulty identifying or setting appropriate boundaries, both in terms of their own and others' behavior. This may result in inappropriately low or loose boundaries in certain situations. Alternatively, the victim may react by enacting particularly high boundaries. This may be in response to feelings of being exposed and vulnerable, reflecting efforts to establish a sense of being separate from and protected against the outside world.

Safety and Revictimization

Many of the difficulties therapists observe in patients who have experienced sexual assault are likely related to issues of safety. A global distrust of others, for example, is one way victims may attempt to reestablish a sense of safety or prevent themselves from being revictimized. However, therapists may also feel frustrated by what they perceive to be patients' *inattention* to safety. Although unquestionably a crucial target for intervention given the high rates of revictimization among sexual assault survivors, even these confusing behaviors can be viewed, paradoxically, as serving a self-protective function. For example, many victims learn to ignore emotions and internal sensations as a way to cope with the emotional flooding that can accompany PTSD. As a result, they may be less attuned to or responsive to signs of danger that may seem clear to others. Furthermore, a reluctance to see oneself as a victim or a need to maintain hope about others may drive a tendency to trust too easily or a decision to remain in an abusive relationship.

Cultural Variances

Victims' reactions to experiences of sexual assault may vary depending on cultural variables such as race/ethnicity and gender (Holzman 1996; Lefley et al. 1993). For example, stigma and societal beliefs about rape victims may be significant obstacles to disclosure for some survivors. Religious and ethnic background may affect whether a victim even identifies her experiences as an assault. Similarly, although the literature on sexual assault among men is relatively small, it does suggest differences in the way men and women react to being sexually assaulted (Rentoul and Appleboom 1997). Issues that men in particular may struggle with include extreme feelings of shame and an accompanying need for secrecy; difficulties seeking out and engaging in care; questioning of gender, sexual identity, and sexual orientation; homophobia; and substance abuse.

Therapist's Gender and Other Characteristics

For both male and female survivors of sexual assault, the therapist's gender is often an issue. Victims may have concerns related to safety, ability to disclose, or inhibition due to gender roles. Providers who are of the same gender as the perpetrator or who share other characteristics of the perpetrator, such as race, mannerisms, or style of dress, may trigger intrusive thoughts or flashbacks for survivors. Many victims may be reluctant or even unable to engage in therapy if required to see a therapist who is of the same sex as their perpetrator; for some, this may be part of a broader difficulty with being in environments dominated by men.

No empirical studies address this issue directly, but it is widely considered best practice in the treatment of victims of sexual trauma to allow them some control in the choice of their therapist's gender. That being said, having a therapist whose gender or other characteristics are reminiscent of the perpetrator's has the potential to be extremely therapeutic. Conceptually, this resemblance is similar to the other types of exposure tasks that will likely be part of a client's PTSD treatment. To the extent that the client can tolerate her emotional reactions to these therapist characteristics, she may ultimately gain a sense of mastery over them. Regardless, the issue of therapist gender is one that should be approached thoughtfully and, as necessary, discussed throughout treatment.

Conclusion

Although extremely rewarding, providing therapy to sexual assault victims can be challenging. In this chapter, we have addressed only a subset of potential issues that bear consideration in working with victims of sexual assault. In negotiating other situations that may arise, the clinician can benefit from adopting the general guiding principle that confusing behaviors reflect, at their core, a victim's attempt to respond to a situation or emotional reaction perceived as overwhelming or threatening. Behind these behaviors is most often an attempt—albeit at times a less-than-optimal attempt—to meet a need, often related to safety, control, or interpersonal connection. Combining this understanding with a thorough psychosocial assessment, evidence-based therapeutic approaches, and sensitivity to the unique issues that may arise during treatment will greatly facilitate effective work with this group of survivors and ultimately their successful recovery from PTSD.

Key Clinical Points

- Rape is more likely to result in a PTSD diagnosis than most other violent crimes.
- When disclosing to others, patients may encounter minimization, questions about credibility, and other rape myths. These negative reactions from others can contribute to subsequent psychopathology and discourage survivors from seeking treatment.
- It is important to screen all patients seeking mental health care for experiences of sexual assault, particularly given some victims' reluctance to spontaneously disclose.
- When working with sexual assault survivors, clinicians should assess various psychosocial factors (e.g., ethnicity/cultural identity; lifetime trauma history; predominant coping strategies) that may shape reactions to the assault. Information about psychological symptoms and general functioning can also provide guidance for treatment planning.
- Self-blame and shame are frequent problems for sexual assault survivors.
- Validating the patient's distress and normalizing the patient's responses to the assault are important early interventions that should be made in conjunction with the assessment process.
- Cognitive-behavioral therapy, specifically prolonged exposure, has demonstrated efficacy in treating PTSD secondary to sexual assault.
- Resolving issues related to trust is likely to be a significant component of therapy, particularly if the patient knew the perpetrator prior to the assault.
- Sex and sexuality are potentially complicated issues for survivors and may be important topics to address during therapy.
- Throughout therapy, providers should help victims regain a sense of control both over their environment and themselves.
- Given high rates of revictimization among sexual assault survivors, clinicians should be attentive to this issue throughout the course of treatment.

References

American Psychiatric Association: Diagnostic and Statistical Manual of Mental Disorders, 4th Edition, Text Revision. Washington, DC, American Psychiatric Association, 2000

Andrews B, Brewin CR, Rose S: Gender, social support, and PTSD in victims of violent crime. J Trauma Stress 16:421–427, 2003

Briere J, Kaltman S, Green BL: Accumulated childhood trauma and symptom complexity. J Trauma Stress 21:223–226, 2008

Campbell R: The psychological impact of rape victims' experiences with the legal, medical, and mental health systems. Psychol Women Q 31:357–370, 2008

Classen C, Field NP, Koopman C, et al: Interpersonal problems and their relationship to sexual revictimization among women sexually abused in childhood. J Interpers Violence 16:495–509, 2001

Cloitre M, Koenen KC, Cohen LR, et al: Skills training in affective and interpersonal regulation followed by exposure: a phase-based treatment for PTSD related to childhood abuse. J Consult Clin Psychol 70:1067–1074, 2002

Crowell NA, Burgess AW (eds): Understanding Violence Against Women. Washington, DC, National Academy Press, 1996

Dickinson LM, deGruy FV 3rd, Dickinson WP, et al: Health-related quality of life and symptom profiles of female survivors of sexual abuse. Arch Fam Med 8:35–43, 1999

DiVasto P: Measuring the aftermath of rape. J Psychosoc Nurs Ment Health Serv 23:33–35, 1985

Elliott DM, Mok DS, Briere J: Adult sexual assault: prevalence, symptomatology, and sex differences in the general population. J Trauma Stress 17:203–211, 2004

Fergusson DM, Boden JM, Horwood LJ: Exposure to childhood sexual and physical abuse and adjustment in early adulthood. Child Abuse Negl 32:607–619, 2008

Filipas HH, Ullman SE: Social reactions to sexual assault victims from various support sources. Violence Vict 16:673–692, 2001

Fisher B, Daigle LE, Cullen FT, et al: Reporting sexual victimization to the police and others: results from a national-level study of college women. Crim Justice Behav 30:6–38, 2003

Foa EB, Rothbaum BO: Treating the Trauma of Rape: Cognitive-Behavioral Therapy for PTSD. New York, Guilford, 1998

Foa EB, Dancu CV, Hembree EA, et al: A comparison of exposure therapy, stress inoculation training and their combination for reducing posttraumatic stress disorder in female assault victims. J Consult Clin Psychol 67:194–200, 1999

Foa EB, Rothbaum BO, Riggs DS, et al: Treatment of posttraumatic stress disorder in rape victims: a comparison between cognitive-behavioral procedures and counseling. J Consult Clin Psychol 59:715–723, 1991

Frazier PA: Perceived control and distress following sexual assault: a longitudinal test of a new model. J Pers Soc Psychol 84:1257–1269, 2003

Hart TC, Rennison C: Reporting Crime to the Police, 1992–2000. Bureau of Justice Statistics Special Report No. NCV–195710. 2003. Available at: http://www.ojp.usdoj.gov/content/pub/pdf/rcp00.pdf. Accessed December 1, 2009.

Holzman CG: Counseling adult women rape survivors: issues of race, ethnicity, and class. Women Ther 19:47–62, 1996

Institute of Medicine: Treatment of Posttraumatic Stress Disorder: An Assessment of the Evidence. Washington DC, National Academies Press, 2008

Kessler RC, Sonnega A, Bromet E, et al: Posttraumatic stress disorder in the National Comorbidity Survey. Arch Gen Psychiatry 52:1048–1060, 1995

Kilpatrick DG: Rape Aftermath Symptom Test, in Dictionary of Behavioral Assessment Techniques. Edited by Bellack HM. New York, Pergamon, 1988, pp 366–367

Kilpatrick DG, Veronen LJ, Resick PA: Psychological sequelae to rape: assessment and treatment strategies, in Behavioral Medicine: Assessment and Treatment Strategies. Edited by Doleys DM, Meredith RI, Ciminero AR. New York, Plenum, 1982, pp 473–497

Kilpatrick DG, Saunders BE, Amick-McMullan A, et al: Victim and crime factors associated with the development of crime-related post-traumatic stress disorder. Behav Ther 20:199–214, 1989

Kilpatrick DG, Edmunds CN, Seymour AK: Rape in America: A Report to the Nation. Arlington, VA, National Victim Center and Medical University of South Carolina, 1992

Kilpatrick DG, Acierno R, Resnick HS, et al: A 2-year longitudinal analysis of the relationships between violent assault and substance use in women. J Consult Clin Psychol 65:834–847, 1997

Kimerling R, Street AE, Gima K, et al: Evaluation of universal screening for military-related sexual trauma. Psychiatr Serv 59:635–640, 2008

Koss MP, Gidycz CA, Wisniewski N: The scope of rape: incidence and prevalence of sexual aggression and victimization in a national sample of higher education students. J Consult Clin Psychol 55:162–170, 1987

Koss MP, Figueredo AJ, Prince RJ: Cognitive mediation of rape's mental, physical, and social health impact: tests of four models in cross-sectional data. J Consult Clin Psychol 70:926–941, 2002

Lefley H, Scott CS, Llabre M, et al: Cultural beliefs about rape and victims' response in three ethnic groups. Am J Orthopsychiatry 63:623–632, 1993

Messman T, Long PJ: Child sexual abuse and its relationship to revictimization in adult women: a review. Clin Psychol Rev 16:397–420, 1996

Rentoul L, Appleboom N: Understanding the psychological impact of rape and serious sexual assault of men: a literature review. J Psychiatr Ment Health Nurs 4:267–274, 1997

Resick PA, Schnicke MK: Cognitive Processing Therapy for Rape Victims: A Treatment Manual. Newbury Park, CA, Sage, 1996

Resick PA, Nishith P, Weaver TL, et al: A comparison of cognitive-processing therapy with prolonged exposure and a waiting condition for the treatment of chronic posttraumatic stress disorder in female rape victims. J Consult Clin Psychol 70:867–879, 2002

Resick PA, Galovski TE, O'Brien Uhlmansiek M, et al: A randomized clinical trial to dismantle components of cognitive processing therapy for posttraumatic stress disorder in female victims of interpersonal violence. J Consult Clin Psychol 76:243–258, 2008

Resnick HS, Newton T: Assessment and treatment of post-traumatic stress disorder in adult survivors of sexual assault, in Treating PTSD: Cognitive-Behavioral Strategies. Edited by Foy DW. New York, Guilford, 1992, pp 99–126

Rothbaum BO, Foa EB, Riggs DS, et al: A prospective examination of post-traumatic stress disorder in rape victims. J Trauma Stress 5:455–475, 1992

Rothbaum BO, Astin MC, Marsteller F: Prolonged exposure versus eye movement desensitization and reprocessing (EMDR) for PTSD rape victims. J Trauma Stress 18:607–616, 2005

Ruch LO, Wang CH: Validation of the Sexual Assault Symptom Scale II (SASS II) using a panel research design. J Interpers Violence 21:1440–1461, 2006

Spitzberg BH: An analysis of empirical estimates of sexual aggression victimization and perpetration. Violence Vict 14:241–260, 1999

Tjaden P, Thoennes N: Prevalence, incidence, and consequences of violence against women: findings from the National Violence Against Women Survey. National Institute of Justice and Centers for Disease Control and Prevention Research in Brief. November 1998. Available at: http://www.ncjrs.gov/pdffiles/172837.pdf. Accessed December 31, 2009.

Tjaden P, Thoennes N: Full Report of the Prevalence, Incidence, and Consequences of Violence Against Women: Findings From the National Violence Against Women Survey (Report NCJ 183781). November 2000. Available at: http://www.ncjrs.gov/pdffiles1/nij/183781.pdf. Accessed December 31, 2009.

Ullman SE: Social reactions, coping strategies, and self-blame attributions in adjustment to sexual assault. Psychol Women Q 20:505–526, 1996

Ullman SE: Social support and recovery from sexual assault: a review. Aggress Violent Behav 4:343–358, 1999

Ullman SE: Psychometric characteristics of the Social Reactions Questionnaire. Psychol Women Q 24:257–271, 2000

Ullman SE, Brecklin LR: Sexual assault history and suicidal behavior in a national sample of women. Suicide Life Threat Behav 32:117–130, 2002

Ullman SE, Brecklin LR: Sexual assault history and health-related outcomes in a national sample of women. Psychol Women Q 27:46–57, 2003

Ullman SE, Filipas HH: Predictors of PTSD symptom severity and social reactions in sexual assault victims. J Trauma Stress 14:369–389, 2001

Ullman SE, Filipas HH, Townsend SM, et al: Psychosocial correlates of PTSD symptom severity in sexual assault survivors. J Trauma Stress 20:821–831, 2007a

Ullman SE, Townsend SM, Filipas HH, et al: Structural models of the relations of assault severity, social support, avoidance coping, self-blame, and PTSD among sexual assault survivors. Psychol Women Q 31:23–37, 2007b

U.S. Department of Justice, Office of Justice Programs, Bureau of Justice Statistics: Criminal Victimization in the United States, 2006 Statistical Tables: National Crime Victimization Survey. Washington, DC, U.S. Department of Justice, 2008

van der Kolk BA, Pelcovitz D, Roth S, et al: Dissociation, somatization, and affect dysregulation: the complexity of adaptation to trauma. Am J Psychiatry 153 (suppl 7):83–93, 1996

13

Military and Veteran Populations

Joshua E. Wilk, Ph.D.

Charles W. Hoge, M.D.

Rates and Risk Factors for PTSD in Combat Veterans

Service members and veterans who have deployed to a combat zone are at much higher risk than the general public for the development of posttraumatic stress disorder (PTSD) (Prigerson et al. 2001). Studies from the wars in Iraq and Afghanistan have confirmed findings from other wars regarding the high risk of developing PTSD and other mental health problems. Hoge et al. (2004) studied U.S. combat Army and Marine infantry units using anonymous surveys either before deployment or 3–4 months following deployment to Iraq or Afghanistan. They found a significant relationship between exposure to combat experiences and the prevalence of PTSD. Depending on the cutoff criteria selected, PTSD prevalence rates were 5%–9% before deployment, 6%–12% after return from Afghanistan, and 12%–20% after return from Iraq.

Since the initial publication of these cross-sectional data, a number of other studies using very different methods, including postdeployment population screening, random telephone surveys, and health care utilization records, have found similar prevalence estimates (Hoge et al. 2006; Milliken et al. 2007; Seal et al. 2007; Smith et al. 2008; Tanielian and Jaycox 2008). Rates of mental health problems in United Kingdom service members have been reported to be lower (Hotopf et al. 2006), but this was likely due to the lower frequency and intensity of combat experiences in southern Iraq where the units were based (Hoge and Castro 2006). Studies have consistently shown that the frequency and intensity of combat experiences are the most important correlates of PTSD and other mental health problems. Additionally, these studies have shown increased rates of other mental health problems, including depression, generalized anxiety disorder, and substance use disorders (Hoge et al. 2004). The aggregate data suggest a substantial burden secondary to combat-related mental health problems.

Moreover, there is a high comorbidity of PTSD with generalized health problems (Boscarino 2004). PTSD is associated with neuroendocrine, autonomic nervous system, and cell-mediated immune dysregulation (Boscarino 2004). One study of infantry soldiers who had returned from Iraq showed that compared with soldiers who screened negative for PTSD, those who screened positive for PTSD were significantly more likely to report missed workdays, an increased number of medical appointments, and high ratings of somatic symptoms (Hoge et al. 2007). These findings were independent of being wounded or injured during combat.

Research on Treatment of Combat-Related PTSD

Given the high prevalence of PTSD and high comorbidity of PTSD with other mental and physical health problems in persons exposed to war, the treatment of PTSD using evidence-based modalities is a high priority. A number of treatment guidelines exist, such as the ones published by the American Psychiatric Association (2004); the Veterans Health Administration, Department of Defense (2004); and the International Society for Traumatic Stress Studies (Foa et al. 2000). All of these guidelines indicate that sufficient evidence has been gathered to recommend either pharmacological or psychotherapeutic approaches. Specifically, selective serotonin reuptake inhibitors (SSRIs) are recommended medications (sertraline and paroxetine have been approved by the U.S. Food and Drug Administration for treatment of PTSD), and cognitive-behavioral therapy (CBT) is recommended as a first-line psychotherapeutic intervention.

In contrast to practice guidelines, the Institute of Medicine (2008) published a comprehensive assessment of the evidence supporting various treatment modalities for PTSD, specifically focused on veteran populations. This report, which used a very high standard to assess the evidence, concluded that exposure therapy was the only treatment category with sufficient quality and confidence of evidence for effectiveness. The committee considered the evidence to be inadequate for all other commonly used psychotherapy or psychopharmacological treatments, including SSRIs, cognitive restructuring, eye movement desensitization and reprocessing (EMDR), coping skills therapy, group therapy, and other modalities.

The Institute of Medicine's (2008) report highlights some fundamental issues with treatment for combat-related PTSD. Notably, the overall effect sizes are modest for all treatment modalities, including exposure therapy. Also, very few studies have involved head-to-head comparisons to determine which components of treatment are most effective.

Most important, limited research has focused specifically on military personnel returning from combat, arguably a group at highest risk. The few studies involving combat veterans have generally included those with longstanding PTSD symptoms existing for years after combat. The limited available data indicate that combat-related PTSD may be more refractory to treatment than PTSD related to other types of traumatic events (Friedman et al. 2007). Clinicians working in the field know that there are unique aspects to treating combat-related PTSD, given the high level of severity and chronicity and the high rate of comorbidity exhibited by many of their patients.

The evidence supporting modalities commonly used in military populations is not based on samples representative of military populations returning from combat. For example, studies supporting available manualized treatment strategies, such as cognitive processing therapy (Resick and Schnicke 1992) and prolonged exposure therapy (Foa and Rothbaum 1998), are based largely on individuals who had single traumatic events (e.g., rape). Therefore, clinicians often have to adapt these modalities for combat veterans who have returned from a long deployment in which they may have experienced multiple significant events. Other issues affecting military populations include stigma associated with mental health treatment, difficulties in accessing treatment or staying in treatment long enough to derive benefit, and the high rate of comorbid conditions.

Assessment and Treatment of Service Members and Veterans With PTSD

In assessing and treating military populations with PTSD, clinicians need to take into account specific considerations, as discussed in this section. Table 13–1 summarizes these considerations.

Assessment

Assessment of service members and veterans with PTSD should include a careful occupational history, including time in military service; occupation within the military; number, location, and length of deployments; combat exposures; and other life stressors resulting from military service. Because a patient may have experienced multiple combat exposures, the clinician should inquire about those that had the most significant impact, bearing in mind that these exposures will be a focus of treatment in later sessions. The clinician should also assess for other types of trauma contributing to PTSD symptoms, including adverse childhood experiences, sexual trauma, motor vehicle accidents, and natural disasters (Cabrera et al. 2007).

The clinician must evaluate the degree to which the patient's difficulties are part of the normal course of readjusting after an intense experience, such as combat, and to what extent they reflect persistent problems that need to be addressed as part of the treatment strategy. A brief PTSD screening instrument, such as the 17-item PTSD Checklist (PCL; Weathers et al. 1993), is a useful part of the assessment process, and the total score on this instrument can be used to gauge the effectiveness of treatment over time. However, high PCL scores are not necessarily consistent with poor social and occupational functioning in combat veterans, because PTSD symptoms such as nightmares and physiological hyperreactivity are commonly experienced after combat, sometimes to a significant degree. In addition, data suggest that reactions to trauma exposure incurred as part of military occupational duties are different from reactions to trauma in other settings. In particular, DSM-IV-TR (American Psychiatric Association 2000) diagnostic Criterion A2 for PTSD (experiencing fear, helplessness, or horror) is often not endorsed by combat veterans despite high levels of exposure to traumatic events and the presence of all symptom criteria (Adler et al. 2008).

The assessment of comorbid mental and physical health conditions is one of the most important components of the assessment of service members and veterans suspected of having PTSD (Hoge et al. 2007; Kessler et al. 1995). Patient evaluation for commonly occurring comorbid conditions, including depression, generalized anxiety, panic disorder, and substance use disorders, should be an integral part of the assessment. Because physical health conditions are important, clinicians should inquire about injuries sustained during deployment (including head injuries), deployment-related health conditions, and chronic pain.

To assess for a history of concussion (i.e., mild traumatic brain injury [TBI]) during deployment, clinicians should ask about injuries resulting in a loss of consciousness, amnesia around the time of the event, or an alteration of consciousness. Additionally, clinicians should assess the number of such injuries; the duration of time unconscious, if any; and the mechanism of injury. This questioning should be followed by a careful assessment of any postconcussive symptoms immediately following the injury event (e.g., headaches, dizziness, tinnitus, nausea, irritability, insomnia, and concentration or memory problems) and the severity and duration of such symptoms.

When these "postconcussive" symptoms persist long after the initial injury, the clinician has greater difficulty assessing and treating patients. The symptoms attributed to concussion or mild TBI are nonspecific and have been shown to strongly correlate with factors such as PTSD, depression, compensation or litigation processes, and negative patient expectations (Carroll et al. 2004; Hoge et al. 2008). Most patients who sustain a concussion or mild TBI have prompt resolution of symptoms within hours or a few days (McCrea et al. 2003); only a small percentage (estimated at less than 5%) have persistent symptoms after 1 year (Iverson et al. 2007; McCrea 2008). Therefore, although these symptoms may be attributed by the patient to a concussion, the patient may have psychological factors such as PTSD or depression or a

Table 13–1. Specific considerations in assessment and treatment of PTSD with military and veteran populations

Assessment	
Occupational history	Deployments
	Combat experiences with most significant impact
	Other military-related stressors
Mental health assessment	Brief PTSD screen (e.g., PTSD Checklist by Weathers et al. 1993)
	Awareness that Criterion A2 experience may be different for trauma that occurred as part of occupation (including combat)
	Other stressors such as adverse childhood experiences, sexual trauma, and motor vehicle accidents
	Co-occurring conditions such as depression, generalized anxiety disorder, and substance abuse
Functional impairment	Social or occupational functioning
	Interview of spouse and/or other close family members
Physical health assessment	Chronic pain, history of injuries (including concussion or mild traumatic brain injury), medications
	Postdeployment symptoms (including postconcussive symptoms)
	Importance of reassurance and promotion of positive expectations for recovery in management of symptoms
Suicidal risk and risky behavior	Ready access to firearms
	Risky driving
	Drinking and driving
	Aggressive behavior

Table 13–1. Specific considerations in assessment and treatment of PTSD with military and veteran populations *(continued)*

Treatment	
Therapeutic alliance	Understand and respect the military experience
	Do not be afraid to ask client for clarification and education regarding military culture
Treatment approach	Use evidence-based modalities, particularly prolonged exposure, cognitive-behavioral therapy, eye movement desensitization and reprocessing, and medications
	Normalize reactions that occur after combat
	Have awareness of the limited research on military populations
	Be flexible and aware that multiple approaches may be necessary
	Address rage, guilt, and grief that may be present
	Address comorbid conditions
	Use case managers and multidisciplinary team approach in complicated cases
Psychoeducation	Educate regarding the nature of PTSD symptoms as physiologically protective reflexes and adaptive in a combat context
	Help patient understand and accept how he or she has changed as a result of combat
Family issues	Address readjustment stress, including potential changes in roles within household
	Include spouse and/or family in treatment
Other considerations	Address stigma
	Address concerns about effect of treatment on occupational functioning and future security clearances
	Address any concerns regarding access or availability of treatment

combination of such conditions. Treatment of cognitive, behavioral, and even physical symptoms attributed to concussion or mild TBI is not likely to be successful unless underlying conditions, such as depression or PTSD, are addressed (Iverson et al. 2007).

Because persistence of symptoms after concussion or mild TBI has been strongly associated with negative expectations regarding recovery (Ferguson et al. 1999), clinicians need to be particularly prudent in how they communicate with patients. By communicating at the outset that these symptoms are due to "brain damage" or are psychological in nature, the clinician may create negative expectations resulting in persistence of symptoms or impairing therapeutic rapport. On the other hand, by communicating that the patient's symptoms are common, the brain has remarkable capacity for healing after concussion, and there are effective treatments for these symptoms (regardless of the etiology), the clinician will both promote positive expectations and communicate that the patient's concerns are being taken seriously.

Additionally, clinicians should assess for suicidal risk, access to firearms, aggression toward others (including intimate partner and children), and risky behaviors such as driving while intoxicated and aggressive driving. Research has found that Operation Iraqi Freedom veterans exposed to combat have an increased propensity for risk taking (Kilgore et al. 2008). Additionally, an assessment of relationships and marital problems is essential. Veterans with combat-related PTSD are at increased risk of aggression in their relationships (Byrne and Riggs 1996). Finally, the clinician should determine what positive or protective factors for treatment the patient may possess, particularly social support. It is helpful to draw on the strength the veteran has already demonstrated in his or her service: courage, honor, service to country, resiliency in combat, cohesion with other unit members, ability to handle extreme levels of stress, and leadership skills.

Interviewing spouses or family members is valuable to the assessment process for two reasons. First, significant others provide different perspectives on the level of symptoms, impairment, and social support. Second, the clinician can assess whether there are current relationship stressors that need to be the focus of treatment (these may actually be a more urgent initial focus than PTSD treatment). Observing interactions between the veteran and his or her family member(s) provides rich information to guide treatment approaches.

Treatment

As with most psychotherapy, a key to working with individuals who have combat-related PTSD is establishing a therapeutic alliance. Working with veterans and service members presents some unique challenges. Unless the clinician has served in the military, the patient may feel that the clinician cannot understand his or her experience. Combat veterans may be reluctant to talk about their experiences to civilian mental health professionals because of the perception that combat experiences are beyond what civilian professionals can comprehend. When working with service members or veterans, mental health professionals must make an effort to show an understanding of and respect for the patient's military service. Clinicians should acknowledge honestly any lack of understanding of military culture and jargon, and should not hesitate to ask patients to help educate them when necessary. Additionally, clinicians should not automatically assume that combat-related trauma is like other forms of trauma.

Developing a treatment plan should address symptoms of PTSD as well as comorbid mental or physical health problems. Despite the large gaps in evidence to guide treatment of combat-related PTSD, a clinician working with an individual service member or veteran must decide how to proceed. Fundamentally, this is a major reason why clinical practice guidelines may differ from assessments of the evidence, such as the Institute of Medicine's (2008) report. In the absence of sufficient evidence, clinical practice guidelines must still provide sufficient recommendations to help guide clinical care. Clinicians need to have training in evidence-based modalities and to understand that these modalities alone may be insufficient for the individual patient.

According to the Institute of Medicine's (2008) report, current evidence indicates that exposure therapy is an essential ingredient of PTSD treatment (Foa et al. 1999). The fundamental element of exposure therapy is the reduction of physiological reactivity through retelling of the traumatic event. Many clinicians, however, disagree with the Institute of Medicine's conclusion and argue that cognitive restructuring through modification of the patient's unhealthy thought processes regarding the traumatic event and his or her safety is as important (e.g., Resick and Schnicke 1992). Still others argue that the most effective treatment involves a combination of approaches (e.g., Bryant et al. 2003, 2008). Research is available to support all three positions.

For example, in a study of female assault survivors by Foa et al. (2005), prolonged exposure therapy alone was compared to prolonged exposure therapy plus cognitive restructuring for the treatment of PTSD. Prolonged exposure therapy utilizes imaginal and in vivo exposure modalities. Compared with wait-list controls, both groups showed significant improvements in PTSD symptoms, which were maintained at up to a 12-month follow-up. The addition of cognitive restructuring resulted in no enhanced outcome.

Conversely, in one of the few dismantling studies of which elements of therapy are most effective, Resick et al. (2008) compared the cognitive restructuring portion of cognitive processing therapy (CPT) with the exposure portion of CPT and with full CPT (both cognitive restructuring and exposure) in 150 adult women with PTSD related to a physical or sexual assault. In the exposure-only component, the participants were alone in a room writing about their worst trauma for 45–60 minutes for five of six 2-hour weekly sessions. At the end of each period, the therapist returned to the room, asked the participant to read the written account aloud, and discussed the participant's emotions regarding the writing. The total number and length of sessions were comparable for all three study groups, although the actual amount of time spent with the therapist was substantially longer for the CPT and cognitive restructuring groups. In contrast to the additive design of the Foa et al. (2005) study, in a dismantling study, components of therapy are examined separately and offered as stand-alone treatments. Resick et al. (2008) argued that in additive studies, treatment components may be condensed in development of the new therapy, and a suboptimal "dose" of each element is given to the patient. The results of the dismantling study showed that full CPT, the cognitive restructuring portion alone, and the exposure portion alone all significantly reduced PTSD symptoms; there was no benefit to combining the elements of CPT over either component in isolation. Those treated with cognitive restructuring alone had significantly greater reduction in PTSD symptoms compared with those who received exposure alone, at posttreatment, but there were no significant differences between groups at 6-month follow-up. It should be noted that the written exposure modality used in CPT is very different in nature from the imaginal and in vivo exposure used in prolonged exposure. It is also noteworthy that the individual writing exposure with substantially reduced therapist time actually showed nearly the same effect as the cognitive restructuring or full CPT. A head-to-head comparison of prolonged exposure and written exposure may help elucidate this matter further.

Finally, Bryant and colleagues conducted two studies comparing prolonged exposure and cognitive restructuring alone to a combination of the two for the treatment of PTSD, with the primary difference being that the first study (Bryant et al. 2003) used only imaginal exposure, whereas the latter (Bryant et al. 2008) use in vivo and imaginal exposure techniques. Contrary to previous studies discussed, both of the studies by Bryant's group found that the combination of cognitive restructuring and prolonged exposure resulted in significantly better outcomes for PTSD than either prolonged exposure or cognitive restructuring alone.

Notably, in all of these studies, cognitive restructuring, prolonged exposure, or the combination of the two significantly outperformed the control condition in the reduction of PTSD symptoms. In addition, a strong evidence base supports the effectiveness of EMDR (Shapiro 1989). The key aspect of EMDR involves asking a patient to process a traumatic event while the clinician moves his or her fingers back and forth in front of the patient's eyes, resulting in alternating, bilateral stimulation. Studies, including head-to-head studies with other evidence-based treatments for PTSD (e.g., Rothbaum et al. 2005), have shown EMDR to be effective for the treatment of PTSD. The mechanism of change in EMDR remains unclear, as does whether EMDR is effective because it is a form of exposure therapy or a stress inoculation technique that reduces the physiological reactivity associated with the traumatic memories. Dismantling studies have not found support for any additional effects of eye movements (e.g., Pitman et al. 1996); however, further research is needed to understand the exact mechanism of EMDR.

Thus, despite the recommendations of the Institute of Medicine (2008), evidence supports the use of exposure, cognitive restructuring, a combination of the two, or EMDR as part of the treatment of PTSD. Unfortunately, this evidence does not come from studies on recently returning soldiers with combat-related trauma. Until more research has been reported with this population, clinicians treating combat-related PTSD should rely on evidence-based treatments and remain flexible in identifying best practices for the individual needs of each patient. Future research may begin to identify strategies for targeting subpopulations of PTSD patients with specific treatments.

Regardless of treatment selection, normalizing reactions frequently occurring after combat is an important component of the therapeutic encounter. Clinicians can help the individual understand that his or her problems are in many ways entirely expected reactions to the traumatic experience. Such help includes education that many of the reactions after combat are physiologically protective reflexes (of the limbic system in the brain) designed to aid with survival. In fact, virtually all symptoms of PTSD are adaptive in a combat setting (e.g., anger, hypervigilance, emotional numbing, heightened physiological reactivity). Clinicians can help service members or veterans with PTSD understand that symptoms exist on a spectrum that includes normal reactions to traumatic events occurring as part of their occupation. The clinician should explain that the difference between "normal" and "abnormal" is not clearly delineated, and that for practical purposes, *abnormal* is simply defined as a symptom or problem that seriously interferes with the person's well-being or functioning. The treatment rationale, therefore, becomes clear: to assist individuals in gaining understanding and acceptance of how they have changed as a result of their experiences, and to help them to gain maximal functioning. Goals include reducing physiological reactivity, improving sleep, reducing anger, and improving relationships, among other things.

Heightened physiological reactivity and avoidance often present challenges to treatment. Many service members who have returned from deployment feel a continuous sense of anxiety about dangers to themselves or their family members. They may be overprotective, be hypervigilant, and carry weapons (Friedman 2006). They may avoid activities they did prior to deployment to avoid putting themselves in situations where their symptoms might be triggered. Such avoidance can lead to profound relationship problems. A combination of psychoeducation, cognitive restructuring, and exposure is helpful in addressing these problems. Clinicians can provide information on how PTSD symptoms have an adaptive physiological and neurobiological basis in a highly threatening environment, such as a war zone, or how emotional numbing and anger are essential survival reactions in combat. These survival mechanisms in combat can become symptoms if they persist and interfere with functioning after returning home. In vivo exposure techniques are particularly important for addressing avoidance associated with physiological hyperarousal to environmental reminders of trauma (Taylor et al. 2003).

Rage, guilt, and grief are important topics for combat veterans; these emotions can interfere with successful therapeutic outcomes if not included as a focus of therapy. The avoidance and emotional numbing symptoms of PTSD can be particularly debilitating to relationships and occupational functioning, and clinicians should be attentive to the possibility that guilt and grief may underlie these reactions. Patients may also have behavioral issues, such as antisocial behaviors or risk-taking behaviors, that present in a manner similar to Axis II personality disorders. Axis II labels should be applied very cautiously because of the uncomplimentary nature of these labels and the potential negative implications such labels may have on establishing and maintaining a strong therapeutic rapport. Focusing directly on the behavioral manifestations of these issues and on reducing problem behaviors, rather than assigning diagnostic labels, can help to maintain a strong therapeutic alliance.

Given that after deployment, service members and veterans often have comorbid PTSD and other mental health problems, particularly depression and substance use disorders, clinicians need to use a range of evidence based treatments beyond those designed for treating PTSD alone. These can include CBT for depression, medication treatment (particularly SSRIs and serotonin-norepinephrine reuptake inhibitors) to address both PTSD and depressive symptoms, and stress inoculation training to reduce physiological reactivity. Sleep disturbance is critically important and can be addressed through sleep hygiene education, psychotherapy including imagery rehearsal, and pharmacological interventions. Comorbid physical health problems, which are strongly associated with both depression and PTSD (Hoge et al. 2007), must be addressed to increase the likelihood of treatment success. This approach requires close coordination with the patient's primary care provider and a careful medication review to ensure that there are no potentially harmful interactions or issues of prescription drug dependence.

Combat-related mental health problems can also be understood within the framework of readjustment and reintegration to life at home after deployment (Friedman 2006). Although most service members readjust successfully and quickly, this readjustment can cause significant problems or go on for a prolonged period of time. Readjustment problems are broader than DSM-IV-TR diagnoses. These problems are addressed by programs such as Battlemind (Thomas et al. 2007), which is developed and disseminated by the U.S. Army.

One of the most valuable contributions of Battlemind is as a risk communication strategy that translates terms familiar to mental health professionals into language that resonates with service members. For example, the state of high situational awareness in a combat environment is comparable to hypervigilance back home. Battlemind also encourages soldiers to draw on their proven strengths. Soldiers are trained to control aggression in the operational environment and ensure that targets are appropriate by following certain procedures and rules of engagement. Therefore, they have proven they possess the skills to avoid indiscriminate aggression back home. The powerful cohesion felt by unit members who depend on each other for survival reflects a vital source of support during the readjustment period after returning home, but can also create conflicts with spouses and loved ones who are also attempting to reconnect after a lengthy separation.

Within the Veterans Affairs (VA) system, Vet Centers offer a community-based approach to readjustment specifically for combat veterans. These centers are staffed by combat veterans and function independently from traditional VA mental health clinics. Many combat veterans receive care for readjustment mental health issues only through Vet Centers. Vet Centers are also available to veterans who have been victims of sexual assault (regardless of eligibility for other services) as well as to family members of deceased service members.

As part of readjustment to noncombat life, a patient should be asked how his or her role in the household may have changed during deployment. Often, a service member returns home to find that his or her spouse has taken over many roles once held by the service member, which can create conflict. Having survived an experience like combat, veterans may not feel it is important to take time to negotiate and work through seemingly trivial home-front issues. The clinician can help to normalize this thinking, but can also insist that the individual learn to address these issues in support of his or her relationships.

The impact of combat-related PTSD symptoms and comorbid disorders can exact a large toll on the family. At the same time, the patient's spouse and family can be vital in the amelioration of these symptoms. Therefore, to minimize the impact of mental health problems on family and social functioning and to muster social support in recovery, clinicians should involve spouses and other family members, with the patient's permission, both to help educate them about the nature of combat-related reactions and to facilitate better understanding of the important treatment focus areas. Additionally, when needed, providing case management services to the patient and family can help to minimize the impact of mental health issues.

Even with a treatment plan addressing these myriad issues, treatment can fail due to a number of obstacles encountered by patients in this population. A frequent impediment to therapy is the stigma associated with mental health issues and treatment in the military (Hoge et al. 2004; Tanielian and Jaycox 2008). Less than half of service members with serious mental health problems report receiving professional help (Hoge et al. 2004), and many who do start treatment fail to follow through on a sufficient number of sessions to achieve a successful outcome. Clinicians need to reassure their patients that treatment will likely improve their occupational functioning rather than interfere with it. Many service members or veterans are concerned that they will not be able to obtain a security clearance if they seek mental health treatment, and clinicians should educate them that new regulations no longer require applicants to acknowledge mental health care for combat-related problems on Department of Defense security questionnaires (Baker 2008).

Other reasons that military personnel do not follow through with treatment include difficulty of accessing care, difficulty getting time off from work, and the fact that current psychotherapy modalities require a considerable number of sessions to be effective. Most of the evidence for CBT in PTSD has been gathered using individual treatments of 10–15 sessions (e.g., Lubin et al. 1998); however, a limited number of studies (e.g., Bisson et al. 2004; Gillespie et al. 2002) have shown efficacy using as few as 4–8 sessions. Clinicians should be aware that treatment may be time limited and adjust treatment plans accordingly. For example, one could plan for 5–6 sessions, followed by a reassessment. Whatever choice a clinician makes with regard to treatment planning, he or she will have to adopt a flexible approach contingent on the competing demands of the patient's situation.

Future Directions

Improving the treatment of combat-related mental health problems will require new clinical research employing rigorous study methodologies, similar to those outlined in the Institute of Medicine's (2008) report. There are numerous gaps in research for treatment of PTSD among service members recently returned from deployment. Although evidence exists that supports

CBT for combat veterans, most of this evidence has been garnered in clinical trials (e.g., Monson et al. 2006) with nonveterans or veterans long after their time of active service. Studies have been heavily weighted toward single-event traumas in which the individual is a victim, rather than multiple events sustained as part of occupational duties. Studies (e.g., Schnurr et al. 2007) have frequently involved individuals who experienced sexual rather than combat-related trauma. Treatment manuals are not necessarily geared toward the issues most relevant for returning service members.

Additionally, most CBT evidence has been gathered using individual treatments of 10–15 sessions. Service members who need treatment often do not receive as many sessions as necessary for a variety of reasons, including understaffing of mental health clinics throughout the military health care system (Department of Defense Task Force on Mental Health 2007), occupational requirements, military training commitments, moves either by the service members or veterans or by their clinicians, and the perceived stigma of receiving care. As a result, treatment modalities that are both effective and more efficient are needed, including approaches that require fewer sessions or that can be delivered in a group rather than individual format. Effective group treatments are especially important, because groups are a common modality used in the VA mental health system. Finally, current evidence does not effectively address the highly prevalent and sometimes equally debilitating conditions that co-occur with combat-related PTSD (American Psychiatric Association 2004; Hoge et al. 2004). With the execution of clinical trials that address these gaps, clinicians treating combat-related PTSD can have further confidence in the evidence base of their treatment plans.

Key Clinical Points

- Frequency and intensity of combat experiences are the most important correlates of PTSD and other mental health problems.
- Combat-related PTSD has a high comorbidity with generalized health problems.
- SSRIs and cognitive-behavioral therapy are the most commonly recommended first-line interventions for combat-related PTSD.

- The stigma of mental health problems and other barriers to care are significant deterrents to treatment in this population.
- The assessment of PTSD should include a detailed trauma history as well as a thorough review for potential comorbidities.
- Assessment for violence and aggression, suicidality, access to firearms, and risky behaviors such as drinking and driving should be included in each evaluation.
- Family and other social supports should be involved in both the evaluation process and the treatment process for individuals suffering from combat-related PTSD.
- Hyperarousal symptoms and sleep difficulties are often a key problem for combat veterans and should be managed aggressively.
- Rage, guilt, and grief are often sources of difficulty and should be a focus for therapy.
- Combat-related mental health problems can often be understood within the framework of readjustment and reintegration into life after deployment and can present major challenges in both the social and occupational arenas for veterans.

References

Adler AB, Wright KM, Bliese PD, et al: A2 diagnostic criterion for combat-related posttraumatic stress disorder. J Trauma Stress 21:301–308, 2008

American Psychiatric Association: Practice Guideline for the Treatment of Patients With Acute Stress Disorder and Posttraumatic Stress Disorder. Washington, DC, American Psychiatric Association, 2004

Baker FW III: DoD changes security clearance question on mental health. American Forces Press Service. 2008. Available at: http://www.defenselink.mil/news/newsarticle.aspx?id=49735. Accessed December 2, 2009.

Bisson J, Shepherd JP, Joy D, et al: Early cognitive-behavioural therapy for post-traumatic stress symptoms after physical injury. Randomised controlled trial. Br J Psychiatry 184:63–69, 2004

Boscarino JA: Posttraumatic stress disorder and physical illness: results from clinical and epidemiological studies. Ann N Y Acad Sci 1032:141–153, 2004

Bryant RA, Moulds ML, Guthrie RM, et al: Imaginal exposure alone and imaginal exposure with cognitive restructuring in treatment of posttraumatic stress disorder. J Consult Clin Psychol 71:706–712, 2003

Bryant RA, Moulds ML, Guthrie RM, et al: A randomized controlled trial of exposure therapy and cognitive restructuring for posttraumatic stress disorder. J Consult Clin Psychol 76:695–703, 2008

Byrne CA, Riggs DS: The cycle of trauma: relationship aggression in male Vietnam veterans with symptoms of posttraumatic stress disorder. Violence Vict 11:213–225, 1996

Cabrera OA, Hoge CW, Bliese PD, et al: Childhood adversity and combat as predictors of depression and post-traumatic stress in deployed troops. Am J Prev Med 33:77–82, 2007

Carroll LJ, Cassidy JD, Peloso PM, et al: Prognosis for mild traumatic brain injury: results of the WHO Collaborating Centre Task Force for mild traumatic brain injury. J Rehabil Med 36 (suppl 43):84–105, 2004

Department of Defense Task Force on Mental Health: An Achievable Vision: Report of the Department of Defense Task Force on Mental Health. Falls Church, VA, Defense Health Board, 2007

Ferguson RJ, Mittenberg W, Barone DF, et al: Postconcussion syndrome following sports-related head injury: expectation as etiology. Neuropsychology 13:582–589, 1999

Foa EB, Rothbaum BO: Treating the Trauma of Rape: Cognitive-Behavioral Therapy for PTSD. New York, Guilford, 1998

Foa EB, Dancu CV, Hembree EA, et al: A comparison of exposure therapy, stress inoculation training, and their combination for reducing posttraumatic stress disorder in female assault victims. J Consult Clin Psychol 67:194–200, 1999

Foa EB, Keane TM, Friedman MJ: Effective Treatments for PTSD. New York, Guilford, 2000

Foa EB, Hembree EA, Cahill SP, et al: Randomized trial of prolonged exposure for posttraumatic stress disorder with and without cognitive restructuring: outcome at academic and community clinics. J Consult Clin Psychol 73:953–964, 2005

Friedman MJ: Posttraumatic stress disorder among military returnees from Afghanistan and Iraq. Am J Psychiatry 163:586–593, 2006

Friedman MJ, Marmar CR, Baker DG, et al: Randomized, double-blind comparison of sertraline and placebo for posttraumatic stress disorder in a Department of Veterans Affairs setting. J Clin Psychol 68:711–720, 2007

Gillespie K, Duffy M, Hackmann A, et al: Community based cognitive therapy in the treatment of posttraumatic stress disorder following the Omagh bomb. Behav Res Ther 40:345–357, 2002

Hoge CW, Castro CA: Post-traumatic stress disorder in UK and US forces deployed to Iraq (letter). Lancet 368:837, 2006

Hoge CW, Castro CA, Messer SC, et al: Combat duty in Iraq and Afghanistan, mental health problems, and barriers to care. N Engl J Med 351:13–22, 2004

Hoge CW, Auchterlonie JL, Milliken CS: Mental health problems, use of mental health services, and attrition from military service after returning from deployment to Iraq or Afghanistan. JAMA 295:1023–1032, 2006

Hoge CW, Terhakopian A, Castro CA, et al: Association of posttraumatic stress disorder with somatic symptoms, health care visits, and absenteeism among Iraq war veterans. Am J Psychiatry 164:150–153, 2007

Hoge CW, McGurk DM, Thomas JL, et al: Mild traumatic brain injury in U.S. soldiers returning from Iraq. N Engl J Med 358:453–463, 2008

Hotopf M, Hull L, Fear NT, et al: The health of UK military personnel who deployed to the 2003 Iraq war: a cohort study. Lancet 367:1731–1741, 2006

Institute of Medicine: Treatment of Posttraumatic Stress Disorder: An Assessment of the Evidence. Washington, DC, National Academics Press, 2008

Iverson GL, Zasler ND, Lange RT: Post-concussive disorder, in Brain Injury Medicine: Principles and Practice. Edited by Zasler ND, Katz DI, Zafonte RD. New York, Demos Medical, 2007, pp 373–405

Kessler RC, Sonnega A, Bromet E, et al: Posttraumatic stress disorder in the National Comorbidity Survey. Arch Gen Psychiatry 52:1048–1060, 1995

Kilgore WD, Cotting DI, Thomas JL, et al: Post-combat invincibility: violent combat experiences are associated with risk-taking propensity following deployment. J Psychiatr Res 42:1112–1121, 2008

Lubin HL, Loris M, Burt J, et al: Efficacy of psychoeducational group therapy in reducing symptoms of posttraumatic stress disorder among multiply traumatized women. Am J Psychiatry 155:1172–1177, 1998

McCrea MA: Mild Traumatic Brain Injury and Postconcussion Syndrome. Oxford, UK, Oxford University Press, 2008, pp 163–167

McCrea MA, Guskiewicz KM, Marshall SW, et al: Acute effects and recovery time following concussion in collegiate football players: the NCAA Concussion Study. JAMA 290:2556–2563, 2003

Milliken CS, Auchterlonie JL, Hoge CW: Longitudinal assessment of mental health problems among active and reserve component soldiers returning from the Iraq war. JAMA 298:2141–2148, 2007

Monson CM, Schnurr PP, Resick PA, et al: Cognitive processing therapy for veterans with military-related posttraumatic stress disorder. J Consult Clin Psychol 74:898–907, 2006

Pitman RK, Orr SP, Altman B, et al: Emotional processing during eye movement desensitization and reprocessing (EMDR) therapy of Vietnam veterans with posttraumatic stress disorder. Compr Psychiatry 37:419–429, 1996

Prigerson HG, Johnson JG, Rosenheck RA: Combat trauma: trauma with highest risk of delayed onset and unresolved posttraumatic stress disorder symptoms, unemployment, and abuse among men. J Nerv Ment Dis 189:99–108, 2001

Resick PA, Schnicke MK: Cognitive processing therapy for sexual assault victims. J Consult Clin Psychol 60:748–756, 1992

Resick PA, Galovski TE, O'Brien Uhlmansiek M, et al: A randomized clinical trial to dismantle components of cognitive processing therapy for posttraumatic stress disorder in female victims of interpersonal violence. J Consult Clin Psychol 76:243–258, 2008

Rothbaum BO, Astin MC, Marsteller F: Prolonged exposure versus eye movement desensitization and reprocessing (EMDR) for PTSD rape victims. J Trauma Stress 18:607–616, 2005

Schnurr PP, Friedman MJ, Engel CC, et al: Cognitive behavioral therapy for posttraumatic stress disorder in women: a randomized controlled trial. JAMA 297:820–830, 2007

Seal KH, Bertenthal D, Miner CR, et al: Bringing the war back home: mental health disorders among 103,788 U.S. veterans returning from Iraq and Afghanistan seen at Department of Veterans Affairs facilities. Arch Intern Med 167:476–482, 2007

Shapiro F: Eye movement desensitization: a new treatment for post-traumatic stress disorder. J Behav Ther Exp Psychiatry 20:211–217, 1989

Smith TC, Ryan MA, Wingard DL, et al: New onset and persistent symptoms of posttraumatic stress disorder self reported after deployment and combat exposures: prospective population-based U.S. military cohort study. BMJ 336:366–371, 2008

Tanielian T, Jaycox LH (eds): Invisible Wounds of War: Psychological and Cognitive Injuries, Their Consequences, and Services to Assist Recovery. Santa Monica, CA, RAND Corporation, 2008

Taylor S, Thordarson DS, Maxfield L, et al: Comparative efficacy, speed, and adverse effects of three PTSD treatments: exposure therapy, EMDR, and relaxation training. J Consult Clin Psychol 71:330–338, 2003

Thomas JL, Castro CA, Adler AB, et al: The efficacy of Battlemind training at immediate post deployment reintegration. Paper presented at the symposium The Battlemind Training System: Supporting Soldiers Throughout the Deployment Cycle (Castro C, Thomas J, co-chairs), American Psychological Association conference, San Francisco, CA, August 2007

Veterans Health Administration, Department of Defense: VA/DoD clinical practice guideline for the management of post-traumatic stress. Version 1.0. Washington, DC, Veterans Health Administration, Department of Defense, 2004

Weathers FW, Litz BT, Herman DS, et al: The PTSD Checklist (PCL): reliability, validity, and diagnostic utility (abstract). International Society for Traumatic Stress Studies. October 1993. Available at: http://www.pdhealth.mil/library/downloads/pcl_sychometrics.doc. Accessed December 2, 2009.

14

Geriatrics

Geoffrey G. Grammer, M.D.
Scott C. Moran, M.D.

The fastest-growing sector of the U.S. population is the group of people over age 65. These generations have witnessed a world war, the Holocaust, and conflicts in Vietnam and Korea (Day 1993). Despite the growing need, very little research into posttraumatic sequelae has been published, and extrapolation of theory and data fails to take into account sociological, psychological, and biological issues that are unique to this age group (Weintraub and Ruskin 1999). The longitudinal course of posttraumatic stress disorder (PTSD) is uncertain for elderly patients. The incidence of PTSD in the elderly population has been estimated at 1.0% by the National Well-Being and Health Study (Andrews et al. 2001; Creamer and Parslow 2008), compared with an estimate of 3.5% in the adult population by the National Comorbidity Survey Replication (Gum et al. 2009). Research in the Netherlands estimated the 6-month prevalence rate of PTSD at 0.9% and of subthreshold PTSD at 13.1% (van Zelst et al. 2003).

As in all geriatric psychiatry, some principles should be followed when treating older patients with PTSD. First, providers must remember that significant physiological and cognitive changes associated with aging must be taken into account in treating older patients. For example, an elder with mild cognitive impairment or dementia may not be able to benefit from cognitive-based therapies. Second, geriatric PTSD remains an understudied phenomenon with large gaps in the scientific literature. Many of the recommendations for treatment of geriatric PTSD in this chapter are based on studies with younger adults, and caution should be used in extrapolating these data to older adults.

Etiologies of Geriatric PTSD

PTSD can have several etiologies and presentations in geriatric populations. The longer one's life experience is, the greater one's chance of enduring or witnessing a traumatic event, yet data have not supported the seemingly obvious conclusion of an escalating risk of development of PTSD in older populations (Creamer and Parslow 2008). The incidence of PTSD may be offset by intrinsic resiliency afforded by the life experience. Just as time adds an increase in risk for trauma, it also allows for cultivation of existential and spiritual beliefs, fostering of interpersonal relationships, and intrapsychic development that may mitigate the effects of adverse life events. PTSD in elderly people may have multiple origins; they may have new-onset PTSD following late-life trauma, delayed-onset PTSD following early-life trauma, or chronic or enduring PTSD persisting into later life (Hiskey et al. 2008a).

Older patients may have new-onset PTSD that results from late-life trauma, such as significant medical illness or injury. The phenomenon of PTSD following myocardial events and intensive care unit stays has been described (Jackson et al. 2007; Wikman et al. 2008). Severe illness, besides being a threat to a person's mortality, may be associated with pain and injury through iatrogenic procedures, such as central line insertion, major surgical interventions, intubation, and arterial blood gas sampling. Sleep deprivation, pharmacological sedatives, and delirium can impair a patient's ability to psychologically negotiate the trauma, amplifying its effects and perhaps contributing to PTSD symptom development.

Earlier trauma may continue to have manifestations decades after an event, due to chronic symptoms associated with PTSD. Public education for psychological health awareness is a relatively recent phenomenon, and older patients may not have a full understanding of their symptoms and the reasons for them. The addition of PTSD to the diagnostic nomenclature did not occur until after the Vietnam War, and although the disorder was earlier described through other terms, it may not have been as conceptually crystallized, particularly if the trauma was not related to combat exposure. Adding to the educational and conceptual limitations is the cultural psychological tolerance of these symptoms by members of the older generation. Given that mental health care is a relatively newer specialty and given the limitations of effective treatments during its formative years, older generations may have been less inclined to describe, discuss, and present for treatment of psychological symptoms (van Zelst et al. 2003).

Some older PTSD patients have significantly delayed onset of symptoms activated by later life events. Growing older may present challenges to mortality and autonomy either through personal illness or through witnessed illness and death within a peer group. This confrontation with mortality may resonate with an earlier life event, leading to threshold symptomatology (Hickey et al. 2008a). In some patients with memory loss due to a dementia process, psychological defense mechanisms may atrophy and more primitive psychological processes may no longer be able to contend with a prior traumatic experience (Ruzich et al. 2005).

In some geriatric patients, PTSD may have been present during their earlier years but then resolved. Although the syndrome may no longer be of clinical concern, contemporary theories help the clinician appreciate the patient's life experience and be vigilant for any reactivation later in life. Other patients, however, have persistent PTSD symptoms that continue to be a source of emotional pain and disability.

In summary, PTSD can be associated with earlier- or later-life trauma and can present at various points during the life cycle. Providers should be mindful of the various unique factors that an older person may present in the context of posttraumatic psychological effects.

Presentation of PTSD

Physiological, psychological, and social aspects that are unique to older persons may alter the presentation of PTSD as it is currently described, thereby clouding diagnostic accuracy and potentially having implications for treatment. Sensitivity in data collection and patient communication must account for these factors in the management of older patients with PTSD.

PTSD has been associated with several biological changes in adults. Compared with younger adults, those over age 65 have both less diurnal variation of and overall levels for serum cortisol, although the clinical relevance of this change is unknown (van der Hal-Van Raalte et al. 2008). Older patients with PTSD may have elevations in serum lipids compared with non-PTSD patients; these elevations may increase the risk of cardiovascular events and further debility (Jakovljevic et al. 2006). As people age, central nervous system dopamine and serotonin levels can decrease, and norepinephrine may increase (Busse et al. 2004). These changes could theoretically alter autonomic hyperactivity seen in some patients with PTSD and may result in varied efficacy of selective serotonin reuptake inhibitor (SSRI) and adrenergic antagonist therapies. A paucity of data to delineate the significance of these findings underscores the need for further research, and extrapolating data from younger study samples has potential pitfalls.

Later life development can be characterized by a need to integrate experiences to negotiate confrontation of mortality. Traumatic experiences and subsequent symptoms in older persons may occur with greater reference context than in younger persons or may become indistinguishable from despair brought on by failure of this stage of development in the life cycle. Either way, symptoms may become clouded in existential challenges intrinsic to this age group.

During the twentieth century, many dramatic historical events occurred. The two world wars encompassed and polarized the globe. Absolute resolve was required for victory, with little room for doubt, debate, or tolerance. Public sacrifice may have been more ubiquitous than in recent conflicts, and a sense of common purpose held a greater importance than the needs of any one individual. This sense of community spread through the following decades, leading to rapid social development toward minority rights and women's equality. Contemporary ambiguities and instantaneous global communications have blurred borders and boundaries. Older persons may find the delineations of the middle parts of the twentieth century more familiar and may not feel well understood by the younger generation. The sense of purpose, control, and integration within social context may mitigate tolerance of or presentation of posttraumatic symptoms (Averill and Beck 2000). Older patients may not be as accepting of having their personal needs attended to in the form of mental health treatment and thus may be less likely to disclose psychiatric distress. Ongoing symptomatology may seem less significant to an older person, and providers should be attuned to the need for helping patients to recognize the need for and to accept assistance. Minimization of symptoms may be rooted not in denial but rather in the notion of self-sacrifice of one's needs as a societal norm.

Pharmacological Treatments

SSRIs and Other Medications

SSRIs are the most extensively studied pharmacological treatment of PTSD and are frequently a first-line therapy (Ursano et al. 2004). Sertraline and paroxetine have been approved by the U.S. Food and Drug Administration for treatment of PTSD, and fluoxetine has shown promise in a randomized trial (Martenyi et al. 2002). Unfortunately, studies involving these agents have not included sufficient numbers of patients over age 65 to adequately assess efficacy or tolerability in this population. Due to an altering risk-benefit ratio as people age, extrapolation of data based on younger patients is potentially flawed. Older patients may be at an elevated risk for hyponatremia secondary to the syndrome of inappropriate antidiuretic hormone secretion (Wilkinson et al. 1999). SSRIs may worsen bleeding risk, especially in patients taking anticoagulation medications, including nonsteroidal anti-inflammatory drugs; this problem is more likely to be encountered in the geriatric population. Paroxetine has significant anticholinergic properties that may exacerbate various medical illnesses, such as urinary retention, chronic constipation, sicca syndrome, dementia syndromes, and visual impairment. Both fluoxetine and paroxetine are inhibitors of cytochrome P450 2D6 and may affect serum levels of other medications that rely on this pathway for metabolism (Wynn et al. 2009).

Though not specifically evaluated in geriatric patients, tricyclic antidepressants for treatment of PTSD have been studied in a few small randomized controlled trials (Southwick et al. 1994). Although imipramine and amitriptyline may offer some symptom relief for patients, their receptor profile may increase the risk of toxicity in elderly individuals. Strong anticholinergic properties have the same pitfalls as mentioned in the previous paragraph. Peripheral alpha-receptor antagonism may potentiate risks of orthostasis and subsequent falls. Antihistaminic properties may cause intractable sedation.

Finally, tricyclic antidepressants may increase mortality in patients with existing ischemic heart disease (Taylor 2008).

Novel antidepressants, such as serotonin-norepinephrine reuptake inhibitors or dopamine-norepinephrine reuptake inhibitors, lack sufficient data demonstrating efficacy in treating PTSD and are not currently recommended. Providers who choose to use these agents should be mindful of potential drug interactions, as seen with nefazodone; orthostasis, as seen with trazodone; and noradrenergic effects of worsening narrow-angle glaucoma, urinary hesitancy, or blood pressure elevations, as might occur with venlafaxine, duloxetine, and desvenlafaxine.

Benzodiazepines are often used in the treatment of PTSD, but few data demonstrate efficacy for this indication. When given benzodiazepines, elderly patients are especially prone to sedation and have an elevated risk of falls with subsequent hip fractures (Cumming and Le Couteur 2003). Use of benzodiazepines for the treatment of PTSD in geriatric populations should be minimal.

The use of antipsychotics, particularly quetiapine, has grown in popularity for the treatment of PTSD, despite a paucity of supportive data (Gao et al. 2006). Their use in the elderly for off-label indications is common, particularly in institutional settings. Atypical antipsychotics are associated with a 1.6- to 1.7-fold increased mortality risk when used in patients with dementia-related psychosis. Observational studies suggest that conventional antipsychotics also hold an elevated mortality risk in elderly patients with dementia-related psychosis. Whether this mortality risk can be extrapolated to all patients over age 65 is unknown, but given the uncertain benefit of antipsychotics in treating PTSD, caution is advisable when considering their use for this condition in the elderly.

Prazosin

The lipophilic alpha-1 antagonist prazosin has received much attention as an effective treatment for certain symptom domains of PTSD. Raskind et al. (2000, 2002) demonstrated the safe use of prazosin in a group of combat veterans ranging in age from 67 to 83 years. In this group, the research demonstrated a significant reduction in scores on the Clinician-Administered PTSD Scale (CAPS) nightmare subscale and the Clinical Global Impression Change Scale (CIG-C) with relatively small dosages of prazosin. Furthermore, the patients did not experience any adverse events, including orthostatic hypotension, from taking the medication. These results persisted as long as patients continued taking the medication. The results for the older veterans were similar to those for other groups of patients studied, including middle-aged combat veterans and young patients with PTSD due to civilian trauma.

Clinicians can consider prazosin as a possibly effective treatment for geriatric patients with PTSD, particularly to help with sleep disturbances and nightmares related to the trauma. Clinicians should be aware, however, that prazosin has several side effects that can be dangerous for older individuals. In particular, orthostatic hypotension due to peripheral alpha-1 antagonism can lead to syncope or falls, which are a leading cause of morbidity and mortality in the elderly population.

Cognitive-Based Therapies

Cognitive-based therapies have proven to be some of the most effective treatments for PTSD (Bisson and Andrew 2007; Monson et al. 2006; Resick and Schnicke 1992). However, very little research has been done on the use of cognitive-behavioral therapy (CBT) or cognitive processing therapy (CPT) in geriatric populations. A Medline search using the terms *CBT* or *CPT* and *geriatric* or *elderly* revealed no studies that specifically examined this population. Although the efficacy of the cognitive-based treatments is well established, clinicians should be very careful regarding using these treatments with older patients. Geriatric patients with preserved cognitive functioning may benefit from CBT or CPT; however, geriatric patients with mild cognitive impairment or dementia may not be able to adapt to and apply the treatments. Further research with geriatric populations to assess the effectiveness of these treatments is warranted.

Exposure-Based Therapies

Exposure-based therapies, whether imaginal or virtual reality–based, demonstrate good effectiveness in the treatment of combat-related PTSD as well as civilian-based PTSD (Bisson and Andrew 2007). Although no studies have been done to demonstrate the effectiveness of exposure-based therapies in a geriatric population, studies using exposure treatments have been done in aging Vietnam veterans. It may be reasonable to try exposure-based treatments in elderly patients. Due to its less technological nature, imaginal exposure may be better tolerated than virtual reality–based exposure by older generations.

Eye Movement Desensitization and Reprocessing

Eye movement desensitization and reprocessing (EMDR) is a psychotherapy technique developed by Shapiro (1996, 2001) to treat trauma-related disorders. As an intervention, it has demonstrated effectiveness in treating PTSD in numerous well-controlled trials and in comparison with other types of psychotherapy, including trauma-focused CBT (Bisson 2007; Bisson and Andrew 2007). EMDR uses a structured eight-phase approach and addresses the past, present, and future aspects of the dysfunctional stored memory. Although much research into this technique has been done in civilian trauma, particularly sexual assault, and combat-related trauma, none of the research evidence focuses exclusively on geriatric patients. Despite this paucity of research with elderly patients, it is reasonable to assume that a cognitively intact older adult with PTSD may benefit from EMDR.

Key Clinical Points

- When treating elderly patients, providers should be aware of the significant physiological changes associated with aging and adjust interventions as necessary.
- Elderly patients are more likely to experience delirium, which may amplify the effects of PTSD and potentially contribute to PTSD symptom development.
- Age-related cognitive changes may lead to the atrophy of psychological defense, with resulting manifestation of previous traumatic experiences.
- Pharmacological interventions for elderly patients should always take into account the physiological changes that occur with age.
- Providers of therapy for elderly patients will likely need to integrate features specific to the geriatric developmental stage, including end-of-life issues.

References

Andrews G, Henderson S, Hall W: Prevalence, comorbidity, disability and service utilisation: overview of the Australian National Mental Health Survey. Br J Psychiatry 178:145–153, 2001

Averill PM, Beck JG: Posttraumatic stress disorder in older adults: a conceptual review. J Anxiety Disord 14:133–156, 2000

Bisson J: Eye movement desensitisation and reprocessing reduces PTSD symptoms compared with fluoxetine at six months post-treatment. Evid Based Ment Health 10:118, 2007

Bisson J, Andrew M: Psychological treatment of post-traumatic stress disorder (PTSD). Cochrane Database Syst Rev CD003388, 2007

Busse EW, Blazer DG, Steffens DC (eds): The American Psychiatric Publishing Textbook of Geriatric Psychiatry, 3rd Edition. Washington, DC, American Psychiatric Publishing, 2004

Creamer M, Parslow R: Trauma exposure and posttraumatic stress disorder in the elderly: a community prevalence study. Am J Geriatr Psychiatry 16:853–856, 2008

Cumming RG, Le Couteur DG: Benzodiazepines and risk of hip fractures in older people: a review of the evidence. CNS Drugs 17:825–837, 2003

Day JC: Population projections of the United States, by age, sex, race, and Hispanic origin: 1993–2050 (Current Population Reports; series P25, no 1104). Washington, DC, U.S. Department of Commerce, Bureau of the Census, 1993

Gao K, Muzina D, Gajwani P, et al: Efficacy of typical and atypical antipsychotics for primary and comorbid anxiety symptoms or disorders: a review. J Clin Psychiatry 67:1327–1340, 2006

Gum AM, King-Kallimanis B, Kohn R: Prevalence of mood, anxiety, and substance-abuse disorders for older Americans in the National Comorbidity Survey-Replication. Am J Geriatr Psychiatry 17:769–781, 2009

Hiskey S, Luckie M, Davies S, et al: The emergence of posttraumatic distress in later life: a review. J Geriatr Psychiatry Neurol 21:232–241, 2008a

Hiskey S, Luckie M, Davies S, et al: The phenomenology of reactivated trauma memories in older adults: a preliminary study. Aging Ment Health 12:494–498, 2008b

Jackson J, Hart R, Gordon S, et al: Post-traumatic stress disorder and post-traumatic stress symptoms following critical illness in medical intensive care unit patients: assessing the magnitude of the problem. Crit Care 11:R27, 2007

Jakovljevic M, Saric M, Nad S, et al: Metabolic syndrome, somatic and psychiatric comorbidity in war veterans with post-traumatic stress disorder: preliminary findings. Psychiatr Danub 18:169–176, 2006

Martenyi F, Brown EB, Zhang H, et al: Fluoxetine versus placebo in posttraumatic stress disorder. J Clin Psychiatry 63:199–206, 2002

Monson CM, Schnurr PP, Resick PA, et al: Cognitive processing therapy for veterans with military-related posttraumatic stress disorder. J Consult Clin Psychol 74:898–907, 2006

Raskind MA, Dobie DJ, Kanter ED, et al: The alpha1-adrenergic antagonist prazosin ameliorates combat trauma nightmares in veterans with posttraumatic stress disorder: a report of 4 cases. J Clin Psychiatry 61:129–133, 2000

Raskind MA, Thompson C, Petrie EC, et al: Prazosin reduces nightmares in combat veterans with posttraumatic stress disorder. J Clin Psychiatry 63:565–568, 2002

Resick PA, Schnicke MK: Cognitive processing therapy for sexual assault victims. J Consult Clin Psychol 60:748–756, 1992

Ruzich MJ, Looi J, Robertson MD: Delayed onset of posttraumatic stress disorder among male combat veterans: a case series. Am J Geriatr Psychiatry 13:424–427, 2005

Shapiro F: Eye movement desensitization and reprocessing (EMDR): evaluation of controlled PTSD research. J Behav Ther Exp Psychiatry 27:209–218, 1996

Shapiro F: Eye Movement Desensitization and Reprocessing: Basic Principles, Protocols and Procedures, 2nd Edition. New York, Guilford, 2001

Southwick SM, Yehuda R, Giller EL Jr, et al: Use of tricyclics and monoamine oxidase inhibitors in the treatment of PTSD: a quantitative review. Progress in Psychiatry 42:293–305, 1994

Taylor D: Antidepressant drugs and cardiovascular pathology: a clinical overview of effectiveness and safety. Acta Psychiatr Scand 118:434–442, 2008

Ursano RJ, Bell C, Eth S, et al: Practice guideline for the treatment of patients with acute stress disorder and posttraumatic stress disorder. Am J Psychiatry 161 (suppl 11):3–31, 2004

van der Hal-Van Raalte EA, Bakermansa-Kranenburg MJ, van Ijzendoorn MH, et al: Diurnal cortisol patterns and stress reactivity in child Holocaust survivors reaching old age. Aging Ment Health 12:630–638, 2008

van Zelst WH, de Beurs E, Beekman A, et al: Prevalence and risk factors of posttraumatic stress disorder in older adults. Psychother Psychosom 72:333–342, 2003

Weintraub D, Ruskin PE: Posttraumatic stress disorder in the elderly: a review. Harv Rev Psychiatry 7:144–152, 1999

Wikman A, Bhattacharyya M, Perkins-Porras L, et al: Persistence of posttraumatic stress symptoms 12 and 36 months after acute coronary syndrome. Psychosom Med 70:764–772, 2008

Wilkinson TJ, Begg EJ, Winter AC, et al: Incidence and risk factors for hyponatraemia following treatment with fluoxetine or paroxetine in elderly people. Br J Clin Pharmacol 47:211–217, 1999

Wynn GH, Oesterheld JR, Cozza KL, et al: Clinical Manual of Drug Interaction Principles for Medical Practice. Washington, DC, American Psychiatric Publishing, 2009

15

Traumatic Brain Injury

Louis M. French, Psy.D.
Grant L. Iverson, Ph.D.
Richard A. Bryant, Ph.D.

Traumatic brain injury (TBI) is a major public health concern. The Centers for Disease Control and Prevention (CDC; 2008) estimated that about 1.1% of the U.S. civilian population, or roughly 3.2 million people, are living with long-term disability due to TBI. These estimates largely reflect those persons who have experienced more severe TBIs. However, much more common is mild TBI (i.e., concussion), which is sometimes excluded from epidemiological studies concerning TBI. Although in the vast majority of cases, these mild TBIs have no obvious enduring consequences, a minority of individuals will have persistent difficulties, which may relate to comorbid conditions. Posttraumatic stress disorder (PTSD) is one possible such condition.

Interest in TBI research has been fueled by the growth in military casualties, resulting largely from the conflicts in Iraq and Afghanistan. The most frequent cause of TBI in service members has been the explosive device. Explosive devices inflict injuries through a number of mechanisms, including metallic fragments, the displacement of the individual through the air, the displacement of objects against the person, or the pressure or thermal blast wave itself. Emotional consequences of the effects of the blast are also possible, either as a result of the injury or because of witnessing other military personnel and/or civilians sustaining injuries.

Overview of Traumatic Brain Injury

TBIs occur as a result of open or closed head injuries. The vast majority of TBIs are closed. TBIs occur as the result of acceleration-deceleration forces, blunt trauma, or both. These injuries occur across a broad spectrum of severity, ranging from very mild and transient effects to catastrophic injuries, which can result in death or long-term disability.

TBIs are often graded by severity using scores on the Glasgow Coma Scale (mild = 13–15; moderate = 9–12; severe = 3–8). However, there is no universal agreement on which specific severity criteria should be used (e.g., duration of loss of consciousness [LOC] and posttraumatic amnesia). A commonly used classification system for mild, moderate, and severe TBI is summarized in Table 15–1. The classification system officially adopted by the U.S. Department of Defense is summarized in Table 15–2.

Although many regions of the brain are vulnerable to the pathophysiology arising from TBI, the anterior portions of the brain (i.e., frontal and temporal regions) are most susceptible to neurological insult. Primary and secondary pathophysiologies contribute to TBI-associated cognitive and neurobehavioral impairment. Primary damage involves axonal injury, vascular injury, contusions, and hemorrhage. Secondary damage arises from the endogenous evolution of cellular damage or from secondary systemic processes, such as hypotension or hypoxia. Endogenous secondary pathophysiologies include 1) ischemia, excitotoxicity, energy failure, and cell death cascades (e.g., necrosis and apoptosis); 2) edema; 3) traumatic axonal injury; and 4) inflammation (Kochanek et al. 2007).

Macroscopic abnormalities within brain tissue or outside the brain (i.e., extra-axial space) can be identified using neuroimaging (e.g., magnetic resonance imaging [MRI]). Such injuries include, but are not limited to,

Table 15–1. Common classification system for traumatic brain injury[a]

Classification	Duration of unconsciousness	Glasgow Coma Scale score	Posttraumatic amnesia
Mild	<30 minutes	13–15[b]	<24 hours
Moderate	30 minutes–24 hours	9–12	1–7 days
Severe	>24 hours	3–8	>7 days

[a]This is not a universally agreed-upon classification system.
[b]Lowest Glasgow Coma Scale score obtained 30 minutes or more postinjury.

Table 15–2. U.S. Department of Defense traumatic brain injury classification system

Classification	Duration of unconsciousness	Alteration of consciousness	Posttraumatic amnesia
Mild	<30 minutes	A moment to 24 hours	<24 hours
Moderate	30 minutes–24 hours	If >24 hours, then severity based on other criteria	1–7 days
Severe	>24 hours		>7 days

hemorrhagic contusions, nonhemorrhagic contusions, hemorrhagic or nonhemorrhagic shearing injuries, herniations, and cerebral edema. Extra-axial manifestations of injury include epidural hematomas, subdural hematomas, subdural hygromas, subarachnoid hemorrhage, intraventricular hemorrhage, and hydrocephalus (Barkley et al. 2007).

A common postacute finding in patients who sustain severe TBIs is white matter atrophy (Bigler 2005; Charness 1993; Huisman et al. 2004; Inglese et al. 2005a; MacKenzie et al. 2002; McAllister et al. 2001; Nakayama et al. 2006). White matter injuries can be identified using quantitative imaging methods targeting the corpus callosum (Adams et al. 1980; Arfanakis et al. 2002; Gorrie et al. 2001; Inglese et al. 2005b; Levin 2003; Levin et al. 1990; Salmond et al. 2006; Sundgren et al. 2004) and other vulnerable regions, such as the genu and splenium (Huisman et al. 2004; Le et al. 2005; Nakayama et al. 2006; Wilde et al. 2006).

Diffusion tensor imaging is a high-resolution MRI technique that exploits the fact that myelin sheaths and cell membranes of white matter tracts restrict the movement of water molecules. Because water molecules often travel the length of axons, the technology can create images of the axons. Studies using diffusion tensor imaging have consistently found decreases in white matter integrity of the corpus callosum in patients following TBI relative to healthy control subjects (Inglese et al. 2005b; Miles et al. 2008; Nakayama et al. 2006; Wilde et al. 2006). Diffusion tensor imaging has been used to assess white matter abnormalities following mild TBI (Rutgers et al. 2008), the length of white matter changes in patients with mild TBI (Rutgers et al. 2008), and the correlation between white matter damage and simple reaction time (Niogi et al. 2007). Researchers have suggested that more severe forms of mild TBI may affect the structural integrity of axons within the genu of the corpus callosum, resulting in reduced functional anisotropy (possibly arising from misalignment of fibers, edema, fiber disruption, or axonal degeneration).

Injuries on the mild end of the mild-TBI spectrum are likely associated with low levels of axonal stretching, resulting in only temporary changes in neurophysiology. Giza and Hovda (2004) described a model, conceptualized as a multilayered neurometabolic cascade, for the complex interwoven cellular and vascular changes following concussive forces applied to the brain. The neurobiology involves ionic shifts, abnormal energy metabolism, diminished cerebral blood flow, and impaired neurotransmission. Fortunately, for the vast majority of affected cells, there appears to be a reversible series of neurometabolic events (Giza and Hovda 2001, 2004; Iverson 2005; Iverson et al. 2007). The ultimate fate of neurons relates to the extent of traumatic axonal injury, which can culminate in secondary axotomy (see Buki and Povlishock 2006 for a summary). In general, however, most injured cells do not undergo secondary axotomy and appear to recover normal cellular function. In other words, for most individuals who sustain a mild TBI, it appears that the brain undergoes dynamic restoration and, in due course, individuals return to normal functioning.

Shared Neurobiology

Other chapters in this textbook describe in some detail the underlying brain changes associated with PTSD. This section will examine some of the relations between purported underlying brain mechanisms associated with PTSD and characteristic structural and biochemical changes associated with TBI.

As noted above, the most frequently affected sites of the brain following traumatic injury are the frontal and temporal lobes. Subcortical structures such as the hippocampus and amygdala, and their cortical connections, are also vulnerable. Previous data have suggested that PTSD is associated with over-activation of the amygdala, due to diminished inhibitory control by the ventromedial prefrontal cortex. Koenigs et al. (2008) reexamined individuals with penetrating TBIs who participated in the Vietnam Head Injury Study during the late 1980s. In the study they underwent two analyses. One of the analyses grouped veterans with brain injuries according to presence or absence of a PTSD diagnosis and then compared pathophysiology between the two groups. The second analysis grouped individuals by lesion location and subsequently compared the prevalence of PTSD between groups.

According to these analyses, lesions in either the ventromedial prefrontal cortex or the amygdala were associated with lower rates of PTSD (perhaps due to a reduction of overall symptom intensity). These findings suggest a somewhat different role of the ventromedial prefrontal cortex than previously reported, since ventromedial prefrontal cortex damage was not associated with greater prevalence of PTSD. However, these findings support the idea of amygdala hyperactivity playing an integral role in the model. Thus, the role of the ventromedial prefrontal cortex is to reactivate emotional states associated with past experiences. Accordingly, treatments aimed at selectively inhibiting the function of the amygdala or the ventromedial prefrontal cortex may be effective in treating PTSD.

Bryant et al. (2008) reported that acute administration of morphine had some independent protective effects against PTSD severity (but not PTSD diagnosis) (see also Saxe et al. 2001). The purported mechanism underlying this effect is morphine attenuating the production of norepinephrine and consequently attenuating the fear conditioning response. However, the influence of morphine on other neurotransmitter systems might also be contributing to this effect. Namely, neurotransmitter changes after TBI are widespread and involve the catecholamines, serotonin, and acetylcholine. One such change is a marked increase in plasma norepinephrine following acute brain injury.

Some data suggest that the early increase in norepinephrine release following cerebral contusion is protective through stabilization of the blood–brain barrier in areas adjacent to the injury site. Accordingly, drugs that interfere with this enhanced noradrenergic function might enhance the damage caused by TBI (Dunn-Meynell et al. 1998). This possibility suggests that strategies utilized to treat one condition (PTSD or TBI) may have unintended consequences on recovery from the other.

TBI and PTSD Comorbidity

The extent to which individuals who have sustained TBIs with associated LOC can also meet criteria for PTSD remains controversial in the literature. Proponents on one side of the debate argue that individuals who cannot recall the traumatic event because of LOC or amnesia should not be able to later recall the event via flashbacks or intrusive recollections. Thus, such individuals with marked amnesia around the time of the event are at relatively low risk for developing PTSD (Bombardier et al. 2006; Levin et al. 2001; Sbordone and Liter 1995).

Some empirical support exists for this viewpoint. For example, Warden and Labbate (2005) followed 47 active-duty service members who sustained moderate TBIs and who had neurogenic amnesia for the event. None developed full criteria for PTSD, although some individuals appeared to develop a PTSD-like anxiety disorder. In a related study, Gil et al. (2005) conducted a prospective examination of 120 civilians who sustained TBIs; individuals who reported amnesia for the event were unlikely to develop PTSD. Similarly, Glaesser et al. (2004) examined 46 patients who had experienced TBI due to accidents with variable extents of unconsciousness. The authors reported that 27% of patients with TBI but no extended LOC developed PTSD, whereas only 3% who were unconscious for more than 12 hours developed the disorder. Furthermore, intrusive memories were more common among participants who had not been unconscious; these participants were also more likely to reexperience symptoms, experience marked psychological distress, and evidence physiological reactivity to antecedent stimuli associated with the traumatic event. Thus, based on limited findings, having neurogenic amnesia for the event appears to provide some protection from developing PTSD (Klein et al. 2003).

Proponents on the opposite side of the debate maintain that the anxiety response is activated in some individuals despite the occurrence of memory impairment. Therefore, according to them, PTSD can exist as a comorbid condition with TBI (Harvey and Bryant 2000; Hickling et al. 1998; Mather et al. 2003; Mayou et al. 2000). From this perspective, PTSD can develop following TBI via several possible mechanisms. First, fear conditioning models of PTSD posit that extreme fear at the time of trauma is conditioned with events and experiences occurring at the time of the event, and these associations between trauma reminders and anxiety responses fuel subsequent PTSD (Rauch et al. 2006). Fear conditioning may occur with varying levels of awareness of the contingency between the trauma and consequences, which may allow for some fear conditioning following TBI. Consistent with this perspective, some evidence suggests that people can develop PTSD following severe TBI, even though these patients do not recall the trauma and do not have intrusive memories of the event (Bryant et al. 2000).

Second, following TBI, people can reconstruct traumatic experiences in ways permitting them to compensate for impaired memory. In one prospective study, patients with mild TBI following motor vehicle accidents were assessed for event memory immediately after the accident and again 2 years later. Although all patients initially reported amnesia of some aspect of the accident, at the 2-year reassessment, 40% reported they had subsequently achieved full recall of the experience (Harvey and Bryant 2001). Supporting this view, case studies have illustrated how reconstructed memories can fuel PTSD. In one case, a man developed PTSD 12 months after his severe TBI when he was directed to resume driving; he developed distressing and intrusive images of his accident based on a newspaper photograph of his wrecked car. Although he was densely amnesic of the accident, he developed a series of images founded on his memory of the photograph (Bryant 1996). The intrusive images of people who reconstruct memories in the absence of recall and of people who have not sustained a TBI and have full recall appear to have little qualitative difference. Bryant and Harvey (1998) compared the intrusive imagery of motor vehicle survivors who 1) had PTSD and no TBI, or 2) had PTSD following severe TBI and reported intrusive memories inconsistent with objective reports of the accident, or 3) had no PTSD. All participants were asked to listen to an audiotape of a car crash sound effect and were then interviewed about cognitive and emotional responses. When these responses were independently rated on a range of constructs, PTSD participants with and without TBI reported comparable levels of vivid imagery, emotional response, involuntariness, and sense of reality. This finding highlights that reconstructed memories in patients who have sustained TBIs can be subjectively compelling and share many of the memory attributes experienced by people with continuous recall of their trauma.

A third possible mechanism for PTSD to develop following TBI is to sustain a TBI and then suffer traumatic experiences following resolution of posttraumatic amnesia. For example, a motor vehicle accident victim may be unconscious at the time of the impact but have full recall of waiting for the ambulance to arrive or of being admitted to an emergency room. These experiences can be sufficiently associated with distressing affect to contribute to PTSD symptoms.

A fourth possible mechanism involves dysfunctional neural functioning secondary to the TBI. Prevailing biological models of PTSD propose exaggerated amygdala response associated with diminished regulation by the medial prefrontal cortex (Rauch et al. 2006). The amygdala is central to the development and expression of conditioned fear reactions, and human and animal studies have shown that learning to inhibit these fear reactions involves inhibition by the medial prefrontal cortex. Consistent with this model, patients with PTSD have diminished medial prefrontal cortex activation during processing of fear (Lanius et al. 2006). As noted above, TBI often involves damage to the prefrontal cortex. An individual's capacity to regulate his or her fear reaction may be impaired after a mild TBI because of damage to the neural networks involved in regulation of anxiety (Bryant 2008).

A final possible mechanism involves the compounding effect of stressors that occur following the precipitating trauma (Bryant and Harvey 1995; L.A. King et al. 1998). The difficulties experienced as a result of TBI may contribute to the development of PTSD.

Relevant to this discussion, Parker (2002) argued that diagnostic categories for comorbid PTSD and TBI in the *Diagnostic and Statistical Manual of Mental Disorders,* 4th Edition, Text Revision (DSM-IV-TR; American Psychiatric Association 2000), are much too narrow. Among his suggested changes was elimination of the criterion requiring memory for the actual event, because PTSD can occur without explicit memory. Likewise, he suggested that the diagnosis of PTSD should not require simultaneous expression of all DSM criteria, A–F. He felt that disability should not necessarily be a defining characteristic because impaired social or occupational functioning may not be present in all affected patients. Rather, he stressed the importance of carefully describing all relevant factors, including the nature of the sustained injury (or injuries), pain, and other symptoms, because these may compound physiological and/or psychological trauma, ultimately reducing the quality of outcomes.

Other authors maintain that substantial overlap of current diagnostic criteria makes accurate diagnosis difficult. Sumpter and McMillan (2006), for example, cautioned readers against misdiagnosing PTSD after TBI. In an examination of a series of individuals with severe TBI, they found a number of overlapping (nonspecific) symptoms, which include insomnia, irritability, and impaired concentration. Given shared symptoms, PTSD can be misdiagnosed when screening only with questionnaires. For example, items such as "avoidance of thoughts or activities" can be interpreted differently within the context of cognitive and functional sequelae of TBI. Although these data suggest that PTSD can be misdiagnosed in persons with more severe TBI, these findings may not be generalizable to milder TBI.

Complicating the diagnostic process is the overall lack of specific criteria for postconcussive symptoms. For example, postconcussive symptoms are endorsed by healthy adults (Gouvier et al. 1988; Iverson and Lange 2003; Kashluba et al. 2006; Machulda et al. 1998; Mittenberg et al. 1992; Sawchyn et al. 2000; Trahan et al. 2001; Wong et al. 1994), by individuals with acute trauma without brain injury (Meares et al. 2008), and by individuals in other clinical groups (Fox et al. 1995; Gasquoine 2000; Iverson and McCracken 1997; Iverson et al. 2007; Lees-Haley and Brown 1993; Mickeviciene et al.

2004; Radanov et al. 1992; Smith-Seemiller et al. 2003). Meares et al. (2008) reported postconcussive symptoms associated with increased levels of posttraumatic stress. These authors suggested that postconcussive symptoms may actually increase the likelihood of developing PTSD because these symptoms interfere with adequate adjustment to the event. This conceptual orientation is consistent with Bryant and Harvey's (1999) model.

Schneiderman et al. (2008) examined a cross-section of military personnel following deployment to Iraq or Afghanistan and reported a 12% rate of mild TBI and an 11% rate of PTSD. Factors associated with PTSD included service in Iraq, female gender, multiple injury mechanisms, and mild TBI. Of the 275 individuals categorized as having sustained a mild TBI while in the theater of operations, 35% reported three or more concurrent neuropsychiatric symptoms, which they attributed to "a possible head injury or concussion." When persons with mild TBI were dichotomized into two levels of severity, those with more severe TBI had more PTSD symptoms. Specifically, PTSD was more common for those individuals reporting three or more neuropsychiatric symptoms, which they attributed to their TBI.

In a review of the U.S. Navy–Marine Corps Combat Trauma Registry, with an associated short-term follow-up (Galarneau et al. 2008), those service members with more severe TBI had higher morbidity and medical utilization. However, mental health conditions were more likely among patients with milder TBI. In those individuals diagnosed with PTSD based on ICD-9 criteria (World Health Organization 1977), the diagnosis accounted for a larger percentage of all mental health conditions among those who had sustained a mild TBI (2.5% of diagnoses) than among those with a moderate to severe TBI (0.2% of diagnoses). According to Gil et al. (2005), risk factors for development of PTSD following TBI include memory of the event, prior psychiatric history, and the development of acute stress symptoms within 1 week of the event.

In those individuals with polytrauma, TBI may affect recovery from other injuries or, conversely, the other injuries and their associated factors may retard the natural recovery from even mild TBI. Minimal extracranial injuries and low pain predict better outcomes for return to work after mild TBI (Stulemeijer et al. 2006). Patients who have both symptoms following mild TBI and symptoms of PTSD often present with significant clinical challenges.

Hoge et al. (2008) examined mild TBI and psychiatric symptoms in U.S. soldiers following a year-long deployment to Iraq. In a survey administered about 3 months after their return, service members answered questions about their deployment, including whether they sustained a mild TBI or other injuries while deployed. PTSD was strongly associated with mild TBI, such that 44% of the soldiers who had injuries with LOC met criteria for PTSD. Of those who met criteria for PTSD, about 27% reported an alteration in consciousness subsequent to the event, about 16% endorsed sustaining other types of injuries, and about 9% reported having no other injuries. Those soldiers who reported mild TBI, especially with LOC, were more likely to report poor general health, more days of missed work, an increased number of medical visits, and a higher number of somatic and postconcussive symptoms than were soldiers with other injuries. Depression was more frequent in those with LOC than in those with other injuries. However, after adjustment for PTSD and depression, the occurrence of mild TBI was no longer significantly associated with these physical concerns (except for headache in the LOC group).

The Hoge et al. (2008) study underscores the important relationship between somatic and psychological symptoms. In an accompanying editorial, Bryant (2008) suggested that—consistent with the model proffered by Kennedy et al. (2007)—damage to the prefrontal cortex in TBI results in disruption of neural networks involved in the regulation of anxiety, making the affected individual more vulnerable to the effects of an emotionally traumatic event. Furthermore, PTSD may also be perpetuated by the impaired cognition of TBI.

Neuropsychological Features

Severe TBIs are associated with persistent neuropsychological impairments, functional disability, and poor return-to-work rates (Dikmen et al. 1993, 1994). Those who sustain severe TBIs are at risk for moderate to severe disability. Despite this risk, a substantial percentage also experience good recovery.

As a rule, the vast majority of recovery from moderate or severe TBI occurs within the first year, with some additional recovery occurring during the second year. Substantial functional improvements due to neuroplasticity are not realistic for most patients after 2 years. However, improvement in functioning can occur through learned accommodations and compensatory strategies.

Neurobehavioral changes associated with TBI include personality changes, emotional dysregulation, apathy, disinhibition, and anosognosia (awareness deficits). Impairments in cognition are most notable in attention, concentration, working memory, speed of processing, and memory (Dikmen et al. 1986, 1995, 2001, 2003; Iverson 2005; Lezak et al. 2004; Mearns and Lees-Haley 1993; Spikman et al. 1999; Whyte et al. 2000). However, cognitive impairment following TBI is difficult to predict. In general, those with severe TBIs are more likely to have some degree of persisting impairment, and those with mild TBIs are less likely to experience persisting impairment (Dikmen et al. 1995, 2001; Schretlen and Shapiro 2003).

Mild TBIs can be associated with obvious cognitive impairment and pronounced postconcussive symptoms in the initial days and sometimes weeks following injury (Bleiberg et al. 2004; Hughes et al. 2004; Lovell et al. 2004; Macciocchi et al. 1996; McCrea et al. 2002, 2003). Due to natural recovery, most patients do not experience measurable cognitive impairment beyond a few months postinjury (e.g., Bijur et al. 1990; Dikmen et al. 1995, 2001; Fay et al. 1993; Gentilini et al. 1985; Goldstein et al. 2001; Lahmeyer and Bellur 1987; Ponsford et al. 2000). Several meta-analyses (Belanger et al. 2005; Binder 1997; Schretlen and Shapiro 2003) and reviews (Carroll et al. 2004; Iverson 2005; Iverson et al. 2007; Ruff 2005) of this literature are available and, as a rule, report very good neuropsychological outcome following mild TBI.

Despite more than two decades of research with diverse clinical groups, it remains unclear whether PTSD results in measurable neurocognitive deficits or diminishment. Some researchers have reported that compared with healthy adults, patients with PTSD perform more poorly on neuropsychological tests (Buckley et al. 2000; Jelinek et al. 2006; Jenkins et al. 2000). The most consistent finding has been worse performance on tests of verbal learning and memory (Bremner et al. 1993, 1995; Sutker et al. 1992; Vasterling et al. 1998; Yehuda et al. 1995). In contrast, some researchers have not found neurocognitive decrements associated with PTSD (Crowell et al. 2002; Stein et al. 1999; Twamley et al. 2004).

Researchers often emphasize methodological issues and problems that might mimic or obscure the true relationship between PTSD and neurocognitive diminishment (Danckwerts and Leathem 2003; Horner and Hamner 2002). Most notably, co-occurring conditions such as depression and substance abuse are also associated with reduced performance on neuropsychological testing; including patients with these comorbidities in clinical samples might result in over-attributing cognitive decrements to PTSD.

In a meta-analysis of the MRI literature, Kitayama et al. (2005) concluded that an association exists between PTSD and smaller hippocampal volume. In a meta-analysis of the memory literature, Brewin et al. (2007) reported that samples of patients with PTSD showed a small decrement in memory functioning (i.e., an effect size of 0.2). Those with PTSD had a slightly greater decrement in verbal memory (i.e., an effect size of 0.3), although the magnitude of this decrement was also small. In both meta-analyses, the cause or causes of these findings remain unclear. Moreover, the methodology did not permit a determination of whether the findings predated the development of PTSD or were a consequence of the PTSD (and comorbid conditions).

Increasingly, researchers are noting that people with PTSD might have lower neuropsychological test scores as a *preexisting* characteristic (Gilbertson et al. 2006; Parslow and Jorm 2007). Additional indirect evidence for preexisting problems with verbal learning and memory can be deduced psychometrically. There is considerable evidence of differences in IQ between people who develop PTSD and those who do not (Brandes et al. 2002; Macklin et al. 1998; Vasterling et al. 2002). That is, those with PTSD are more likely to have average or below-average IQs, whereas people exposed to traumatic events who do not develop PTSD are more likely to have high-average or superior IQs. Evidence also indicates that reduced hippocampal volume is a preexisting factor that heightens an individual's propensity to develop PTSD once exposed to trauma. A study of hippocampal volumes in monozygotic twins discordant for PTSD and trauma exposure provided initial supporting evidence (Gilbertson et al. 2002). This study revealed comparable reductions in hippocampal volume in both the twin with PTSD and in the non-trauma-exposed twin relative to healthy non-PTSD twin pairs, suggesting the possibility of a genetic contribution to variation in hippocampal volume. From this evidence, the authors proposed that smaller hippocampal volume is a preexisting risk factor for severe chronic PTSD rather than a consequence of trauma exposure.

These findings have led to speculation that a higher IQ is "protective" against developing PTSD, or that intelligence represents a vulnerability-protective dimension (Vasterling et al. 2002). If people who develop PTSD actually have lower IQs than trauma-exposed people who do not develop PTSD, then those who develop PTSD would also be expected to have lower pretrauma learning and memory scores. This assumption is based on a medium-sized positive correlation between intelligence and memory.

Without question, assessing cognition in people with a history of mild TBI, PTSD, or both is extraordinarily complex in regard to 1) subjective symptoms, 2) objective test results, and 3) determining the cause of any particular finding. Complicating the picture, people with a history of mild TBI, PTSD, or both can also have comorbid depression, substance abuse, or chronic pain. Moreover, individuals with PTSD can have preexisting lower scores on intellectual and neuropsychological tests. PTSD itself should not lower intelligence scores. Therefore, it is essential to interpret neuropsychological test scores in people with PTSD carefully, not by simply comparing them to normative data adjusted for age, but by considering patients' educational attainment and level of intelligence. These factors can have a substantial impact on the interpretation of neuropsychological test results.

Substance Abuse, PTSD, and Traumatic Brain Injury

The relationship between TBI and substance abuse is an important one, representing a number of complex, interrelated factors. Intoxication is a risk factor for TBI in that TBI can result from unintentional alcohol-related causes, such as motor vehicle accidents or falls. Other alcohol-related TBIs can result from more "intentional" causes, such as assault while intoxicated (i.e., intoxication of the victim and/or the perpetrator), domestic violence, and suicide attempts (Rutland-Brown et al. 2006). A TBI can exacerbate previous substance abuse problems or lead to behavioral and personality changes, which contribute to alcohol or drug misuse.

Prior history of a substance abuse disorder is a risk factor for greater morbidity (Corrigan 1995) and excessive substance use following TBI (Horner et al. 2005). Substance use disorders following TBI adversely affect neuropsychological functioning, subjective well-being, and employment, and increase involvement with the criminal justice system (Corrigan et al. 1997; Kreutzer et al. 1991, 1996; Sherer et al. 1999).

Because injuries to the frontal and temporal lobes may diminish self-control and increase impulsivity, the structural changes associated with TBI may contribute to substance abuse. The relationship of PTSD to substance abuse may be indirect, occur through the TBI mechanism, or be more direct. Corrigan and Cole (2008) suggested that one of the key features of PTSD, hyperarousal, may lead to substance abuse problems. In this model, hyperarousal leads to hypervigilance, which in turn leads to avoidance of stimuli associated with high levels of distress. This in turn leads to emotional numbing and social detachments. All of these factors can lead to substance abuse through attempts to self-medicate anxiety, avoid traumatic memories, or increase emotional numbing and detachment.

Military Aspects

The current conflicts in Iraq and Afghanistan have provided a population of individuals affected by both mild TBI and PTSD. Therefore, careful examination is possible of a group of relatively "clean" individuals who, by definition, are employed at the time of injury, have at least normal-range intellectual functioning and schooling, and in many cases have had careful and thorough medical examinations prior to injury. Although some aspects of emotional trauma may differ in military and nonmilitary populations, in terms of the types of exposures, the military population makes up a relatively large group that meets criteria for both PTSD and TBI.

This military population potentially comprises two different populations of interest: those who require medical evacuation for their injuries and those who do not. The latter group may be identified in the theater of operations as suffering from stress symptoms (Forsten and Schneider 2005) or mild TBI (French et al. 2008) and may or may not receive specific treatment while deployed. During the normal postdeployment medical screening process (Terrio et al. 2009), these individuals are asked about symptoms they may be experiencing. A clinician is then able to do a more careful evaluation and try to identify the etiology of the current symptoms. In some cases, these symptoms may be related to the emotional stress of deployment, the residual effects of a mild TBI, or other clinical concerns. In the medically evacuated group, the injuries or symptoms are of sufficient severity to require evacuation to a more definitive level of care. In some cases of mild TBI, the evacuation may be based on other bodily injuries.

Regardless of the injury type, psychiatric care through the hospital-based consultation-liaison service is part of the standard of care in large military treatment facilities (Wain et al. 2005). According to Zatzick et al. (2007), in a large study of injured trauma survivors across the United States, those hospitalized for physical injuries had an increased risk of PTSD. In this sample, initially high levels of postinjury emotional distress as well as physical pain were most strongly associated with an increased risk of symptoms consistent with PTSD.

In a study of rates of PTSD and depression among soldiers who were seriously injured and required medical evacuation and hospitalization at Walter Reed Army Medical Center, approximately 4% had PTSD and/or depression at 1 month postinjury. These rates increased to 12.2% for PTSD and 8.9% for depression at 4 months, and 12% and 9.3%, respectively, at 7 months. High levels of self-reported physical problems at 1 month postinjury were significantly predictive of PTSD and depression at 7 months. The majority of soldiers with PTSD or depression at 7 months did not have those conditions at 1 month (Grieger et al. 2006). This relationship between PTSD and physical injury has been previously reported by Koren et al. (2005) in a study of rates of PTSD in injured Israeli war veterans. In that study, the findings clearly indicated that bodily injury is a risk factor for PTSD, with approximately eight times greater odds of developing PTSD following traumatic injury than following injury-free emotional trauma. More recently, Gaylord et al. (2008) examined the relationship between PTSD and TBI in a group of 76 burned military service members. In that study, the incidence rates of PTSD and mild TBI were 32% and 41%, respectively; 18% screened positive for both conditions. (For a summary of studies reporting on comorbid PTSD and TBI rates in Operation Iraqi Freedom and Operation Enduring Freedom service members, see Table 15–3.) In those acutely hospitalized for physical trauma, general recovery was enhanced through the identification and treatment of comorbid psychological conditions, including PTSD, because psychological condition is well known to affect recovery from trauma (Holbrook et al. 1999; Michaels et al. 2000).

The use of explosive devices in terror attacks can lead to co-occurring TBI and PTSD in victims. A study done in Israel (Schwartz et al. 2007) found that despite high rates of PTSD (about 50%) in those who experienced TBI either from terror-related attacks or through more traditional mechanisms, the rates of PTSD based on the circumstances were not significantly different between the groups. Furthermore, both groups showed similar outcomes as measured by return-to-work and rehabilitation gains. These findings were surprising considering that the victims of terror attacks had more severe injuries overall.

Table 15–3. Summary of studies reporting on comorbid PTSD and TBI rates in Operation Iraqi Freedom (OIF) and Operation Enduring Freedom (OEF) veterans

			Rate			
Author	*N*	Population	PTSD	TBI	Both	Neither
Gaylord et al. 2008	76	OIF/OEF veterans; medically evacuated for burns	32.0%	41.0%	18.0%	46.0%
Hoge et al. 2008	2,525	Surveyed OIF veterans; not medically evacuated	13.9%	15.2%	Not reported	Not reported
Lew et al. 2007	62	VA PRC outpatients with TBI; 89% OIF/OEF veterans	71.0%	NA	Not reported	NA
Schneiderman et al. 2008	2,235	Surveyed OIF/OEF veterans in Washington, D.C., area; not medically evacuated	11.0%	12.0%	Not reported	Not reported
Tanielian and Jaycox 2008	1,965	Surveyed OIF deployed	13.8%	19.5%	1.1%	69.3%
Vasterling 2006	1,457	Surveyed OIF deployed	11.6%	7.6%[a]	Not reported	Not reported

Note. NA=not applicable; TBI=traumatic brain injury; VA PRC=Veterans Affairs Polytrauma Rehabilitation Center.

[a]As defined by loss of consciousness>5 minutes.

Treatment Considerations

Cognitive or neurobehavioral impairments associated with TBI might influence the efficacy of treatments for anxiety, PTSD, and depression. For example, psychotherapeutic or educational strategies often require intact cognition, which may not always be present in individuals with TBI. Those with cognitive impairment may take longer to benefit from educational information and psychotherapeutic interventions. Even more subtle attentional or memory difficulties might affect learning or other aspects of the treatment process. One case study of a man with coexisting PTSD, TBI, and dysexecutive difficulties suggested that some forms of therapy, such as those involving exposure, could have adverse outcomes in individuals with these conditions (N.S. King 2002); the author suggested that interventions in those with brain injuries should initially focus on nonexposure aspects of treatment (e.g., anxiety management skills or cognitive restructuring) before any exposure-based work.

In a comprehensive Cochrane review of the literature for psychological treatment of anxiety in people with TBI (Soo and Tate 2007), the authors concluded that some evidence supports the effectiveness of cognitive-behavioral therapy (CBT) for treatment of acute stress following mild TBI, and of CBT combined with neurorehabilitation for generalized anxiety in those who sustained TBI of mild to moderate severity. For example, one study provided either CBT or supportive counseling to 24 patients with acute stress disorder following mild TBI (Bryant et al. 2003). Exposure therapy was amended to focus on those aspects of the traumatic experience that the patients were able to recall. Consistent with the previous studies, fewer participants receiving CBT (8%) than those receiving supportive counseling (58%) met criteria for PTSD at 6-month follow-up. Tiersky et al. (2005) provided a comprehensive outpatient neuropsychological rehabilitation program targeting persistent or psychological dysfunction, emotional distress, and accompanying functional disabilities. The results provided preliminary evidence that intensive outpatient treatment, consisting of both CBT and cognitive remediation, improved patients' persistent emotional distress following mild TBI and had possible beneficial effects on related cognitive difficulties.

When working with patients who have sustained a TBI, clinicians need to evaluate physical, cognitive, and emotional symptoms and problems. Clinicians should avoid being overly focused on one domain, such as emotional functioning, and should not neglect other symptoms causing significant distress. Regardless of the etiologies of particular symptoms, a thorough treatment strategy views all patient-reported symptoms as areas for possible intervention.

Some possible comorbid symptoms and conditions that should be addressed for a person to recover well include chronic pain (Rudy et al. 2003; Young 2007), headache (Walker et al. 2005), auditory or other sensory dysfunction (Lew et al. 2007), and sleep changes (Thaxton and Myers 2002). For patients with mild TBI, treatment strategies with the strongest scientific support are those emphasizing education related to symptoms, expected clinical course of recovery, and basic stress management techniques (Borg et al. 2004; Mittenberg et al. 1996; Ponsford et al. 2002).

Relatively few randomized controlled trials have examined pharmacological agents in the treatment of the neurobehavioral consequences of TBI. A few thorough reviews have been published (e.g., Lee et al. 2003; Warden et al. 2006), but this area clearly needs additional work. Clinicians trying to ameliorate behavioral, emotional, and cognitive symptoms associated with TBI must make decisions about pharmacotherapy based mainly on clinical experience and judgment (Tenovuo 2006). Typical pharmacological treatments for anxiety are often used, although benefits are complicated by sensitivity to drug-induced side effects (Warden and Labbate 2005). Benzodiazepines have been used but may be problematic due to adverse effects on motor coordination, concentration, and memory. In general, such treatments should be administered on a short-term basis and at the lowest possible dosages (Warden and Labbate 2005). Selective serotonin reuptake inhibitors (SSRIs) have shown some benefit in the treatment of depression after TBI (Fann et al. 2000), although randomized controlled trials are needed. Warden et al. (2006) cautioned about the use of SSRIs in patients with brain injury because they may worsen preexisting apathy related to frontal injuries or introduce side effects potentially more problematic than the anxiety itself. When used, SSRI treatment should begin at the lowest possible dosage. Antipsychotic medications appear to benefit anxiety associated with psychosis. However, patients with brain injury may be particularly sensitive to extrapyramidal side effects. In general, antipsychotics, especially older high-potency neuroleptics, should not be used as first-line agents for anxiety.

Conclusion

Researchers have shown considerable interest in the comorbidity of TBI and PTSD. The literature on the development of PTSD in patients with TBI is mixed. Individuals who sustain moderate or severe TBIs are likely at less risk for developing PTSD than those who sustain mild TBIs. Some evidence suggests that amnesia for the event is associated with a lower prevalence of PTSD; however, other evidence indicates that PTSD can occur in those with more severe TBIs, because following injury, individuals may have islands of memory for the traumatic experience, psychological trauma may occur following resolution of posttraumatic amnesia, and some fear conditioning can occur despite an altered mental state. In recent studies involving soldiers and veterans, data suggest that sustaining a mild TBI may be associated with increased risk for PTSD (Hoge et al. 2008; Schneiderman et al. 2008).

PTSD and TBI might affect similar neural systems. PTSD appears to be associated with impaired functioning of the medial prefrontal cortex, which limits regulation of the amygdala. Theoretically, traumatic injury to these prefrontal and subcortical networks could precipitate posttraumatic stress symptoms.

From a psychological perspective, the extent to which people catastrophize a traumatic experience and its aftermath is related to the development of PTSD (Ehlers and Clark 2000). Inappropriate cognitive strategies after trauma are a major predictor of PTSD (Ehlers et al. 1998). Injuries to the brain can impair cognitive resources and thus compromise one's capacity to engage in the optimal cognitive strategies to manage the aftermath of a psychological trauma. Furthermore, in those with impaired cognition, this process can be even more difficult and typical treatment strategies may be less effective.

In patients with TBI, regardless of its severity, careful attention must be paid to comorbid conditions. These conditions, whether related to the associated physical effects of trauma or to the emotional sequelae, may complicate the clinical picture, the overall recovery, and/or the treatment strategies employed. Careful screening, as well as an understanding of the interplay between the physical and emotional factors involved in these injuries, is necessary.

Key Clinical Points

- Although the spectrum of possible injury from a TBI is wide, the frontal and temporal regions of the brain are most susceptible to this neurological insult.
- Diffusion tensor imaging has consistently found decreases in white matter integrity of the corpus callosum in patients who have sustained a TBI.
- For most persons who sustain a mild TBI, neurons undergo dynamic restoration and return to normal functioning over time.
- TBI may cause amygdala hyperactivity, possibly via ventromedial prefrontal cortex reactivation of emotional states associated with past experiences.
- Loss of consciousness from a TBI (neurogenic amnesia) may provide some protection from subsequent PTSD, although the validity of this finding remains unclear, as does the mechanism.
- Diagnostic overlap between TBI and PTSD, particularly the lack of specific criteria for mild TBI or postconcussive syndrome, makes the understanding of the relationship between these two disorders very uncertain.
- Individuals with mild TBI and persistent symptoms are more likely to report poor general health, increased medical symptoms and health care utilization, more days of missed work, and higher comorbidity with other mental health disorders, although the relationships among these factors remain unclear.
- Most recovery from a TBI occurs within the first year, with some additional recovery occurring during the second year. Any further recovery is primarily through learned accommodation and compensatory strategies.
- Neurobehavioral changes from a TBI can include personality changes, emotional dysregulation, apathy, disinhibition, and a variety of cognitive impairments.
- Cognitive impairments resulting from a TBI are important considerations in treatment planning, given that most nonpharmacological interventions require that the patient have intact cognition.

- Given the often very complex nature of symptoms experienced by individuals with a TBI, it is vital that providers evaluate all domains of functioning and provide treatment strategies for any areas of deficit.
- Although some evidence supports the use of a few pharmacological agents such as SSRIs and antipsychotics in patients with a TBI, it is important to note the limited research in this area as well as the increased likelihood of medication side effects within this population.

References

Adams JH, Graham DI, Scott G, et al: Brain damage in fatal non-missile head injury. J Clin Pathol 33:1132–1145, 1980

American Psychiatric Association: Diagnostic and Statistical Manual of Mental Disorders, 4th Edition, Text Revision. Washington, DC, American Psychiatric Association, 2000

Arfanakis K, Haughton VM, Carew JD, et al: Diffusion tensor MR imaging in diffuse axonal injury. AJNR Am J Neuroradiol 23:794–802, 2002

Barkley JM, Morales D, Hayman LA, et al: Static neuroimaging in the evaluation of TBI, in Brain Injury Medicine: Principles and Practice. Edited by Zasler ND, Katz DI, Zafonte RD. New York, Demos Medical Publications, 2007, pp 129–148

Belanger HG, Curtiss G, Demery JA, et al: Factors moderating neuropsychological outcomes following mild traumatic brain injury: a meta-analysis. J Int Neuropsychol Soc 11:215–227, 2005

Bigler ED: Structural imaging, in Textbook of Traumatic Brain Injury. Edited by Silver JM, McAllister TW, Yudofsky SC. Washington, DC, American Psychiatric Publishing, 2005, pp 79–105

Bijur PE, Haslum M, Golding J: Cognitive and behavioral sequelae of mild head injury in children. Pediatrics 86:337–344, 1990

Binder LM: A review of mild head trauma, part II: clinical implications. J Clin Exp Neuropsychol 19:432–457, 1997

Bleiberg J, Cernich AN, Cameron K, et al: Duration of cognitive impairment after sports concussion. Neurosurgery 54:1073–1080, 2004

Bombardier CH, Fann JR, Temkin N, et al: Posttraumatic stress disorder symptoms during the first six months after traumatic brain injury. J Neuropsychiatry Clin Neurosci 18:501–508, 2006

Borg J, Holm L, Peloso PM, et al: Non-surgical intervention and cost for mild traumatic brain injury: results of the WHO Collaborating Centre Task Force on Mild Traumatic Brain Injury. J Rehabil Med (43 suppl):76–83, 2004

Brandes D, Ben-Schachar G, Gilboa A, et al: PTSD symptoms and cognitive performance in recent trauma survivors. Psychiatry Res 110:231–238, 2002

Bremner JD, Scott TM, Delaney RC, et al: Deficits in short-term memory in posttraumatic stress disorder. Am J Psychiatry 150:1015–1019, 1993

Bremner JD, Randall P, Scott TM, et al: Deficits in short-term memory in adult survivors of childhood abuse. Psychiatry Res 59:97–107, 1995

Brewin CR, Kleiner JS, Vasterling JJ, et al: Memory for emotionally neutral information in posttraumatic stress disorder: a meta-analytic investigation. J Abnorm Psychol 116:448–463, 2007

Bryant RA: Posttraumatic stress disorder, flashbacks, and pseudomemories in closed head injury. J Trauma Stress 9:621–629, 1996

Bryant RA: Disentangling mild traumatic brain injury and stress reactions. N Engl J Med 358:525–527, 2008

Bryant RA, Harvey AG: Psychological impairment following motor vehicle accidents. Aust J Public Health 19:185–188, 1995

Bryant RA, Harvey AG: Traumatic memories and pseudomemories in posttraumatic stress disorder. Appl Cogn Psychol 12:81–88, 1998

Bryant RA, Harvey AG: Postconcussive symptoms and posttraumatic stress disorder after mild traumatic brain injury. J Nerv Ment Dis 187:302–305, 1999

Bryant RA, Marosszeky JE, Crooks J, et al: Posttraumatic stress disorder after severe traumatic brain injury. Am J Psychiatry 157:629–631, 2000

Bryant RA, Moulds M, Guthrie R, et al: Treating acute stress disorder following mild traumatic brain injury. Am J Psychiatry 160:585–587, 2003

Bryant RA, Creamer M, O'Donnell M, et al: A study of the protective function of acute morphine administration on subsequent posttraumatic stress disorder. Biol Psychiatry 65:438–440, 2009

Buckley TC, Blanchard EB, Neill WT: Information processing and PTSD: a review of the empirical literature. Clin Psychol Rev 20:1041–1065, 2000

Buki A, Povlishock JT: All roads lead to disconnection? Traumatic axonal injury revisited. Acta Neurochir (Wien) 148:181–194, 2006

Carroll LJ, Cassidy JD, Peloso PM, et al: Prognosis for mild traumatic brain injury: results of the WHO Collaborating Centre Task Force on Mild Traumatic Brain Injury. J Rehabil Med 36 (suppl 43):84–105, 2004

Centers for Disease Control and Prevention: Traumatic Brain Injury. April 1, 2008. Available at: http://www.cdc.gov/TraumaticBrainInjury/index.html. Accessed February 25, 2010.

Charness ME: Brain lesions in alcoholics. Alcohol Clin Exp Res 17:2–11, 1993

Corrigan JD: Substance abuse as a mediating factor in outcome from traumatic brain injury. Arch Phys Med Rehabil 76:302–309, 1995

Corrigan JD, Cole TB: Substance use disorders and clinical management of traumatic brain injury and posttraumatic stress disorder. JAMA 300:720–721, 2008

Corrigan JD, Smith-Knapp K, Granger CV: Validity of the Functional Independence Measure for persons with traumatic brain injury. Arch Phys Med Rehabil 78:828–834, 1997

Crowell TA, Kieffer KM, Siders CA, et al: Neuropsychological findings in combat-related posttraumatic stress disorder. Clin Neuropsychol 16:310–321, 2002

Danckwerts A, Leathem J: Questioning the link between PTSD and cognitive dysfunction. Neuropsychol Rev 13:221–235, 2003

Dikmen S, McLean A Jr, Temkin NR, et al: Neuropsychologic outcome at one-month postinjury. Arch Phys Med Rehabil 67:507–513, 1986

Dikmen S, Machamer J, Temkin N: Psychosocial outcome in patients with moderate to severe head injury: 2-year follow-up. Brain Inj 7:113–124, 1993

Dikmen S, Temkin NR, Machamer JE, et al: Employment following traumatic head injuries. Arch Neurol 51:177–186, 1994

Dikmen S, Machamer JE, Winn R, et al: Neuropsychological outcome 1-year post head injury. Neuropsychology 9:80–90, 1995

Dikmen S, Machamer J, Temkin N: Mild head injury: facts and artifacts. J Clin Exp Neuropsychol 23:729–738, 2001

Dikmen S, Machamer JE, Powell JM, et al: Outcome 3 to 5 years after moderate to severe traumatic brain injury. Arch Phys Med Rehabil 84:1449–1457, 2003

Dunn-Meynell AA, Hassanain M, Levin BE: Norepinephrine and traumatic brain injury: a possible role in post-traumatic edema. Brain Res 800:245–252, 1998

Ehlers A, Clark DM: A cognitive model of posttraumatic stress disorder. Behav Res Ther 38:319–345, 2000

Ehlers A, Mayou RA, Bryant B: Psychological predictors of chronic posttraumatic stress disorder after motor vehicle accidents. J Abnorm Psychol 107:508–519, 1998

Fann JR, Uomoto JM, Katon WJ: Sertraline in the treatment of major depression following mild traumatic brain injury. J Neuropsychiatry Clin Neurosci 12:226–232, 2000

Fay GC, Jaffe KM, Polissar NL, et al: Mild pediatric traumatic brain injury: a cohort study. Arch Phys Med Rehabil 74:895–901, 1993

Forsten R, Schneider B: Treatment of the stress casualty during Operation Iraqi Freedom One. Psychiatr Q 76:343–350, 2005

Fox DD, Lees-Haley PR, Ernest K, et al: Post-concussive symptoms: base rates and etiology in psychiatric patients. Clin Neuropsychol 9:89–92, 1995

French LM, McCrea M, Baggett MR: The Military Acute Concussion Evaluation (MACE). J Spec Oper Med 8:68–77, 2008

Galarneau MR, Woodruff SI, Dye JL, et al: Traumatic brain injury during Operation Iraqi Freedom: findings from the United States Navy-Marine Corps Combat Trauma Registry. J Neurosurg 108:950–957, 2008

Gasquoine PG: Postconcussional symptoms in chronic back pain. Appl Neuropsychol 7:83–89, 2000

Gaylord KM, Cooper DB, Mercado JM, et al: Incidence of posttraumatic stress disorder and mild traumatic brain injury in burned service members: preliminary report. J Trauma 64 (suppl 2):S200–S206, 2008

Gentilini M, Nichelli P, Schoenhuber R, et al: Neuropsychological evaluation of mild head injury. J Neurol Neurosurg Psychiatry 48:137–140, 1985

Gil S, Caspi Y, Ben-Ari IZ, et al: Does memory of a traumatic event increase the risk for posttraumatic stress disorder in patients with traumatic brain injury? A prospective study. Am J Psychiatry 162:963–969, 2005

Gilbertson MW, Shenton ME, Ciszewski A, et al: Smaller hippocampal volume predicts pathologic vulnerability to psychological trauma. Nat Neurosci 5:1242–1247, 2002

Gilbertson MW, Paulus LA, Williston SK, et al: Neurocognitive function in monozygotic twins discordant for combat exposure: relationship to posttraumatic stress disorder. J Abnorm Psychol 115:484–495, 2006

Giza CC, Hovda DA: The neurometabolic cascade of concussion. J Athl Train 36:228–235, 2001

Giza CC, Hovda DA: The pathophysiology of traumatic brain injury, in Traumatic Brain Injury in Sports. Edited by Lovell MR, Echemendia RJ, Barth JT, et al. Lisse, The Netherlands, Swets & Zeitlinger, 2004, pp 45–70

Glaesser J, Neuner F, Lügehetmann R, et al: Posttraumatic stress disorder in patients with traumatic brain injury. BMC Psychiatry 4:5, 2004

Goldstein FC, Levin HS, Goldman WP, et al: Cognitive and neurobehavioral functioning after mild versus moderate traumatic brain injury in older adults. J Int Neuropsychol Soc 7:373–383, 2001

Gorrie C, Duflou J, Brown J, et al: Extent and distribution of vascular brain injury in pediatric road fatalities. J Neurotrauma 18:849–860, 2001

Gouvier WD, Uddo-Crane M, Brown LM: Base rates of post-concussional symptoms. Arch Clin Neuropsychol 3:273–278, 1988

Grieger TA, Cozza SJ, Ursano RJ, et al: Posttraumatic stress disorder and depression in battle-injured soldiers. Am J Psychiatry 163:1777–1783; quiz 1860, 2006

Harvey AG, Bryant RA: Two-year prospective evaluation of the relationship between acute stress disorder and posttraumatic stress disorder following mild traumatic brain injury. Am J Psychiatry 157:626–628, 2000

Harvey AG, Bryant RA: Reconstructing trauma memories: a prospective study of "amnesic" trauma survivors. J Trauma Stress 14:277–282, 2001

Hickling EJ, Gillen R, Blanchard EB, et al: Traumatic brain injury and posttraumatic stress disorder: a preliminary investigation of neuropsychological test results in PTSD secondary to motor vehicle accidents. Brain Inj 12:265–274, 1998

Hoge CW, McGurk D, Thomas JL, et al: Mild traumatic brain injury in U.S. soldiers returning from Iraq. N Engl J Med 358:453–463, 2008

Holbrook TL, Anderson JP, Sieber WJ, et al: Outcome after major trauma: 12-month and 18-month follow-up results from the Trauma Recovery Project. J Trauma 46:765–773, 1999

Horner MD, Hamner MB: Neurocognitive functioning in posttraumatic stress disorder. Neuropsychol Rev 12:15–30, 2002

Horner MD, Ferguson PL, Selassie AW, et al: Patterns of alcohol use 1 year after traumatic brain injury: a population-based, epidemiological study. J Int Neuropsychol Soc 11:322–330, 2005

Hughes DG, Jackson A, Mason DL, et al: Abnormalities on magnetic resonance imaging seen acutely following mild traumatic brain injury: correlation with neuropsychological tests and delayed recovery. Neuroradiology 46:550–558, 2004

Huisman TA, Schwamm LH, Schaefer PW, et al: Diffusion tensor imaging as potential biomarker of white matter injury in diffuse axonal injury. AJNR Am J Neuroradiol 25:370–376, 2004

Inglese M, Bomsztyk E, Gonen O, et al: Dilated perivascular spaces: hallmarks of mild traumatic brain injury. AJNR Am J Neuroradiol 26:719–724, 2005a

Inglese M, Makani S, Johnson G, et al: Diffuse axonal injury in mild traumatic brain injury: a diffusion tensor imaging study. J Neurosurg 103:298–303, 2005b

Iverson GL: Outcome from mild traumatic brain injury. Curr Opin Psychiatry 18:301–317, 2005

Iverson GL, Lange RT: Examination of "postconcussion-like" symptoms in a healthy sample. Appl Neuropsychol 10:137–144, 2003

Iverson GL, McCracken LM: "Postconcussive" symptoms in persons with chronic pain. Brain Inj 11:783–790, 1997

Iverson GL, Lange RT, Gaetz M, et al: Mild TBI, in Brain Injury Medicine: Principles and Practice. Edited by Zasler ND, Katz DI, Zafonte RD. New York, Demos Medical Publications, 2007, pp 333–371

Jelinek L, Jacobsen D, Kellner M, et al: Verbal and nonverbal memory functioning in posttraumatic stress disorder (PTSD). J Clin Exp Neuropsychol 28:940–948, 2006

Jenkins MA, Langlais PJ, Delis DA, et al: Attentional dysfunction associated with posttraumatic stress disorder among rape survivors. Clin Neuropsychol 14:7–12, 2000

Kashluba S, Casey JE, Paniak C: Evaluating the utility of ICD-10 diagnostic criteria for postconcussion syndrome following mild traumatic brain injury. J Int Neuropsychol Soc 12:111–118, 2006

Kennedy JE, Jaffee MS, Leskin GA, et al: Posttraumatic stress disorder and posttraumatic stress disorder-like symptoms and mild traumatic brain injury. J Rehabil Res Dev 44:895–920, 2007

King LA, King DW, Fairbank JA, et al: Resilience-recovery factors in post-traumatic stress disorder among female and male Vietnam veterans: hardiness, postwar social support, and additional stressful life events. J Pers Soc Psychol 74:420–434, 1998

King NS: Perseveration of traumatic re-experiencing in PTSD: a cautionary note regarding exposure based psychological treatments for PTSD when head injury and dysexecutive impairment are also present. Brain Inj 16:65–74, 2002

Kitayama N, Vaccarino V, Kutner M, et al: Magnetic resonance imaging (MRI) measurement of hippocampal volume in posttraumatic stress disorder: a meta-analysis. J Affect Disord 88:79–86, 2005

Klein E, Caspi Y, Gil S: The relation between memory of the traumatic event and PTSD: evidence from studies of traumatic brain injury. Can J Psychiatry 48:28–33, 2003

Kochanek PM, Clark RSB, Jenkins LW: TBI: pathobiology, in Brain Injury Medicine: Principles and Practice. Edited by Zasler ND, Katz DI, Zafonte RD. New York, Demos Medical Publications, 2007, pp 81–96

Koenigs M, Huey ED, Raymont V, et al: Focal brain damage protects against posttraumatic stress disorder in combat veterans. Nat Neurosci 11:232–237, 2008

Koren D, Norman D, Cohen A, et al: Increased PTSD risk with combat-related injury: a matched comparison study of injured and uninjured soldiers experiencing the same combat events. Am J Psychiatry 162:276–282, 2005

Kreutzer JS, Wehman PH, Harris JA, et al: Substance abuse and crime patterns among persons with traumatic brain injury referred for supported employment. Brain Inj 5:177–187, 1991

Kreutzer JS, Witol AD, Marwitz JH: Alcohol and drug use among young persons with traumatic brain injury. J Learn Disabil 29:643–651, 1996

Lahmeyer HW, Bellur SN: Cardiac regulation and depression. J Psychiatr Res 21:1–6, 1987

Lanius RA, Bluhm R, Lanius U, et al: A review of neuroimaging studies in PTSD: heterogeneity of response to symptom provocation. J Psychiatr Res 40:709–729, 2006

Le TH, Mukherjee P, Henry RG, et al: Diffusion tensor imaging with three-dimensional fiber tractography of traumatic axonal shearing injury: an imaging correlate for the posterior callosal "disconnection" syndrome: case report. Neurosurgery 56:189, 2005

Lee HB, Lyketsos CG, Rao V: Pharmacological management of the psychiatric aspects of traumatic brain injury. Int Rev Psychiatry 15:359–370, 2003

Lees-Haley PR, Brown RS: Neuropsychological complaint base rates of 170 personal injury claimants. Arch Clin Neuropsychol 8:203–209, 1993

Levin HS: Neuroplasticity following non-penetrating traumatic brain injury. Brain Inj 17:665–674, 2003

Levin HS, Williams DH, Valastro M, et al: Corpus callosal atrophy following closed head injury: detection with magnetic resonance imaging. J Neurosurg 73:77–81, 1990

Levin HS, Brown SA, Song JX, et al: Depression and posttraumatic stress disorder at three months after mild to moderate traumatic brain injury. J Clin Exp Neuropsychol 23:754–769, 2001

Lew HL, Jerger JF, Guillory SB, et al: Auditory dysfunction in traumatic brain injury. J Rehabil Res Dev 44:921–928, 2007

Lezak MD, Howieson DB, Loring DW: Neuropsychological Assessment, 4th Edition. New York, Oxford University Press, 2004

Lovell MR, Collins MW, Iverson GL, et al: Grade 1 or "ding" concussions in high school athletes. Am J Sports Med 32:47–54, 2004

Macciocchi SN, Barth JT, Alves W, et al: Neuropsychological functioning and recovery after mild head injury in collegiate athletes. Neurosurgery 39:510–514, 1996

Machulda MM, Bergquist TF, Ito V, et al: Relationship between stress, coping, and post concussion symptoms in a healthy adult population. Arch Clin Neuropsychol 13:415–424, 1998

MacKenzie JD, Siddiqi F, Babb JS, et al: Brain atrophy in mild or moderate traumatic brain injury: a longitudinal quantitative analysis. AJNR Am J Neuroradiol 23:1509–1515, 2002

Macklin ML, Metzger LJ, Litz BT, et al: Lower precombat intelligence is a risk factor for posttraumatic stress disorder. J Consult Clin Psychol 66:323–326, 1998

Mather FJ, Tate RL, Hannan TJ: Post-traumatic stress disorder in children following road traffic accidents: a comparison of those with and without mild traumatic brain injury. Brain Inj 17:1077–1087, 2003

Mayou RA, Black J, Bryant B: Unconsciousness, amnesia and psychiatric symptoms following road traffic accident injury. Br J Psychiatry 177:540–545, 2000

McAllister TW, Sparling MB, Flashman LA, et al: Neuroimaging findings in mild traumatic brain injury. J Clin Exp Neuropsychol 23:775–791, 2001

McCrea M, Kelly JP, Randolph C, et al: Immediate neurocognitive effects of concussion. Neurosurgery 50:1032–1040, 2002

McCrea M, Guskiewicz KM, Marshall SW, et al: Acute effects and recovery time following concussion in collegiate football players: the NCAA Concussion Study. JAMA 290:2556–2563, 2003

Meares S, Shores EA, Taylor AJ, et al: Mild traumatic brain injury does not predict acute postconcussion syndrome. J Neurol Neurosurg Psychiatry 79:300–306, 2008

Mearns J, Lees-Haley PR: Discriminating neuropsychological sequelae of head injury from alcohol-abuse-induced deficits: a review and analysis. J Clin Psychol 49:714–720, 1993

Michaels AJ, Michaels CE, Smith JS, et al: Outcome from injury: general health, work status, and satisfaction 12 months after trauma. J Trauma 48:841–850, 2000

Mickeviciene D, Schrader H, Obelieniene D, et al: A controlled prospective inception cohort study on the post-concussion syndrome outside the medicolegal context. Eur J Neurol 11:411–419, 2004

Miles L, Grossman RI, Johnson G, et al: Short-term DTI predictors of cognitive dysfunction in mild traumatic brain injury. Brain Inj 22:115–122, 2008

Mittenberg W, DiGiulio DV, Perrin S, et al: Symptoms following mild head injury: expectation as aetiology. J Neurol Neurosurg Psychiatry 55:200–204, 1992

Mittenberg W, Tremont G, Zielinski RE, et al: Cognitive-behavioral prevention of postconcussion syndrome. Arch Clin Neuropsychol 11:139–145, 1996

Nakayama N, Okumura A, Shinoda J, et al: Evidence for white matter disruption in traumatic brain injury without macroscopic lesions. J Neurol Neurosurg Psychiatry 77:850–855, 2006

Niogi SN, Mukherjee P, McCandliss BD: Diffusion tensor imaging segmentation of white matter structures using a Reproducible Objective Quantification Scheme (ROQS). Neuroimage 35:166–174, 2007

Parker RS: Recommendations for the revision of DSM-IV diagnostic categories for co-morbid posttraumatic stress disorder and traumatic brain injury. NeuroRehabilitation 17:131–143, 2002

Parslow RA, Jorm AF: Pretrauma and posttrauma neurocognitive functioning and PTSD symptoms in a community sample of young adults. Am J Psychiatry 164:509–515, 2007

Ponsford J, Willmott C, Rothwell A, et al: Factors influencing outcome following mild traumatic brain injury in adults. J Int Neuropsychol Soc 6:568–579, 2000

Ponsford J, Willmott C, Rothwell A, et al: Impact of early intervention on outcome following mild head injury in adults. J Neurol Neurosurg Psychiatry 73:330–332, 2002

Radanov BP, Dvorak J, Valach L: Cognitive deficits in patients after soft tissue injury of the cervical spine. Spine 17:127–131, 1992

Rauch SL, Shin LM, Phelps EA: Neurocircuitry models of posttraumatic stress disorder and extinction: human neuroimaging research—past, present, and future. Biol Psychiatry 60:376–382, 2006

Rudy TE, Lieber SJ, Boston JR, et al: Psychosocial predictors of physical performance in disabled individuals with chronic pain. Clin J Pain 19:18–30, 2003

Ruff R: Two decades of advances in understanding of mild traumatic brain injury. J Head Trauma Rehabil 20:5–18, 2005

Rutgers DR, Toulgoat F, Cazejust J, et al: White matter abnormalities in mild traumatic brain injury: a diffusion tensor imaging study. AJNR Am J Neuroradiol 29:514–519, 2008

Rutland-Brown W, Langlois JA, Thomas KE, et al: Incidence of traumatic brain injury in the United States, 2003. J Head Trauma Rehabil 21:544–548, 2006

Salmond CH, Menon DK, Chatfield DA, et al: Diffusion tensor imaging in chronic head injury survivors: correlations with learning and memory indices. Neuroimage 29:117–124, 2006

Sawchyn JM, Brulot MM, Strauss E: Note on the use of the Postconcussion Syndrome Checklist. Arch Clin Neuropsychol 15:1–8, 2000

Saxe G, Stoddard F, Courtney D, et al: Relationship between acute morphine and the course of PTSD in children with burns. J Am Acad Child Adolesc Psychiatry 40:915–921, 2001

Sbordone RJ, Liter JC: Mild traumatic brain injury does not produce post-traumatic stress disorder. Brain Inj 9:405–412, 1995

Schneiderman AI, Braver ER, Kang HK: Understanding sequelae of injury mechanisms and mild traumatic brain injury incurred during the conflicts in Iraq and Afghanistan: persistent postconcussive symptoms and posttraumatic stress disorder. Am J Epidemiol 167:1446–1452, 2008

Schretlen DJ, Shapiro AM: A quantitative review of the effects of traumatic brain injury on cognitive functioning. Int Rev Psychiatry 15:341–349, 2003

Schwartz I, Tuchner M, Tsenter J, et al: Cognitive and functional outcomes of terror victims who suffered from traumatic brain injury. Brain Inj 22:255–263, 2008

Sherer M, Bergloff P, High W Jr, et al: Contribution of functional ratings to prediction of longterm employment outcome after traumatic brain injury. Brain Inj 13:973–981, 1999

Smith-Seemiller L, Fow NR, Kant R, et al: Presence of post-concussion syndrome symptoms in patients with chronic pain vs mild traumatic brain injury. Brain Inj 17:199–206, 2003

Soo C, Tate R: Psychological treatment for anxiety in people with traumatic brain injury. Cochrane Database Syst Rev CD005239, 2007

Spikman JM, Timmerman ME, Zomeren van AH, et al: Recovery versus retest effects in attention after closed head injury. J Clin Exp Neuropsychol 21:585–605, 1999

Stein MB, Hanna C, Vaerum V, et al: Memory functioning in adult women traumatized by childhood sexual abuse. J Trauma Stress 12:527–534, 1999

Stulemeijer M, van der Werf SP, Jacobs B, et al: Impact of additional extracranial injuries on outcome after mild traumatic brain injury. J Neurotrauma 23:1561–1569, 2006

Sumpter RE, McMillan TM: Errors in self-report of post-traumatic stress disorder after severe traumatic brain injury. Brain Inj 20:93–99, 2006

Sundgren PC, Dong Q, Gomez-Hassan D, et al: Diffusion tensor imaging of the brain: review of clinical applications. Neuroradiology 46:339–350, 2004

Sutker PB, Allain AN Jr, Johnson JL, et al: Memory and learning performances in POW survivors with history of malnutrition and combat veteran controls. Arch Clin Neuropsychol 7:431–444, 1992

Tanielian T, Jaycox LH (eds): Invisible Wounds of War: Psychological and Cognitive Injuries, Their Consequences, and Services to Assist Recovery. Santa Monica, CA, RAND Corp, 2008

Tenovuo O: Pharmacological enhancement of cognitive and behavioral deficits after traumatic brain injury. Curr Opin Neurol 19:528–533, 2006

Terrio H, Brenner LA, Ivins B, et al: Traumatic brain injury screening: preliminary findings in a US Army Brigade Combat Team. J Head Trauma Rehabil 24:14–23, 2009

Thaxton L, Myers MA: Sleep disturbances and their management in patients with brain injury. J Head Trauma Rehabil 17:335–348, 2002

Tiersky LA, Anselmi V, Johnston MV, et al: A trial of neuropsychologic rehabilitation in mild-spectrum traumatic brain injury. Arch Phys Med Rehabil 86:1565–1574, 2005

Trahan DE, Ross CE, Trahan SL: Relationships among postconcussional-type symptoms, depression, and anxiety in neurologically normal young adults and victims of brain injury. Arch Clin Neuropsychol 16:435–445, 2001

Twamley EW, Hami S, Stein MB: Neuropsychological function in college students with and without posttraumatic stress disorder. Psychiatry Res 126:265–274, 2004

Vasterling JJ, Brailey K, Constans JI, et al: Attention and memory dysfunction in posttraumatic stress disorder. Neuropsychology 12:125–133, 1998

Vasterling JJ, Duke LM, Brailey K, et al: Attention, learning, and memory performances and intellectual resources in Vietnam veterans: PTSD and no disorder comparisons. Neuropsychology 16:5–14, 2002

Vasterling JJ, Proctor SP, Amoroso P, et al: Neuropsychological outcomes of army personnel following deployment to the Iraq war. JAMA 296:519–529, 2006

Wain H, Bradley J, Nam T, et al: Psychiatric interventions with returning soldiers at Walter Reed. Psychiatr Q 76:351–360, 2005

Walker WC, Seel RT, Curtiss G, et al: Headache after moderate and severe traumatic brain injury: a longitudinal analysis. Arch Phys Med Rehabil 86:1793–1800, 2005

Warden DL, Labbate LA: Posttraumatic stress disorder and other anxiety disorders, in Textbook of Traumatic Brain Injury. Edited by Silver JM, McAllister TW, Yudofsky SC. Washington, DC, American Psychiatric Publishing, 2005, pp 231–243

Warden DL, Gordon B, McAllister TW, et al: Guidelines for the pharmacologic treatment of neurobehavioral sequelae of traumatic brain injury. J Neurotrauma 23:1468–1501, 2006

Whyte J, Schuster K, Polansky M, et al: Frequency and duration of inattentive behavior after traumatic brain injury: effects of distraction, task, and practice. J Int Neuropsychol Soc 6:1–11, 2000

Wilde EA, Chu Z, Bigler ED, et al: Diffusion tensor imaging in the corpus callosum in children after moderate to severe traumatic brain injury. J Neurotrauma 23:1412–1426, 2006

Wong JL, Regennitter RP, Barrios F: Base rate and simulated symptoms of mild head injury among normals. Arch Clin Neuropsychol 9:411–425, 1994

World Health Organization: International Classification of Diseases, 9th Revision. Geneva, World Health Organization, 1977

Yehuda R, Keefe RS, Harvey PD, et al: Learning and memory in combat veterans with posttraumatic stress disorder. Am J Psychiatry 152:137–139, 1995

Young JA: Pain and traumatic brain injury. Phys Med Rehabil Clin N Am 18:145–163, vii–viii, 2007

Zatzick DF, Rivara FP, Nathens AB, et al: A nationwide US study of post-traumatic stress after hospitalization for physical injury. Psychol Med 37:1469–1480, 2007

16

Sociocultural Considerations

Laurence J. Kirmayer, M.D., F.R.C.P.C.
Cécile Rousseau, M.D., M.Sc.
Toby Measham, M.D., M.Sc.

Over the past three decades, *trauma* has emerged as a cultural keyword broadly applied to various forms of human suffering (Fassin and Rechtman 2009). Psychiatric interest in trauma has emphasized the construct of posttraumatic stress disorder (PTSD), which describes a common syndrome of trauma response centered on fear conditioning and related psychobiological processes. This construct may have some universal applicability, but the focus on PTSD must be widened to recognize the multiple biosocial, cultural, and political processes that are essential aspects of traumatic suffering, as well as resilience and recovery (Kirmayer et al. 2007).

In this chapter, we provide an overview of sociocultural considerations related to the diagnostic assessment and treatment of patients with trauma exposure and PTSD. The assessment of trauma in cross-cultural perspective requires attention to a variety of social and cultural contexts, including kin relations, political structures, religious beliefs, and local conceptions of health and illness (Marsella 2008). This attention has become increasingly important in light of the experience of displaced and refugee populations and the growing diversity of multicultural societies due to globalization. We begin this chapter by reviewing some of the universal and culture-specific dimensions of responses to "trauma," and then discuss approaches to clinical assessment and treatment interventions. We conclude by considering how trauma services may be culturally adapted to render them more appropriate to diverse clinical situations.

Trauma in Cultural Context

The *Diagnostic and Statistical Manual of Mental Disorders*, 4th Edition, Text Revision (DSM-IV-TR) of the American Psychiatric Association (2000) frames acute stress disorder and PTSD as the core pathological responses to traumatic events. PTSD can be diagnosed in culturally diverse settings (de Jong et al. 2001), and similar syndromes are recognized in some indigenous systems of diagnosis and healing. However, such local categories and concepts of illness and illness behaviors related to traumatic experiences often traverse DSM categories, include symptoms not recognized in conventional nosology, and cannot be mapped onto PTSD or other DSM categories (Eisenbruch 1991; Fox 2003).

Views of trauma within psychiatry have undergone significant shifts over time (Leys 2000), and diagnostic criteria for acute stress disorder and PTSD represent the outcomes of complex social, moral, and political debates, as well as empirical research (Young 1995). Historically, various sets of psychological and somatic symptoms have been associated with traumatic events during different wars (Jones 2006). Across Western categories of trauma syndromes (e.g., railway spine, shell shock, combat fatigue, acute stress reaction), variations have occurred in the type and frequency of medically unexplained somatic symptoms (Jones 2006; Mayer 2007). Even currently accepted core features of PTSD, such as flashbacks, were absent or at least unrecognized until a particular historical moment (Jones et al. 2003). This discrepancy across cultures and over time calls into question the universality of the syndrome of PTSD as currently configured and raises the possibility that for people from other cultural backgrounds, different syndromes that fit their own descriptive frameworks may better capture the covariation of posttraumatic distress (Summerfield 1999). Indigenous diagnostic constructs overlap only partially with PTSD as currently described (Fox 2003). Of course, the absence of popular or professional descriptions of particular symptoms or syndromes does not mean they are not present. Evidence suggests that a history of PTSD symptoms often can be identified among people who are not aware of the diagnostic category (Kagee 2004). Cultural idioms of distress are important, however, because they influence patients' help-seeking and coping and may constitute clinical problems in their own right.

Culture influences not only a patient's symptom experience and expression but also the ways that physicians categorize and interpret a patient's distress (Kirmayer and Bhugra 2009). Existing nosology describes specific physiological and psychological responses in the face of trauma but does not emphasize issues of shame, anger, and existential concerns that may be paramount for many trauma survivors. The experience of traumatic suffering is both personally and socially value-laden. Accidents, disasters, domestic violence, political violence, torture, forced migration, war, and genocide all have specific meanings that influence their psychiatric clinical expression and social consequences, as well as the processes of recovery or restitution (Kirmayer et al. 2010; Marsella 2008).

Silove (2007) outlined a range of processes involved in situations of severe trauma and human rights violations. These include biocultural systems involved in establishing and maintaining basic needs. Traumatic disruptions of each of these systems mobilize specific adaptive responses at restoration and, when these fail, may result in specific types of problems (see Table 16–1). Although not all of these issues correspond to specific DSM-IV-TR diagnostic categories, they may constitute important targets for clinical attention. Each issue needs to be understood in a patient's cultural context and resolved in ways that reflect the culturally based values, patterns of coping and interpersonal interaction, and family and community resources available to the individual.

The dilemma with the current emphasis on PTSD, therefore, is that although the diagnosis may capture a universal pattern of fear conditioning, anxiety, and avoidance behavior, this pattern is only a limited aspect of the range of clinical problems that can be directly related to trauma exposure. Other dimensions of trauma experience based on specific social and cultural meanings and dynamics require comparable clinical attention.

Table 16–1. Problems resulting from traumatic disruptions to the meeting of basic needs

Need	Resulting problems
Personal safety	Anxiety disorders and PTSD
Secure interpersonal attachments	Grief, homesickness, and depression
A sense of justice and fairness in social relations	Chronic anger, bitterness, mistrust, and preoccupation with revenge
A valued social role or identity	Alienation, helplessness, and aimlessness
Existential meaning in life	Demoralization, isolation, and despair

Source. Adapted from Silove D: "Adaptation, Ecosocial Safety Signals, and the Trajectory of PTSD," in *Understanding Trauma: Integrating Clinical, Biological, and Cultural Perspectives.* Edited by Kirmayer LJ, Lemelson R, Barad M. New York, Cambridge University Press, 2007, pp. 242–258. Used with the permission of Cambridge University Press.

Assessment

Assessment and treatment of trauma-related symptoms and syndromes require attention to the social and cultural contexts of the patient's history and current life situation (Kirmayer et al. 2008). The Outline for Cultural Formulation in DSM-IV-TR (Appendix I) provides a way to organize basic information about a patient's social and cultural context that is relevant to diagnostic assessment and treatment planning (American Psychiatric Association 2000). This outline summarizes information on four broad domains: patient's cultural identity; cultural explanations of the illness; cultural factors related to psychosocial environment and levels of functioning; and cultural elements that may affect the clinician-patient relationship. These domains are discussed in the following subsections. Several publications provide suggestions for how to collect the information needed to develop a cultural formulation (Group for the Advancement of Psychiatry 2002; Lim 2006; Mezzich et al. 2009).

Cultural Identity

Identity is based on the individual's sense of affiliation with different socially defined groups, roles, and statuses embedded in a biographical narrative. Identity is drawn from participation in an in-group and defined against the backdrop of those viewed as "other." Situations of violent conflict and even isolated traumatic events may intensify these group boundaries and identifications, making culturally constructed notions of gender, race, ethnicity, and religion more salient. Trauma often challenges an individual's sense of identity. The acute experience of life-threatening violence may induce derealization and depersonalization, leading to subsequent efforts to reaffirm identity through culturally familiar signs and symbols. Cultural identities also may be linked to collective trauma because, depending on political circumstances, they may make the individual a target for violence and subsequently recast him or her as a "victim," "bystander," or "perpetrator." The aftermath of trauma poses complex individual and social problems of reconfiguring identity in ways that are morally acceptable and that sustain the individual's self-esteem and self-efficacy.

Illness Explanations

Illness explanations may be based on previous experiences with similar symptoms and syndromes that serve as prototypes, causal attributions, and notions about the underlying processes, course, and outcome of a condition (Kirmayer and Sartorius 2009). These explanations are related to perceptions of appropriate treatment and expected prognosis, which in turn shape coping style, help-seeking behavior, and treatment adherence.

A variety of culture-related symptoms and syndromes may predominate in the clinical presentation of patients from specific cultures. For example, somatoform symptoms may be common in cultural contexts where bodily idioms of distress provide acceptable modes of expressing suffering (Kirmayer 1996). Similarly, dissociative symptoms, which often accompany acute and chronic stress syndromes, may be more common in settings where religious and healing ritual practices employ dissociation. These symptoms may be part of culture-related syndromes, folk diagnostic categories, or cultural idioms of distress. Syndromes, folk and biomedical diagnoses, and idioms of distress may also function as explanations for symptoms and suffering.

Idioms of distress are local ways of talking about troubles and suffering that are intelligible to others within a community. Table 16–2 presents some folk categories and idioms of distress that are nonspecific but may be associated with trauma-related syndromes. Cultural idioms may overlap only partially with psychiatric diagnoses. For example, in Central America, the terms *nervios* and *susto* may refer, respectively, to a state of generalized anxiety and to

Table 16–2. Some folk illness categories and idioms of distress that may be associated with trauma

Culture	Category or idiom	Symptoms	Source
Afghan	*jigar khun*	Form of sadness, (inclusive of emotional grief from loss of family members in war), response to painful experience	Miller et al. 2006
	asabi	Feeling stressed/overwhelmed; nervous	Miller et al. 2006
	fishar-e-bala *fishar-e-payin* (at times interpreted by individual as high and low blood pressure, respectively)	State of agitation and intense emotion, and state of low energy/motivation, respectively	Miller et al. 2006
Central American, Caribbean, South American	*nervios*	Nervousness, anxiety, malaise	Guarnaccia et al. 2003
	ataque de nervios	Shouting, crying uncontrollably; fainting, loss of consciousness	Lewis-Fernandez et al. 2002
	susto	Any illness attributed to sudden fright	Jenkins 1991
	espanto	Any illness attributed to sudden fright	Tousignant 1979
	calor	Sensations of heat	Jenkins 1991
Khmer (Cambodian)	*kyol goeu* ("wind overload")	Orthostatic panic attacks	Hinton et al. 2001

Table 16–2. Some folk illness categories and idioms of distress that may be associated with trauma *(continued)*

Culture	Category or idiom	Symptoms	Source
Latino (United States)	*triste* (sad) *enojada* (angry) *nerviosa* (nervous) *miedo* (scared) stress	Somatic symptoms Poor concentration	Eisenman et al. 2008
Somali	*murug*	Ranges from sadness to "craziness"; symptoms such as headache, anorexia, tearfulness, anhedonia, flashbacks, and physical illnesses such as alopecia and hypertension	Carroll 2004
	waali	"Madness," "craziness" due to severe trauma; may be characterized by anger, aimless wandering, disorganized speech, unpredictable violence	Carroll 2004
Vietnamese	*bi trúng gió* ("hit by wind"): weak heart; burst cerebral vessels; ripped brain nerves	Orthostatic panic attacks	Hinton et al. 2007

an acute reaction of fear to a startling event or stressor. However, *nervios* may also commonly refer to other forms of emotional malaise, and *susto* may function as an explanation for a wide range of ailments that are attributed to exposure to a sudden fright. Because the meanings of these idioms vary across different cultural communities as well as for individuals, the clinician must explore how they relate to a particular patient's symptoms. Symptom interpretations and illness labels can determine the pattern of psychological, somatic, or moral idioms of distress (Kirmayer 2001).

Cultural variation is evident in the ways that symptoms are attributed to specific causes. Cultural and individual differences in cognitive appraisals of symptomatology can influence the symptom experience, the manifestations and course of psychopathology, and the modes of help-seeking and coping with distress (Kirmayer and Bhugra 2009). Among Cambodian and Vietnamese refugees, for example, a variety of culturally specific panic syndromes may co-occur with PTSD (Hinton et al. 2001, 2007). These culturally specific panic attacks may focus on worries about a neck "vessel" rupturing or on symptoms of dizziness due to orthostatic hypotension. Culturally based attributions of sensations and symptoms can therefore form an essential part of the vicious circles constituting syndromes of panic, hypochondriacal worry, and other forms of anxiety (Kirmayer and Blake 2009; Kirmayer and Sartorius 2007).

The sociocultural significance of traumatic events and symptoms also leads to diverse strategies of coping. For example, the belief that suffering is inevitable or that one's life is predetermined as part of a larger pattern of karma may lead some Southeast Asians not to seek health care for disabling symptoms (Boehnlein 2007). Cultural notions of sickness may be linked to broader notions about the self, personhood, emotions, moral agency, the body, and the universe that can influence the goals and process of psychosocial and psychotherapeutic interventions (Kirmayer 2007).

Psychosocial Environment

The psychosocial environment includes sources of stress and social support as well as the culturally valued roles and relationships that define an individual's expected and actual level of functioning. Lack of social support is the single strongest predictor of risk for PTSD after trauma exposure (Brewin et al. 2000; Charuvastra and Cloitre 2008). For immigrants and refugees, the individual and family migration trajectory and the resettlement situation are crucial determinants of health status (see Table 16–3). The impact of trauma depends not only on the nature and severity of the threat, assault and subsequent injury and loss, but also on the personal and collective meaning of the events (see Table 16–4).

Trauma can have a profound impact on the family. Parental mental health problems increase the likelihood of psychological problems in children. Trauma may be difficult to discuss within the family because of the suffering it triggers for other members and because of individual and collective values about the acceptability or appropriateness of disclosing trauma, as well as concerns about how to discuss trauma with children. Specific forms of trauma may have strong social and culturally determined meanings associated with gender roles and family dynamics. For example, political rape is intended to attack the viability of the family and community by damaging the status of women.

The risk of trauma exposure in migrants depends on their region of origin and migratory path. By definition, refugees are people who have faced severe threats in their countries of origin and many experience violence during their

Table 16–3. Determinants of health status and outcomes in refugees

Individual and family migration
Displacement issues
Forced migration
Loss
Resettlement issues
Citizenship status
Family reunification
Discrimination
Socioeconomic conditions
Recognition of education and occupational status
Opportunities for meaningful work

Source. Beiser 2006; Porter 2007.

Table 16–4. Personal and collective meaning of trauma

Perceptions of the agent and cause of the trauma
• Natural catastrophe
• Accident or human error
• Individual act of violence
• Organized political violence
Relationship between perpetrator and victim
Past history and current relations between the social groups (ethnic, cultural, religious, political) of the perpetrator and victim

flight or in refugee camps. Disruption of social networks and separation from or loss of family members are common consequences of forced migration and are associated with an increased risk for subsequent mental health problems. The quality of the individual's reception and adaptation in the country of safe haven after migration is among the strongest predictors of long-term mental health (Beiser 2006; Porter 2007). A sense of being exiled, fears of repatriation, social and economic uncertainty, unemployment or underemployment in jobs not commensurate with the migrant's education and skills, and ongoing concerns about the situation for loved ones left behind are all risk factors for PTSD and other adjustment problems.

Refugees and other migrants may have experienced torture, which can have profound physical and psychological impact on the person. Some risk factors for exposure to torture are listed in Table 16–5 (Piwowarczyk et al. 2000). Psychological torture may have more severe and long-lasting effects than the physical violence of torture. Religious faith, a sense of commitment to a political cause, and psychological preparedness for torture may provide some protection against adverse psychological effects. Some of the various psychological responses to torture are listed in Table 16–6 (Weinstein et al. 2001).

Clinician-Patient Relationship

The clinician-patient relationship is shaped by cultural expectations that begin before the clinical encounter and influence the subsequent conversation. Patients who have experienced severe trauma or torture may evoke strong coun-

Table 16–5. Risk factors for exposure to torture

Refugee or asylum seeker status
Involvement in a political opposition group
Relative of a torture survivor
History of arrest or detention
Prisoner of war
Migrant from a country with political instability, police corruption, or an oppressive government or regime
Civil war or strife
Genocide
Member of a vulnerable minority group

Source. Adapted from Piwowarczyk L, Moreno A, Grodin M: "Health Care of Torture Survivors." *Journal of the American Medical Association* 284:539–541, 2000.

tertransference reactions in clinicians ranging from denial to overidentification and can lead to avoidance or vicarious traumatization (McCann and Pearlman 1990) and "burnout" (Pross 2006). Although there are differing views on the evidence for vicarious traumatization, intrusive traumatic symptoms have been observed in mental health caregivers (Sabin-Farrell and Turpin 2003). Professionals must recognize their own vulnerability and identify strategies to manage distress and seek professional support or counseling when needed.

In addition to these well-recognized issues of emotional reactions when working with trauma patients, intercultural work adds another layer of complexity based on the identity of patient and clinician. Collective histories of colonialism, racism, violence and exploitation may influence the development of a working alliance based on trust and confidence in the clinician's benevolence and integrity.

Cultural Formulation

The overall cultural formulation synthesizes the clinically relevant aspects of the patient's social and cultural context and experience with an aim to making an accurate diagnosis. This formulation provides a more complete assessment of the patient's problems and concerns that may not correspond to any psy-

Table 16–6. Psychological responses to torture

Posttraumatic stress disorder
Chronic somatic symptoms and syndromes
• Headaches
• Musculoskeletal pain
• Irritable bowel syndrome
• Neurasthenia or fatigue syndromes
• Other unexplained medical symptoms and conditions
Depression
Substance abuse
Neuropsychological impairment
Psychosis
Enduring personality changes
Anxiety
Dissociative disorders

Source. Adapted from Weinstein HM, Dansky L, Iacopino V: "Torture and War Trauma Survivors in Primary Care Practice." *Western Journal of Medicine* 165:112–118, 1996. Used with permission.

chiatric disorder but that nevertheless require clinical attention. The formulation also aims to identify culturally based strengths and resources pertinent to the treatment plan.

Process of Assessment

The clinician needs to be aware of cultural issues potentially associated with specific types of trauma. The traumatic event may not be seen as an issue of illness but rather in terms of its social, moral or political meanings. These meanings have a substantial effect on the risk for psychopathology and the response to treatment. People from different ethnocultural communities have their own collective histories, living conditions, and social, moral and political concerns that form the backdrop for their personal trauma experience.

Clinicians working with immigrants and refugees should familiarize themselves with the living conditions, political conflicts, and cultures of their patients, as well as the types of trauma their patients may have endured. Cultures change with migration and over time, so the clinician should have knowledge of local cultural communities and current issues and concerns. Clinicians should also be aware of their own personal and professional cultural assumptions and the way that they are likely to be received by patients from different backgrounds. However, because wide variation exists within ethnocultural groups, this general knowledge may not apply to any given patient and should be used to generate hypotheses and lines of inquiry to explore in the assessment process.

It is important to clarify at the outset why the assessment is taking place. Diagnostic assessment may be performed at the request of the patient, another referring clinician or professional, or other agencies. For children, the request is usually from a parent, school, day care center, or child welfare service. Common reasons for assessment among asylum seekers include relief or management of symptoms, such as sleep disturbance, chronic pain, anxiety, or depression; psychosocial support (material, instrumental, and economic assistance with finances, housing, and employment); and documentation of the premigration trauma exposure and subsequent impact to support a claim for refugee status.

When a cultural difference exists between clinician and patient, in particular if the patient belongs to a minority group or has a precarious migration status, the patient's apprehensions of being discriminated against, misunderstood, or simply not believed may interfere with trust and disclosure. Memory and concentration problems are common in patients with PTSD, anxiety, depression, and dissociative disorders. These problems may slow the process of obtaining the history and may affect an individual's ability to keep appointments and follow treatment instructions. Assessment requires patience, flexibility, and the consensual use of family and friends to obtain additional information and support.

Engagement of the family is particularly important for children and adolescents. Observing family interactions provides crucial information about clinically relevant issues such as conflicts, supports, and resources. Interviewing family members separately can allow each person to speak more freely about concerns. However, the approach to the family must respect cultural notions of hierarchy and authority to maintain collaboration with key members of the system.

Establishing and maintaining an alliance between the clinician and the patient is essential for adequate assessment and treatment. Talking about trauma can trigger or exacerbate symptoms, and the clinical setting itself can become a reminder of trauma. Every effort should be made to avoid retraumatizing the patient. Insensitive exploration of traumatic experiences may prevent the patient from seeking subsequent mental health care.

For survivors of torture or other traumas, the clinical situation may present reminders of their past. Exploration of the trauma history should be conducted gently and respectfully. Communication with a patient should be empathetic and sensitive so that the interview does not resemble an interrogation and the interview context is perceived as safe and secure. Traumatized patients may have difficulties developing trust in general and particularly toward authority figures, such as staff of government services or physicians, who may remind them of those involved in torture in their place of origin. Patients may not be familiar with the role of the mental health professional, and this role should be clearly explained along with the rules of confidentiality. Sufficient time should be allowed to create a working alliance. Some patients may try to shield the professional from the potential negative effects of their trauma experience, so it should be clearly communicated that the clinician is willing to listen and allow enough time for the story to unfold at a comfortable pace.

The interview can proceed chronologically, with the clinician asking about life in the refugee's home country before leaving, the process of flight (particularly, who accompanied the patient in migration and who was left behind), dangers experienced during migration, experiences in a refugee camp, and subsequent challenges faced in resettlement. Documentation of torture to support an application for refugee status or other medicolegal, forensic, or human rights advocacy should include attention to both physical and psychological forms of violence and their impact on current health (Office of the United Nations High Commissioner for Human Rights 2004; World Medical Association 2007).

Some current guidelines recommend the routine use of a brief screening instrument for PTSD as part of the initial health care assessment for refugees and asylum seekers (National Collaborating Centre for Mental Health 2005). Few studies have compared the efficacy of current screening instruments either within or across most cultural groups, and insufficient evidence is available to recommend any specific screen for particular cultural groups (Hollifield et al. 2002).

The Harvard Trauma Questionnaire is a self-report measure designed to obtain a history of trauma exposure and the cardinal symptoms of DSM-IV-TR PTSD (Mollica et al. 2004). This questionnaire has been translated into many languages, including Arabic, Bosnian, Croatian, Japanese, Khmer, Laotian, and Vietnamese, and has been widely used in research (Shoeb et al. 2007). The instrument must be adapted to specific cultural groups and should not be used as a substitute for a skillful clinical interview that is guided by the patient's comfort level. Checklists or structured interviews focused on posttraumatic symptoms should be used only as adjuncts to a flexible clinical interview because they fail to capture the range of refugee experiences (Lustig et al. 2004).

Language is a central issue in cross-cultural clinical work. Reporting of symptoms and referral to mental health services may be improved when there is concordance in language between patient and clinician (Bischoff et al. 2003). In many clinical settings, an informal interpreter (often a family member or friend) is used to explore health issues. However, disclosing traumatic experience in the presence of relatives, family members, or children can be very difficult and highly transgressive. The interpreter may also be at risk for vicarious traumatization. The interpreter's distress may prevent a patient from expressing concerns, and the situation may violate the patient's right to confidentiality. For these reasons, interviews should always be conducted with formally trained interpreters, if the patient's language ability is not adequate to express concerns and explore solutions. Table 16–7 summarizes basic issues in working with interpreters.

Although the use of trained interpreters is strongly recommended, the clinician must carefully appraise the acceptability of an interpreter to the patient. Ethnic match is not always the best solution. Due to intraethnic conflict, as well as issues of shame and honor that may be evoked by the disclosure of traumatic events, some patients may prefer interpreters who are not part of their own community or do not share their ethnic background.

Working with interpreters and culture brokers can be essential for obtaining the information needed to make a diagnostic assessment, forge a treatment alliance, and deliver effective interventions. These mediators may help to better attune clinicians to views and understandings of traumatic suffering that take into account the following as important constituents of trauma response: the relevance of differing concepts of personhood, styles of emotional expression, the sociomoral meaning of suffering, and the politics of traumatic memory.

Table 16–7. Assessment of trauma and PTSD in cultural context

Use of an interpreter

- Clarify the acceptability of the interpreter for the patient and/or family (gender, religion, ethnic identity).
- If trauma is suspected, discuss beforehand with the interpreter to foster a warm climate.
- Debrief the interpreter after the interview to provide support and prevent vicarious traumatization.

History of the traumatic events

- Invite disclosure by acknowledging the possibility of the trauma and your readiness to hear about it.
- Do not push disclosure. Try to understand the resistance (cultural taboos and social consequences of disclosure, unsafe assessment environment, traumatic avoidance linked to overwhelming trauma).

Use of the cultural formulation

- Use to elicit cultural idioms of distress related to trauma (e.g., *susto*, *espanto*, "hit by wind").
- Use to understand the multiple meanings associated with the trauma and associated events (personal, familial, traditional, religious, political, etc.).
- Use to document the help-seeking trajectory and reconstruction path favored by the patient, family, and/or community.
- Use to identify resources in individual, family, and community that can be mobilized as part of an intervention.

Finally, eliciting the core symptoms of PTSD or some other trauma-related syndrome does not mean the patient and clinician have arrived at a shared understanding of the nature of the patient's suffering or the clinical problem. Reflecting the clinical diagnostic formulation back to the patient, clarifying divergent interpretations, and negotiating areas of consensus are important to ensure ongoing collaboration in treatment and follow-up.

Treatment

Most people with acute trauma-related symptoms will recover spontaneously over time. Little evidence supports pharmacological treatments as being useful in the acute posttraumatic period, and psychological debriefing is not recommended and may be harmful (Institute of Medicine 2008; Wessley et al. 2008). The potential for harm may be more likely in social and cultural settings where open expression of strong emotions is discouraged or where serious interpersonal or political risks are associated with disclosure.

Pharmacotherapy may have a role in the management of PTSD symptoms and comorbid conditions (e.g., depression, anxiety, psychosis). Commonly used medications include antidepressants (selective serotonin reuptake inhibitors or serotonin-norepinephrine reuptake inhibitors), beta-blockers (for hyperarousal symptoms), alpha-adrenergic antagonists (for sleep disturbance and nightmares), benzodiazepines, and atypical antipsychotics. In addition to ethnocultural differences in the frequency and tolerance of side effects, the use of medications also may have culture-specific meanings that influence treatment adherence. Biological differences across different populations in pharmacokinetics and pharmacodynamics may influence the potential benefits and adverse effects experienced by the individual in treatment. Cultural differences in diet or the concomitant use of herbal medicines may induce or inhibit cytochrome P450 enzymes, altering drug metabolism. Inherited or induced variations in drug metabolism may require adjustment of dosage or change in medication. A lack of response to medication or complaints of side effects should alert the clinician to the possibility of incorrect dosing and can be followed up by measuring medication blood levels.

Trauma-focused cognitive-behavioral treatment can help patients with severe and disabling PTSD. Current guidelines for the treatment of trauma and PTSD emphasize the value of psychological interventions, including trauma-focused cognitive-behavioral therapy (CBT) and exposure therapy (American Psychiatric Association 2004; National Collaborating Centre for Mental Health 2005). CBT and other therapies can be administered successfully with the aid of interpreters (d'Ardenne et al. 2007).

For persistent PTSD and trauma-related symptoms, only exposure therapy has a strong evidence base (Institute of Medicine 2008). Exposure therapy does not involve "erasing" fear conditioning but rather developing alternative responses that gradually generalize (Bouton and Waddell 2007). The learning theory on which exposure therapy is based should be universally applicable, but the actual delivery depends on effective clinical communication and engagement. Because limited evidence exists for the cross-cultural applicability of current approaches, the clinician would do well to consider cultural modification, adaptation, or alternative treatments. The development of new coping strategies depends on culturally mediated processes of self-regulation of cognition and emotion. Employing culturally adapted strategies for intervention (e.g., reconnection with religious or other community activities that offer both social support and specific coping skills) is likely to be more acceptable to and effective for patients. However, such recommendations depend on careful inquiry into the individual patient's cultural identity and practices and his or her relationship to the local community (Drozdek and Wilson 2007).

The development of cultural adaptations of evidence-based treatments involves consulting with the individual and the community with the goal of tailoring the trauma intervention to local context and culture. This process helps communities to articulate concerns and develop a sense of ownership of the interventions; it can also set up a network that can be used for patient monitoring, support, and social integration. Examples of cultural adaptation include the use of local idioms of distress (e.g., *nervios*) in the language of therapy and the incorporation of traditional healing practices, as well as spiritual or religious activities (e.g., prayer, meditation) (Ngo et al. 2008).

Relaxation and self-soothing methods related to yoga, meditation, prayer or other spiritual and religious practices may be applicable both within and across cultures (Somasundaram 2008). There are important convergences between the practice of Buddhist mindfulness meditation and current CBT methods. Such CBT interventions may be well accepted, with modifications, for patients from Buddhist backgrounds (Hinton et al. 2005). Similarly, yoga and other forms of meditation or prayer may provide important methods of self-soothing and symptom management. Traditional practices not only are useful supplements to conventional psychiatric treatments but may constitute the core of effective intervention in many cases.

Patients often make use of multiple sources of help and may be using home remedies, traditional medicines and healers, and religious or spiritual helpers both from their own traditions and from the many forms of complementary and alternative medicine available in most urban settings. In some cases, referral to an appropriate traditional healer with a positive community reputation may be useful. This suggestion should be presented as a complement or adjunct to conventional mental health care, not as a mutually exclusive alternative. Clinicians should consider how such treatments may interact

Table 16–8. Treatment of PTSD in refugee families

Phase 1: Ensure that safety has been attained. Consider the following:

- Has the patient's asylum claim been accepted?
- Is survival (housing, food, health) in the host country ensured?
- Is the patient worried about the safety of family members in the country of origin?

If safety has not yet been attained, do the following:

1. Provide practical, family and social support.
2. Advocate to obtain migration status for patient and family.
3. Refer to community organizations for assistance with basic needs.
4. Alleviate the most disturbing symptoms.

Phase 2 (once basic safety has been attained): Propose trauma treatment, respecting patient preferences. Consider the following:

- Trauma-focused psychological treatment (culturally adapted)
- Specific therapy for sleep disorder (cognitive-behavioral therapy or pharmacotherapy)
- Symptomatic treatment of anxiety or other symptoms
- Pharmacotherapy (not a first-line treatment choice)

Phase 3: Support ongoing integration in host country (employment, schooling, language, family reunification).

with conventional therapies (e.g., herb-drug interactions, differing approaches to disclosure) and should help the client to make informed decisions on management.

Refugees

British guidelines for the treatment of trauma-related symptoms in refugees suggest a 3-step phased model of care (see Table 16–8). Phase 1 aims to ensure safety from persecution and to facilitate provision of accommodation and other basic needs. To assist during this phase, clinicians should familiarize themselves with immigration law, welfare rights, and relevant social, economic, and political issues. Supportive counseling, psychoeducation, and medication may be offered. Phase 2 usually occurs after basic safety has been established and addresses persistent symptoms through trauma-focused therapy. Phase 3 focuses on integration into the host society (National Collaborating Centre for Mental Health 2005).

In the development of a treatment plan for refugee patients, clinicians should first assess whether a basic level of safety has been attained. Asylum seekers risk being sent back to their countries of origin. This presents a potential trauma repetition because asylum refusal may be perceived as an impending death sentence. The precariousness of the patient's migration status is a strong predictor of anxiety and depressive symptoms (Momartin et al. 2006). During Phase 1, practical family and social supports are the main interventions, and trauma-focused therapy is not recommended. Clinicians should adapt the treatment plan to the most immediate needs of their patients. In this initial phase, advocacy and help in the fulfillment of basic needs are key. Detention and proceedings for determination of refugee status may lead to retraumatization. Resolution of patients' immigration status may lead to amelioration of symptoms (Davis 2006; Momartin et al. 2006).

During Phase 2, the clinician recommends trauma-focused psychological interventions. These interventions should accommodate the patient's personal preferences and be culturally appropriate. The types of psychological treatment that have been evaluated with traumatized patients from diverse cultural backgrounds include CBT, narrative exposure therapy (Bichescu et al. 2007; Neuner et al. 2004), and testimonial therapy (Igreja et al. 2004). Several cultural adaptations of evidence-based psychological trauma treatments for adults and children have been developed and evaluated to various degrees (Hinton et al. 2005; Neuner et al. 2004; Tol et al. 2008).

Phase 3 concerns social integration, and at this point the response of the receiving society is paramount. Because social relationships and unemployment in the host country have such a strong effect on mental health symptoms and quality of life (Carlsson et al. 2006), social integration should be addressed early and in an ongoing way.

Controversy continues over the appropriateness of exposure methods in the treatment of survivors of torture (Basoglu 2006). Most experts recommend an emphasis on a long-term supportive relationship rather than intensive therapy, which may be retraumatizing (Kinzie 2007). The long-term outcome of multimodal treatment of severe trauma, including torture, is not yet clear. A longitudinal 10-year follow-up of torture survivors who received psychological (CBT) and pharmacological treatment in Copenhagen found no long-term benefit of the treatment (Carlsson et al. 2006). Carlsson and colleagues suggest that the intervention did not sufficiently take into account the social and familial factors, which are key in the resettlement process. The treatment of refugees and immigrants who have suffered trauma should include interventions addressing the global sense of safety, social integration, and well-being (and reunification) of families.

Child and Adolescent Refugees

Interventions aimed at children and adolescents need to consider their well-being within multiple systems, including family, school and community. Culturally sensitive community-based and preventive intervention programs can help refugee children and their families. A growing literature supports the usefulness of school-based interventions to reduce the psychological effect of trauma both in developing countries and in multiethnic societies receiving immigrants and refugees (Ehntholt et al. 2005; Kataoka et al. 2003; Rousseau and Guzder 2008). These interventions may be directed to children identified as more symptomatic through screening (Tol et al. 2008) or delivered to a global school population (Rousseau et al. 2009). The more general intervention may be less stigmatizing for children. School-based programs combine creative and play activities, elements of CBT, and other counseling techniques. Cultural adaptation in multiethnic schools is challenging because of the diversity of students; however, students may benefit from learning about each other's cultural backgrounds (Miller and Rasco 2004).

Mental health clinic–based treatment models can offer further assistance to those children and families whose symptoms and functional impairments cannot be fully addressed by preventive intervention programs. Multiple treatment modalities, including family, individual, and group psychotherapies, have been used with refugee children and adolescents. Despite the relatively high prevalence of PTSD in refugee youth, very few systematic treatment studies are available. However, psychotherapeutic approaches available for adults may potentially be modified for use with younger patients, and psychosocial interventions may be very cost-efficient with mothers and young children. Case series studies offer preliminary support for the value of modified CBT, group CBT, narrative exposure therapy, testimonial psychotherapy, and eye movement desensitization and reprocessing with children and adolescents (Ehntholt and Yule 2006). No pharmacological agents have been recommended for the treatment of PTSD among children and adolescents.

Creative arts therapies may be useful in working with young people who have difficulty articulating their experiences, either due to language differences or traumatic content. Creative expression can help children and adolescents construct meaning and come to terms with traumatic experiences (Rousseau et al. 2004). Different art modalities and types of therapy may be best suited and most acceptable for specific cultures, age groups, and individuals. The empirical evidence base for creative arts therapies is limited, but there are good theoretical rationales for their use in working with trauma (Johnson 2009).

Conclusion

Current diagnostic and treatment approaches to trauma and PTSD require careful rethinking before they can be applied across cultures. The meanings of trauma, modes of symptom expression and coping, and significance of disclosure and treatment interventions all vary substantially. The basic approach to trauma assessment must be supplemented by working with interpreters and culture brokers and by systematic exploration of the cultural meanings of the trauma itself, its context, and subsequent symptoms. Treatment interventions must be tailored to the patient, family, and community. Cultural traditions and communities represent important sources of resilience and resources for making sense of trauma and developing coping and intervention strategies.

Health care systems and services must provide the resources necessary to conduct effective intercultural work. Trained interpreters and culture brokers or mediators knowledgeable about the local cultural communities are essential members of the health care team. Although working across cultures, particularly with interpreters and culture brokers, requires additional time, this investment is necessary to avoid errors in diagnosis and to ensure a working alliance that will increase the likelihood of effective follow-up and treatment. Key elements of a successful intercultural clinical service are summarized in Table 16–9 (Kinzie 2004, pp. 268–269).

The predicament of traumatized patients raises both practical and ethical issues in diagnosis and treatment. Narratives of trauma may link the medical problem of suffering with injustices in the larger society. Work with trauma

Table 16–9. Keys to a successful intercultural clinical service

Goals	Strategies
Provide relief of symptoms and co-morbid conditions	Treat somatic syndromes (chronic pain, irritable bowel syndrome, fatigue), anxiety, depression, substance abuse
Provide medical care	Arrange for physical assessment, treatment, and follow-up concurrent with psychiatric care
Establish effective clinical communication	Use trained interpreters and culture brokers Elicit feedback from patients to ensure mutual understanding and response to concerns
Develop culturally competent staff	Employ appropriately skilled clinical staff with training in intercultural work Provide training in culture and mental health to all staff, including interpreters and cultural brokers
Facilitate access to services	Minimize wait times Provide flexible hours, child care, and transportation Provide outreach and follow-up (e.g., telephone, home visits) Address stigma issues (e.g., situate mental health services in general medical setting)
Improve continuity of care	Facilitate community links between services (e.g., outpatient clinics and crisis services)
Build credibility with community	Learn from community Develop ongoing dialogue with community members and leaders Contribute to public education and mental health literacy Engage community in direction and governance of health care programs, services, and institutions

Source. Kinzie 2007; Kirmayer et al. 2003.

patients often requires that clinicians accept the role of advocate for vulnerable groups. For collective trauma that occurs in zones of war or oppressive political regimes, clinicians may play an essential role in highlighting injustices and raising awareness about ethical issues and human rights that may be important contributors to individual and collective recovery.

Key Clinical Points

- Biosocial, cultural, and political processes must be understood as essential aspects of the overall construct of PTSD.
- The psychological and somatic consequences of trauma are mediated by cultural models that have cognitive, intepersonal, and social dimensions.
- Cultural context influences the experience and expression of symptoms by patients as well as the categorization and interpretation of symptoms by providers.
- The DSM-IV-TR Outline for Cultural Formulation provides a structure for assessing multiple domains, including the patient's cultural identity; illness explanations; psychosocial stressors, psychosocial supports, and functional status; and the clinician-patient interaction.
- The overall cultural formulation synthesizes the clinically relevant aspects of a patient's social and cultural context and experience with the aim of making an accurate diagnosis.
- Cultural issues such as viewing traumatic events in terms of social or political meaning rather than through illness can substantially affect the dynamics of a clinician's interactions with a patient.
- Clinicians working with cultures other than their own should familiarize themselves with living conditions, political conflicts, and other aspects of culture to provide a more thorough backdrop for the evaluation.
- Cultural norms of hierarchy and authority that are not followed by clinicians may significantly disrupt the therapeutic alliance.
- Language barriers and other intercultural confusions are likely to occur during evaluations across cultures and should be addressed empathically and with patience.
- Interventions should take into account intraethnic variations in pharmacokinetics and pharmacodynamics as well as cultural norms regarding psychotherapy.
- Utilization of culturally appropriate interventions, such as yoga, meditation, or spiritual practices, either individually or in conjunction with

conventional psychiatric practice, may help alleviate concerns about cultural differences.

- Assessments and treatments should be tailored to the patient, family, and community in order to achieve the greatest efficacy.

References

American Psychiatric Association: Diagnostic and Statistical Manual of Mental Disorders, 4th Edition, Text Revision. Washington, DC, American Psychiatric Association, 2000

American Psychiatric Association: Practice Guideline for the Treatment of Patients With Acute Stress Disorder and Posttraumatic Stress Disorder. Washington, DC, American Psychiatric Association, 2004

Basoglu M: Rehabilitation of traumatised refugees and survivors of torture. BMJ 333:1230–1231, 2006

Beiser M: Longitudinal research to promote effective refugee resettlement. Transcult Psychiatry 43:56–71, 2006

Bichescu D, Neuner F, Schauer M, et al: Narrative exposure therapy for political imprisonment-related chronic posttraumatic stress disorder and depression. Behav Res Ther 45:2212–2220, 2007

Bischoff A, Bovier PA, Rrustemi I, et al: Language barriers between nurses and asylum seekers: their impact on symptom reporting and referral. Soc Sci Med 57:503–512, 2003

Boehnlein JK: Religion and spirituality after trauma, in Understanding Trauma: Integrating Clinical, Biological, and Cultural Perspectives. Edited by Kirmayer LJ, Lemelson R, Barad M. New York, Cambridge University Press, 2007, pp 259–274

Bouton ME, Waddell J: Some biobehavioral insights into persistent effects of emotional trauma, in Understanding Trauma: Integrating Clinical, Biological, and Cultural Perspectives. Edited by Kirmayer LJ, Lemelson R, Barad M. New York, Cambridge University Press, 2007

Brewin CR, Andrews B, Valentine JD: Meta-analysis of risk factors for posttraumatic stress disorder in trauma-exposed adults. J Consult Clin Psychol 68:748–766, 2000

Carlsson JM, Olsen DR, Mortensen EL, et al: Mental health and health-related quality of life: a 10-year follow-up of tortured refugees. J Nerv Ment Dis 194:725–731, 2006

Carroll J: *Murug, Waali,* and *Gini*: expression of distress in refugees from Somalia. J Clin Psychiatry 6:119–125, 2004

Charuvastra A, Cloitre M: Social bonds and posttraumatic stress disorder. Annu Rev Psychol 59:301–328, 2008

Davis RM: PTSD symptom changes in refugees. Torture 16:10–19, 2006

d'Ardenne P, Ruaro L, Cestari L, et al: Does interpreter-mediated CBT with traumatized refugee people work? A comparison of patient outcomes in East London. Behav Cogn Psychother 35:293–301, 2007

de Jong JT, Komproe IH, Van Ommeren M, et al: Lifetime events and posttraumatic stress disorder in 4 postconflict settings. JAMA 286:555–562, 2001

Drozdek B, Wilson JP (eds): Voices of Trauma: Treating Psychological Trauma Across Cultures. New York, Springer, 2007

Ehntholt KA, Yule W: Practitioner review: assessment and treatment of refugee children and adolescents who have experienced war-related trauma. J Child Psychol Psychiatry 47:1197–1210, 2006

Ehntholt KA, Smith PA, Yule W: School-based cognitive-behavioural therapy group intervention for refugee children who have experienced war-related trauma. Clin Child Psychol Psychiatry 10:235–250, 2005

Eisenbruch M: From post-traumatic stress disorder to cultural bereavement: diagnosis of Southeast Asian refugees. Soc Sci Med 33:673–680, 1991

Eisenman DP, Meredith LS, Rhodes H, et al: PTSD in Latino patients: illness beliefs, treatment preferences, and implications for care. J Gen Intern Med 23:1386–1392, 2008

Fassin D, Rechtman R: The Empire of Trauma: An Inquiry Into the Condition of Victimhood. Princeton, NJ, Princeton University Press, 2009

Fox SH: The Mandinka nosological system in the context of post-trauma syndromes. Transcult Psychiatry 40:488–506, 2003

Group for the Advancement of Psychiatry: Cultural Assessment in Clinical Psychiatry. Washington, DC, American Psychiatric Publishing, 2002

Guarnaccia PJ, Lewis-Fernández R, Marano MR: Toward a Puerto Rican popular nosology: *nervios* and *ataque de nervios.* Cult Med Psychiatry 27:339–366, 2003

Hinton D, Um K, Ba P: *Kyol goeu* ("wind overload"), part I: a cultural syndrome of orthostatic panic among Khmer refugees. Transcult Psychiatry 38:403–432, 2001

Hinton DE, Chhean D, Pich V, et al: A randomized controlled trial of cognitive-behavior therapy for Cambodian refugees with treatment-resistant PTSD and panic attacks: a cross-over design. J Trauma Stress 18:617–629, 2005

Hinton DE, Hinton L, Tran M, et al: Orthostatic panic attacks among Vietnamese refugees. Transcult Psychiatry 44:515–544, 2007

Hollifield M, Warner TD, Lian N, et al: Measuring trauma and health status in refugees: a critical review. JAMA 288:611–621, 2002

Igreja V, Kleihn WC, Schreuder BJN, et al: Testimony method to ameliorate post-traumatic stress symptoms. Br J Psychiatry 184:251–257, 2004

Institute of Medicine: Treatment of Posttraumatic Stress Disorder: An Assessment of the Evidence. Washington, DC, National Academies Press, 2008

Jenkins JH: The state construction of affect: political ethos and mental health among Salvadoran refugees. Cult Med Psychiatry 15:139–165, 1991

Johnson DR: Commentary: examining underlying paradigms in the creative arts therapies of trauma. The Arts in Psychotherapy 36:114–120, 2009

Jones E: Historical approaches to post-combat disorders. Phil Trans R Soc Lond B Biol Sci 361:533–542, 2006

Jones E, Vermaas RH, McCartney H, et al: Flashbacks and post-traumatic stress disorder: the genesis of a 20th-century diagnosis. Br J Psychiatry 182:158–163, 2003

Kagee A: Do South African former detainees experience post-traumatic stress? Circumventing the demand characteristics of psychological assessment. Transcult Psychiatry 41:323–336, 2004

Kataoka SH, Stein BD, Jaycox LH, et al: A school-based mental health program for traumatized Latino immigrant children. J Am Acad Child Adolesc Psychiatry 42:311–318, 2003

Kinzie D: Cross-cultural treatment of PTSD, in Treating Psychological Trauma and PTSD. Edited by Wilson J, Friedman MJ, Lindy J. New York, Guilford, 2004, pp 255–277

Kinzie D: PTSD among traumatized refugees, in Understanding Trauma: Integrating Clinical, Biological, and Cultural Perspectives. Edited by Kirmayer LJ, Lemelson R, Barad M. New York, Cambridge University Press, 2007, pp 194–206

Kirmayer LJ: Confusion of the senses: implications of ethnocultural variations in somatoform and dissociative disorders for PTSD, in Ethnocultural Aspects of Post-Traumatic Stress Disorders: Issues, Research and Clinical Applications. Edited by Marsella AJ, Friedman MJ, Gerrity ET, et al. Washington, DC, American Psychological Association, 1996, pp 131–164

Kirmayer LJ: Cultural variations in the clinical presentation of depression and anxiety: implications for diagnosis and treatment. J Clin Psychiatry 62 (suppl 13):22–28, 2001

Kirmayer LJ: Psychotherapy and the cultural concept of the person. Transcult Psychiatry 44:232–257, 2007

Kirmayer LJ, Bhugra D: Culture and mental illness: social context and explanatory models, in Psychiatric Diagnosis: Patterns and Prospects. Edited by Salloum IM, Mezzich JE. New York, Wiley, 2009, pp 29–37

Kirmayer LJ, Blake C: Theoretical perspectives on the cross-cultural study of panic disorder, in Culture and Panic Disorder. Edited by Hinton D, Good BJ. Stanford, CA, Stanford University Press, 2009, pp 35–56

Kirmayer LJ, Sartorius N: Cultural models and somatic syndromes, in Somatic Presentations of Mental Disorders: Refining the Research Agenda for DSM-V. Edited by Dimsdale JE, Patel V, Xin Y, et al. Arlington, VA, American Psychiatric Publishing, 2009, pp 23–46

Kirmayer LJ, Lemelson R, Barad M: Introduction: inscribing trauma in culture, brain, and body, in Understanding Trauma: Integrating Clinical, Biological, and Cultural Perspectives. Edited by Kirmayer LJ, Lemelson R, Barad M. New York, Cambridge University Press, 2007, pp 1–20

Kirmayer LJ, Rousseau C, Jarvis GE, et al: The cultural context of clinical assessment, in Psychiatry, 3rd Edition. Edited by Tasman A, Maj M, First MB, et al. New York, Wiley, 2008, pp 54–66

Kirmayer LJ, Kienzler H, Afana A, et al: Trauma and disasters in social and cultural context, in Principles of Social Psychiatry, 2nd Edition. Edited by Bhugra D, Morgan C. New York, Wiley-Blackwell, 2010, pp 155–177

Lewis-Fernandez R, Garrido-Castillo P, Bennasar MC, et al: Dissociation, childhood trauma, and *ataque de nervios* among Puerto Rican psychiatric outpatients. Am J Psychiatry 159:1603–1605, 2002

Leys R: Trauma: A Genealogy. Chicago, IL, University of Chicago Press, 2000

Lim R (ed): Clinical Manual of Cultural Psychiatry. Arlington, VA, American Psychiatric Publishing, 2006

Lustig SL, Kia-Keating M, Knight WG, et al: Review of child and adolescent refugee mental health. J Am Acad Child Adolesc Psychiatry 43:24–36, 2004

Marsella AJ (ed): Ethnocultural Perspectives on Disasters and Trauma: Foundations, Issues, and Applications. New York, Springer, 2008

Mayer E: Somatic manifestations of traumatic stress, in Understanding Trauma: Integrating Clinical, Biological, and Cultural Perspectives. Edited by Kirmayer LJ, Lemelson R, Barad M. New York, Cambridge University Press, 2007, pp 142–170

McCann IL, Pearlman LA: Vicarious traumatization: a framework for understanding the psychological effects of working with victims. J Trauma Stress 3:131–149, 1990

Mezzich JE, Caracci G, Fabrega H, et al: Cultural formulation guidelines. Transcult Psychiatry 46:383–405, 2009

Miller KE, Rasco LM: An ecological framework for addressing the mental health needs of refugee communities, in The Mental Health of Refugees: Ecological Approaches to Healing and Adaptation. Edited by Miller KE, Rasco LM. Mahwah, NJ, Erlbaum, 2004, pp 1–64

Miller KE, Omidian P, Quraishy AS, et al: The Afghan Symptom Checklist: a culturally grounded approach to mental health assessment in a conflict zone. Am J Orthopsychiatry 76:423–433, 2006

Mollica RF, McDonald LS, Massagli MP, et al: Measuring Trauma, Measuring Torture: Instructions and Guidance on the Utilization of the Harvard Program in Refugee Trauma's Versions of the Hopkins Symptom Checklist-25 (HSCL-25) and the Harvard Trauma Questionnaire (HTQ). Cambridge, MA, Harvard Program in Refugee Trauma, 2004

Momartin S, Steel Z, Coello M, et al: A comparison of the mental health of refugees with temporary versus permanent protection visas. Med J Aust 185:357–361, 2006

National Collaborating Centre for Mental Health: Post-traumatic Stress Disorder: The Management of PTSD in Adults and Children in Primary and Secondary Care (National Clinical Practice Guideline Vol 26). London, Gaskell and the British Psychological Society, 2005

Neuner F, Schauer M, Klaschik C, et al: A comparison of narrative exposure therapy, supportive counseling, and psychoeducation for treating posttraumatic stress disorder in an African refugee settlement. J Consult Clin Psychol 72:579–587, 2004

Ngo V, Langley A, Kataoka SH, et al: Providing evidence-based practice to ethnically diverse youths: examples from the Cognitive Behavioral Intervention for Trauma in Schools (CBITS) program. J Am Acad Child Adolesc Psychiatry 47:858–862, 2008

Office of the United Nations High Commissioner for Human Rights: Istanbul Protocol: Manual on the Effective Investigation and Documentation of Torture and Other Cruel, Inhuman or Degrading Treatment or Punishment. Geneva, Switzerland, United Nations, 2004

Piwowarczyk L, Moreno A, Grodin M: Health care of torture survivors. JAMA 284:539–541, 2000

Porter M: Global evidence for a biopsychosocial understanding of refugee adaptation. Transcult Psychiatry 44:418–439, 2007

Pross C: Burnout, vicarious traumatization and its prevention. Torture 16:1–9, 2006

Rousseau C, Guzder J: School-based prevention programs for refugee children. Child Adolesc Psychiatr Clin N Am 17:533–549, 2008

Rousseau C, Singh A, Lacroix L, et al: Creative expression workshops for immigrant and refugee children. J Am Acad Child Adolesc Psychiatry 43:235–238, 2004

Rousseau C, Benoit M, Lacroix L, et al: Evaluation of a sandplay program for preschoolers in a multiethnic neighborhood. J Child Psychol Psychiatry 50:743–750, 2009

Sabin-Farrell R, Turpin G: Vicarious traumatization: implications for the mental health of health workers? Clin Psychol Rev 23:449–480, 2003

Shoeb M, Weinstein H, Mollica R: The Harvard Trauma Questionnaire: adapting a cross-cultural instrument for measuring torture, trauma and posttraumatic stress disorder in Iraqi refugees. Int J Soc Psychiatry 53:447–463, 2007

Silove D: Adaptation, ecosocial safety signals, and the trajectory of PTSD, in Understanding Trauma: Integrating Clinical, Biological, and Cultural Perspectives. Edited by Kirmayer LJ, Lemelson R, Barad M. New York, Cambridge University Press, 2007, pp 242–258

Silove D, Steel Z, Watters C: Policies of deterrence and the mental health of asylum seekers. JAMA 284:604–611, 2000

Somasundaram D: Psychosocial aspects of torture in Sri Lanka. International Journal of Culture and Mental Health 1:10–23, 2008

Summerfield D: A critique of seven assumptions behind psychological trauma programmes in war-affected areas. Soc Sci Med 48:1449–1462, 1999

Tol WA, Komproe IH, Susanty D, et al: School-based mental health intervention for children affected by political violence in Indonesia. JAMA 300:655–662, 2008

Tousignant M: *Espanto:* a dialogue with the gods. Cult Med Psychiatry 3:347–361, 1979

Weinstein CS, Fucetola R, Mollica R: Neuropsychological issues in the assessment of refugees and victims of mass violence. Neuropsychol Rev 11:131–141, 2001

Wessely S, Bryant RA, Greenberg N, et al: Does psychoeducation help prevent post traumatic psychological distress? Psychiatry 71:287–302, 2008

World Medical Association: World Medical Association resolution on the responsibility of physicians in the documentation and denunciation of acts of torture or cruel or inhuman or degrading treatment. 2007. Available at: http://www.wma.net/en/30publications/10policies/t1/index.html. Accessed March 9, 2010.

Young A: The Harmony of Illusions: Inventing Post-traumatic Stress Disorder. Princeton, NJ, Princeton University Press, 1995

Index

Page numbers printed in **boldface** type refer to tables or figures.